W9-BVQ-097

Contents

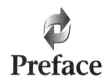

Preface

This textbook comprises debates on controversial issues on health and society. Each issue consists of opposing viewpoints presented in a YES–NO format. Most of the questions that are included here relate to health topics of modern concern, such as universal health insurance, abortion, and drug use and abuse. The authors of these selections take strong stands on specific issues and provide support for their positions. While we may not agree with a particular point of view, each author clearly defines his or her stand on the issues.

This book is divided into six units containing related issues. Each issue is preceded by an Introduction, which sets the stage for the debate, gives historical background on the subject, provides learning outcomes, and provides a context for the controversy. Each issue concludes with further exploration of the issue, which offers a summary of the debate and some concluding observations and suggests further readings on the subject. The summary also raises further points, since most of the issues have more than two sides.

Contributors to this volume are identified, which gives information on the physicians, professors, journalists, theologians, and scientists whose views are debated here.

Taking Sides: Clashing Views in Health and Society, 11th edition, is a tool to encourage critical thought on important health issues. Readers should not feel confined to the views expressed in the selections. Some readers may see important points on both sides of an issue and may construct for themselves a new and creative approach, which may incorporate the best of both sides or provide an entirely new vantage point for understanding.

Changes to this edition: The 11th edition of *Taking Sides: Clashing Views in Health and Society* includes some important changes from previous editions: for some issues, I have kept the topic from the past edition but have replaced one or both of the selections in order to make the topic more current or more clearly focus the controversy. I also added new topics and selections that reflect current controversies in health and society.

Eileen Daniel
SUNY College

Editor of This Volume

Eileen Daniel, a registered dietitian and licensed nutritionist, is a professor in the Department of Health Science and associate vice provost for academic affairs at the State University of New York College at Brockport. She received a BS in nutrition and dietetics from the Rochester Institute of Technology, an MS in community health education from SUNY College at Brockport, and a PhD in health education from the University of Oregon. A member of the American Dietetics Association, the New York State Dietetics Society, and other professional and community organizations, she has published over 40 articles in professional journals on issues of health, nutrition, and health education. She is the editor of *Annual Editions: Health*.

Acknowledgments

Special thanks to John, Diana, and Jordan. Also, thanks to my colleagues at the State University of New York College at Brockport for all their helpful contributions. I was also assisted in preparing this edition by the valuable suggestions from the adopters of *Taking Sides* who filled out comment cards and questionnaires. Many of your recommendations were incorporated into this edition. Finally, I appreciate the assistance of David Welsh and the staff at McGraw Hill for all their help.

Academic Advisory Board Members

Members of the Academic Advisory Board are instrumental in the final selection of articles for each edition of TAKING SIDES. Their review of articles for content, level, and appropriateness provides critical direction to the editor and staff. We think that you will find their careful consideration well reflected in this volume.

Douglas Abbott
University of Nebraska, Lincoln

Harold Abramowitz
Charles Drew University

Isaac Addai
Lansing Community College

David Anderson
George Mason University

Steven Applewhite
University of Houston

Judith Ary
North Dakota State University

Faye Avard
Mississippi Valley State University

Alice Baldwin-Jones
The City College of New York

Barry Brock
Barry University

Elaine Bryan
Georgia Perimeter College

Cynthia Cassell
University of North Carolina, Charlotte

Jeanne Clerc
Western Illinois University

Marilyn Coleman
University of Missouri

Scarlett Conway
University of South Carolina Upstate

J. Sunshine Cowan
University of Central Oklahoma

Susan Crowley
North Idaho College

Peter Cruise
Mary Baldwin College

Michelle D'abundo
University of North Carolina, Wilmington

Evia L. Davis
Langston University

Geoffrey Davison
Lyndon State College

Cherie de Sues-Wilson
American Career College

Joanne Demyun
Eastern University

Karen Dennis
Illinois State University

Kathi Deresinski
Triton College

Diane Dettmore
Fairleigh Dickinson University

Jonathan Deutsch
Kingsborough Community College

Johanna Donnenfield
Scottsdale Community College

Karen Dorman
St. Johns University

Wilton Duncan
ASA College

William Dunscombe
Union County College

Neela Eisner
Cuyahoga Community College

Ifeanyi Emenike
Benedict College

Marie Emerson
Washington County Community College

Brad Engeldinger
Sierra College

David Evans
Pennsylvania College of Technology

Susan Farrell
Kingsborough Community College

Jenni Fauchier
Metropolitan Community College

Christine Feeley
Adelphi University

Catherine Felton
Central Piedmont Community College

Patrice Fike
Barry University

Virginia S. Fink
University of Colorado, Denver

Paul Finnicum
Arkansas State University

Eunice Flemister
Hostos Community College, Cuny

Deborah Flynn
Southern Conn State University

Mary Flynn
Brown University

Amy Frith
Ithaca College

Bernard Frye
University of Texas, Arlington

Stephen Gambescia
Drexel University

Kathie Garbe
University of North Carolina, Asheville

Jeff Goodman
Union College

Aleida Gordon
California State Polytechnic University, Pomona

Jerome G. Greene, Jr.
Mississippi Valley State University

Deborah Gritzmacher
Clayton State University

Dana Hale
Itawamba Community College

Jeffrey Hampl
Arizona State University

Michele Haywood
Potomac College

Leslie Hellstrom
Tidewater Community College

George Hertl
Northwest Mississippi Community College

Martha Highfield
California State University, Northridge

Marc D. Hiller
University of New Hampshire

Cathy Hix-Cunningham
Tennessee Technological University

Loreen Huffman
Missouri Southern State University

Kevin Hylton
University of Maryland, Baltimore County

Allen Jackson
Chadron State College

Leslie Jacobson
Brooklyn College

Pera Jambazian
California State University, Los Angeles

Barry Johnson
Davidson County Community College

Marcy Jung
Fort Lewis College

Melissa Karolides
San Diego City College

Leroy Keeney
York College of Pennsylvania

John Kowalczyk
University of Minnesota, Duluth

Sylvette La Touche-Howard
University of Maryland, College Park

Leslie Lamb
Dowling College

Robert Lavery
Montclair State University

Jennifer Leach
Lehigh Valley College

Hans Leis
Louisiana College

Craig Levin
National American University

Linda Levin-Messineo
Carlow University

Karen Lew
University of Miami

Michelle Lewis
Fairleigh Dickinson University

Xiangdong Li
New York City College of Technology

Fredanna M'Cormack
Coastal Carolina University

Cindy Manjounes
Lindenwood University

Hal Marchand
Western Illinois University

Willis McAleese
Idaho State University

Michael McDonough
Berkeley College

James McNamara
Alverno College

Julie Merten
University Of North Florida

James Metcalf
George Mason University

Eric Miller
Kent State University

Lloyd Mitchell III
Elizabeth City State University

Kara Montgomery
University of South Carolina

Martha Olson
Iowa Lakes Community College

Anna Page
Johnson County Community College

Judy Peel
North Carolina State University

Tina M. Penhollow
Florida Atlantic University

Jane Petrillo
Kennesaw State University

Regina Pierce
Davenport University

Roger Pinches
William Paterson University

Roberta L. Pohlman
Wright State University

M. Paige Powell
University of Alabama, Birmingham

Elizabeth Quintana
West Virginia University

Leon Ragonesi
California State University, Dominguez Hills

Ralph Rice
Wake Forest University School of Medicine

Leigh Rich
Armstrong Atlantic State University

Andrea Salis
Queensborough Community College

Kathryn Schneider
Pacific Union College

Elizabeth Schneider
Keiser University, Ft. Lauderdale

Allan Simmons
Jackson State University

Donna Sims
Fort Valley State University

Carrie Lee Smith
Millersville University

Cynthia Smith
Central Piedmont Community College

Kathleen Smyth
College of Marin

Debbie Sowers
Eastern Kentucky University

Stephen Sowulewski
J. Sargeant Reynolds Community College

Caile Spear
Boise State University

Diane Spokus
Penn State University, University Park

Betsy Stern
Milwaukee Area Technical College

Craig Stillwell
Southern Oregon University

Susan Stockton
University of Central Missouri

Meg Stolt
John Jay College

Lori Stolz
Oakland City University

Winona Taylor
Bowie State University

Michael Teague
University of Iowa

Julie Thurlow
University of Wisconsin, Madison

Theresa Tiso
Stony Brook University

Terry Weideman
Oakland Community College

Peggie Williamson
Central Texas College

Mary Alice Wolf
Saint Joseph College

Correlation Guide

The *Taking Sides* series presents current issues in a debate-style format designed to stimulate student interest and develop critical thinking skills. Each issue is thoughtfully framed with an issue summary, an issue introduction, and a postscript. The pro and con essays—selected for their liveliness and substance—represent the arguments of leading scholars and commentators in their fields.

Taking Sides: Clashing Views in Health and Society, 11/e is an easy-to-use reader that presents issues on important topics such as *health insurance*, *drug testing*, and *government regulation in health care*. For more information on *Taking Sides* and other *McGraw-Hill Create™* titles, visit www.mcgrawhillcreate.com.

This convenient guide matches the issues in **Taking Sides: Clashing Views in Health and Society, 11/e** with the corresponding chapters in two of our best-selling McGraw-Hill Education Health textbooks by Insel/Roth and Payne/Hahn/Lucas.

Taking Sides: Health and Society, 11/e	Core Concepts in Health, 13/e by Insel/Roth	Understanding Your Health, 12/e by Payne/Hahn/Lucas
Does the Affordable Health Care Violate Religious Freedom by Requiring Employers' Health Insurance Plans to Cover Birth Control?	**Chapter 6:** Contraception **Chapter 20:** Conventional and Complementary Medicine	**Chapter 16:** Managing Your Fertility **Chapter 18:** Becoming an Informed Health Care Consumer
Should Health Care Be Rationed in the U.S.?	**Chapter 20:** Conventional and Complementary Medicine	**Chapter 18:** Becoming an Informed Health Care Consumer
Should Prescription Drugs Be Advertised Directly to Consumers?	**Chapter 9:** Drug Abuse and Addiction	**Chapter 7:** Making Decisions About Drug Use **Chapter 18:** Becoming an Informed Health Care Consumer
Are We Winning the War on Cancer?	**Chapter 16:** Cancer	**Chapter 11:** Living with Cancer
Should Marijuana Be Legalized for Medicinal Purposes?	**Chapter 9:** Drug Abuse and Addiction	**Chapter 7:** Making Decisions About Drug Use
Is the Use of "Smart" Pills for Cognitive Enhancement Dangerous?	**Chapter 9:** Drug Abuse and Addiction	**Chapter 7:** Making Decisions About Drug Use **Chapter 18:** Becoming an Informed Health Care Consumer
Should Embryonic Stem Cell Research Be Permitted?		
Should Addiction to Drugs Be Labeled a Brain Disease?	**Chapter 1:** Taking Charge of Your Health **Chapter 9:** Drug Abuse and Addiction	**Chapter 1:** Shaping Your Health **Chapter 7:** Making Decisions About Drug Use
Do Religion and Prayer Benefit Health?	**Chapter 3:** Psychological Health	**Chapter 2:** Achieving Psychological Health
Is It Necessary for Pregnant Women to Completely Abstain from All Alcoholic Beverages?	**Chapter 8:** Pregnancy and Childbirth **Chapter 10:** Alcohol Use and Alcoholism	**Chapter 8:** Taking Control of Alcohol Use **Chapter 16:** Managing Your Fertility
Should Pro-Life Health Providers Be Allowed to Deny Prescriptions on the Basis of Conscience?	**Chapter 6:** Contraception **Chapter 7:** Abortion	**Chapter 16:** Managing Your Fertility
Should the Cervical Cancer Vaccine for Girls Be Compulsory?	**Chapter 5:** Sex and Your Body **Chapter 16:** Cancer **Chapter 18:** Sexually Transmitted Diseases	**Chapter 13:** Preventing Infectious Diseases
Do Ultrathin Models and Actresses Influence the Onset of Eating Disorders?	**Chapter 14:** Weight Management	**Chapter 6:** Maintaining a Healthy Weight
Is There a Valid Reason for Routine Infant Male Circumcision?	**Chapter 5:** Sex and Your Body **Chapter 17:** Immunity and Infection	**Chapter 13:** Preventing Infectious Diseases
Is There a Link Between Vaccination and Autism?	**Chapter 17:** Immunity and Infection **Chapter 19:** Environmental Health	**Chapter 13:** Preventing Infectious Diseases **Chapter 20:** The Environment and Your Health
Do Cell Phones Cause Cancer?	**Chapter 19:** Environmental Health	**Chapter 20:** The Environment and Your Health
Will Hydraulic Fracturing (Fracking) Negatively Affect Human Health and the Environment?	**Chapter 19:** Environmental Health	**Chapter 20:** The Environment and Your Health

Is Breastfeeding the Best Way to Feed Babies?	**Chapter 8:** Pregnancy and Childbirth	**Chapter 17:** Becoming a Parent
Are Restrictions on Sugar and Sugary Beverages Justified?	**Chapter 12:** Nutrition Basics **Chapter 14:** Weight Management	**Chapter 5:** Understanding Nutrition and Your Diet **Chapter 6:** Maintaining a Healthy Weight
Is Weight-Loss Maintenance Possible?	**Chapter 14:** Weight Management	**Chapter 6:** Maintaining a Healthy Weight
Are Energy Drinks with Alcohol Dangerous Enough to Ban?	**Chapter 9:** Drug Use and Addiction **Chapter 10:** Alcohol Use and Alcoholism	**Chapter 7:** Making Decisions About Drug Use **Chapter 8:** Taking Control of Alcohol Use

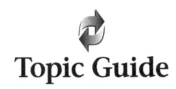

Topic Guide

This topic guide suggests how the issues in this book relate to the subjects covered in your course. You may want to use the topics listed on these pages to search the web more easily.

All the issues that relate to each topic are listed below the bold-faced term.

Alcohol/Alcoholism

Are Energy Drinks with Alcohol Dangerous Enough to Ban?
Is It Necessary for Pregnant Women to Completely Abstain from All Alcoholic Beverages?

Autism

Is There a Link Between Vaccination and Autism?

Birth Control

Does the Affordable Health Care Violate Religious Freedom by Requiring Employers' Health Insurance Plans to Cover Birth Control?
Should Pro-Life Health Providers Be Allowed to Deny Prescriptions on the Basis of Conscience?

Breastfeeding

Is Breastfeeding the Best Way to Feed Babies?

Caffeine

Are Energy Drinks with Alcohol Dangerous Enough to Ban?

Cancer

Are We Winning the War on Cancer?
Do Cell Phones Cause Cancer?
Should the Cervical Cancer Vaccine for Girls Be Compulsory?

Circumcision

Is There a Valid Reason for Routine Infant Male Circumcision?

Dieting and Weight Control

Do Ultrathin Models and Actresses Influence the Onset of Eating Disorders?
Is Weight-Loss Maintenance Possible?

Drugs, Addiction, and Alcohol

Are Energy Drinks with Alcohol Dangerous Enough to Ban?
Is It Necessary for Pregnant Women to Completely Abstain from All Alcoholic Beverages?
Is the Use of "Smart" Pills for Cognitive Enhancement Dangerous?
Should Addiction to Drugs Be Labeled a Brain Disease?
Should Marijuana Be Legalized for Medicinal Purposes?
Should Prescription Drugs Be Advertised Directly to Consumers?

Environmental Health

Do Cell Phones Cause Cancer?
Will Hydraulic Fracturing (Fracking) Negatively Affect Human Health and the Environment?

Health Care

Does the Affordable Health Care Violate Religious Freedom by Requiring Employers' Health Insurance Plans to Cover Birth Control?
Should Health Care Be Rationed in the U.S.?
Should Pro-Life Health Providers Be Allowed to Deny Prescriptions on the Basis of Conscience?

Nutrition

Are Restrictions on Sugar and Sugary Beverages Justified?
Is Weight-loss Maintenance Possible?

Pregnancy

Is It Necessary for Pregnant Women to Completely Abstain from All Alcoholic Beverages?

Prescription Drugs

Should Prescription Drugs Be Advertised Directly to Consumers?
Should Pro-Life Health Providers Be Allowed to Deny Prescriptions on the Basis of Conscience?

Rationing

Should Health Care Be Rationed in the U.S.?

Religion and Health

Do Religion and Prayer Benefit Health?
Does the Affordable Health Care Violate Religious Freedom by Requiring Employers' Health Insurance Plans to Cover Birth Control?

Stem Cells

Should Embryonic Stem Cell Research Be Permitted?

Sugar

Are Restrictions on Sugar and Sugary Beverages Justified?

Vaccination

Is There a Link Between Vaccination and Autism?
Should the Cervical Cancer Vaccine for Girls Be Compulsory?

Women's Health

Do Ultrathin Models and Actresses Influence the Onset of Eating Disorders?
Is Breastfeeding the Best Way to Feed Babies?
Is It Necessary for Pregnant Women to Completely Abstain from All Alcoholic Beverages?
Should the Cervical Cancer Vaccine for Girls Be Compulsory?

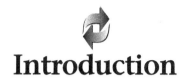

Introduction

What Is Health?

Traditionally, being healthy meant being free of illness. If an individual did not have a disease, then he or she was considered healthy. The overall health of a nation or specific population was determined by data measuring illness, disease, and death rates. Today, this rather negative view of assessing individual health, and health in general, is changing. A healthy person is one who is not only free from disease but also fully well.

Being well, or wellness, involves the interrelationship of many dimensions of health: physical, emotional, social, mental, and spiritual. This multifaceted view of health reflects a holistic approach, which includes individuals taking responsibility for their own well-being.

Our health and longevity are affected by the many choices we make every day: medical reports tell us that if we abstain from smoking, drugs, excessive alcohol, fat, and cholesterol consumption and get regular exercise, the rate of our disease and disability will significantly decrease. These reports, while not totally conclusive, have encouraged many people to make positive lifestyle changes. Millions of people have quit smoking, alcohol consumption is down, and more and more individuals are exercising regularly and eating low-fat diets. While these changes are encouraging, many people who have been unable or unwilling to make these changes are left feeling worried and/or guilty over continuing their negative health behaviors.

But disagreement exists among the experts about the exact nature of positive health behaviors, which causes confusion. For example, some scientists claim that overweight Americans should make efforts to lose weight, even if it takes many tries. Many Americans have unsuccessfully tried to lose weight by eating a low-fat diet though the experts debate which is best: a low-fat, high-carbohydrate diet or a low-carbohydrate diet, which includes ample protein and fat. Other debatable issues include whether or not people utilize conventional medicine or seek out alternative therapies.

Health status is also affected by society and government. Societal pressures have helped pass smoking restrictions in public places, mandatory safety belt legislation, and laws permitting condom distribution in public schools. The government plays a role in the health of individuals as well, although it has failed to provide minimal health care for many low-income Americans.

Unfortunately, there are no absolute answers to many questions regarding health and wellness issues. Moral questions, controversial concerns, and individual perceptions of health matters all can create opposing views. As you evaluate the issues in this book, you should keep an open mind toward both sides. You may not change your mind regarding the morality of abortion or the limitation of health care for the elderly or mentally handicapped, but you will still be able to learn from the opposing viewpoint.

The Health Care Industry

In the United States, approximately 40 million Americans have no health insurance, there has been a resurgence in infectious diseases such as TB, and antibiotic-resistant strains of bacterial infections threaten thousands of Americans, all putting pressure on the current system along with AIDS, diabetes, and other chronic diseases. Those enrolled in government programs such as Medicaid often find few, if any, physicians who will accept them as patients since reimbursements are so low and the paperwork is so cumbersome. On the other hand, Americans continue to live longer and longer, and for most of us, the health care available is among the best in the world. While many Americans agree that there are some situations in which limited health care dollars should be rationed, it's unclear by whom or how these decisions should be made. Other issues in this unit address the debate over the value of direct marketing prescription drugs. While many lifesaving medications have been developed in recent years, they come at a high price. Should consumers pay for the advertising of drugs to enrich pharmaceutical companies?

Health and Society

This unit introduces current issues related to health from a societal perspective. The controversial issues of whether or not schools should be required to track the body mass index of students and report those data to parents, the debate over the "war" on cancer, whether marijuana should be legalized, and whether embryonic stem cell research should be allowed are addressed. Stem cell technology offers the *potential* to cure or treat diseases such as Parkinson's and multiple sclerosis and others. While there are pros and cons to the use of stem cells, ethical and moral questions also arise.

Mind–Body Relationships

Important issues related to the relationship between mind and body are discussed in this unit. Millions of Americans use and abuse drugs that alter their minds and affect their bodies. These drugs range from illegal substances, such as crack cocaine and opiates, to the widely used legal drugs, such as alcohol and tobacco. Increasingly, prescription drugs obtained either legally or not are becoming substances of abuse. Use of these substances can lead to physical and psychological addiction and the related problems of family dysfunction, reduced worker productivity, and crime. Are addictions within the control of individuals who abuse drugs? Or are they an actual disease of the brain, which needs treatment? The role of spirituality in the prevention and treatment of disease is discussed in this unit. Many studies have found that religion and prayer play a role in recovery from sickness. Should health providers encourage spirituality for their patients? Does prayer really help to prevent disease and hasten recovery from illnesses?

Sexuality and Gender Issues

There is much advice given to pregnant women to help ensure they have healthy babies. Research indicates that women who avoid drugs, alcohol, and tobacco reduce the risk of complications. If a pregnant woman does not consume any alcohol, her child will not be born with fetal alcohol syndrome. For some women, however, avoiding alcohol during pregnancy is particularly difficult and they question whether or not it's safe to have a moderate amount of alcohol. For years, physicians and other health providers have cautioned that even one drink consumed at the wrong time could negatively affect the outcome of the pregnancy. This obviously created much concern for women, especially those who drank before they knew they were pregnant.

Other issues debate the conscience clause relative to health providers and whether or not the cervical cancer vaccine for girls should be mandatory. Should pro-life doctors and pharmacists have the right to refuse to prescribe and/or dispense birth control or morning after pills if their beliefs and conscience do not support the use of these drugs? Two selections are debates over the role, if any, ultrathin models and actresses play in the onset of eating disorders. On one side, researchers claim that the promotion of an ultrathin ideal body produces an environment that favors eating disorders. The other side argues that eating disorders predate the ultrathin ideal. Also in this unit is an argument over the validity of routine male circumcision.

Public Health Issues

Debate continues over fundamental matters surrounding many health concerns. Topics addressed in this unit include issues related to immunizations and a possible link to autism, and the ongoing debate over the health impacts of "fracking." While this process of natural gas extraction offers considerable economic benefits, there appears to be a downside related to water pollution and potential human health concerns.

The threat of bioterrorism has resurrected the risk of smallpox, thought to have been eradicated in the late 1970s. Should all parents be forced to have their children immunized against smallpox, which carries certain risks? At the turn of the century, millions of American children developed childhood diseases such as tetanus, polio, measles, and pertussis (whooping cough). Many of these children died or became permanently disabled because of these illnesses. Today, vaccines exist to prevent all of these conditions; however, not all children receive their recommended immunizations. Some do not get vaccinated until the schools require them, and others are allowed exemptions. More and more, parents are requesting exemptions for some or all vaccinations based on fears over their safety and/or their effectiveness. The pertussis vaccination seems to generate the biggest fears. Reports of serious injury to children following the whooping cough vaccination (usually given in a combination of diphtheria, pertussis, and tetanus, or DPT) have convinced many parents to forgo immunization. As a result, the rates of measles and pertussis have been climbing after decades of decline. Is it safer to be vaccinated than to risk getting the disease? Is there a relationship between vaccination and the development of autism? Is the research linking the two valid? Also included in this unit are the health issues linked to breastfeeding. Is it the best way to feed babies? What about women who are unable to nurse their babies? Two authors disagree on this concern.

In September 2012, New York City's Board of Health voted to ban the sale of sugary drinks in containers larger than 16 ounces in restaurants and other venues, in a move meant to combat obesity and encourage residents to live healthier lifestyles. That topic is debated in this unit. Are restrictions on sugar and sugary beverages justified? Finally, the topic of a theoretical relationship between cell phone usage and cancer is addressed. As the number of cell phones continues to rise, questions about their safety are raised.

Consumer Health

This unit introduces questions about particular issues related to consumer choices about health issues or products. As Americans grow increasingly overweight, the most effective means of weight control continues to be debated. Along with that debate is the controversy over whether or not it's possible to lose weight and actually keep it off. The risk associated with the use of alcoholic energy drinks is an increasingly important topic and many college students consume this beverage.

Will the many debates presented in this book ever be resolved? Some issues may resolve themselves because of the availability of resources. For instance, health care rationing in the United States, as it is in the United Kingdom, may be legislated simply because there are increasingly limited resources to go around. An overhaul of the health care system to provide care for all while keeping costs down seems inevitable, as most Americans agree that the system should be changed. Other controversies may require the test of time for resolution. The debates over the health effects of global warming and the long-term benefits of medical marijuana may also take years to be fully resolved.

Other controversies may never resolve themselves. There may never be a consensus over the right of health providers to be allowed to deny care based on their beliefs, the abortion issue, rationing health care, or the cancer–cell phone connection. This book will introduce you to many ongoing controversies on a variety of sensitive and complex health-related topics. In order to have a good grasp of one's own viewpoint, it is necessary to be familiar with and understand the points made by the opposition.

Eileen Daniel
SUNY Brockport

Unit 1

UNIT

The Health Care Industry

*T*he United States currently faces many challenging health and health care concerns, including lack of universal health insurance for all its citizens. Unlike other major industrialized nations, the United States doesn't have a single payer plan to fund national health coverage, and over 40 million Americans are without health insurance. We also don't have a formal means of rationing health care, which exists in other developed nations. We do have a for-profit health care system that includes direct marketing of prescription drugs to Americans. For over 20 years, drug companies have advertised prescription medications on television, in newspapers, magazines, and online.

Does the Affordable Health Care Act Violate Religious Freedom by Requiring Health Care Plans to Cover Birth Control? by Daniel

13

Selected, Edited, and with Issue Framing Material by:
Eileen Daniel, *SUNY College at Brockport*

ISSUE

Does the Affordable Health Care Violate Religious Freedom by Requiring Employers' Health Insurance Plans to Cover Birth Control?

YES: **Wesley J. Smith**, from "What About Religious Freedom: The Other Consequences of Obamacare," *The Weekly Standard* (October 29, 2012)

NO: **Aram A. Schvey**, from "Much Ado About Nothing?" *Human Rights* (January 2013)

Learning Outcomes

After reading this issue, you should be able to:

- Discuss the provisions of the Affordable Care Act.
- Assess the impact of the Act on religious liberty.
- Discuss the importance of access to affordable birth control.

ISSUE SUMMARY

YES: Senior fellow in the Discovery Institute's Center on Human Exceptionalism Wesley J. Smith believes birth control cases are just the beginning for far more intrusive violations of religious liberty to come, for example, requiring businesses to provide free abortions to their employees.

NO: Attorney and Policy Counsel for Foreign Policy and Human Rights at the Center for Reproductive Rights Aram A. Schvey argues that access to affordable contraception is a cornerstone of women's independence and equality and that the Affordable Care Act does not violate religious freedom.

$\mathbf{T}$he Patient Protection and Affordable Care Act (PPACA), also known as "Obamacare" (common usage) or the Affordable Care Act, is a federal statute signed into law by President Obama in the spring of 2010. The Act aims to both increase the rate of Americans with health insurance and lower the overall costs of health care. The PPACA includes several components including mandates, subsidies, and tax credits to help and encourage employers and individuals to increase the coverage rate. Additional reforms seek to improve health care outcomes and streamline the delivery of health care. The Congressional Budget Office predicts that the PPACA will reduce both future deficits and spending for Medicare.

Polls indicate support of health care reform in general, but became more negative in regards to specific plans during legislative debates. While the Act was ultimately signed into law in 2010, it remains controversial with opinions falling along party lines. Opinions are clearly divided by age and party affiliation, with a solid majority

of seniors and Republicans opposing the bill while a solid majority of Democrats and those younger than 40 in favor. In a 2010 poll conducted by CNN, 62 percent of respondents said they thought the PPACA would "increase the amount of money they personally spend on health care," 56 percent said the bill "gives the government too much involvement in health care," and only 19 percent said they thought they and their families would be better off with the legislation.

The Act mandates that insurance companies cover all applicants at the same rates regardless of preexisting conditions or gender. In addition, a controversial provision mandates that all insurance policies cover birth control without a co-pay as part of preventive care. The Act requires that all insurance policies cover *all* forms of basic preventive care without a co-pay, including wellwoman, well-baby, and well-child visits, as well as other basic prevention care for men and women. This coverage is intended to save costs and promote public health. Basic preventive, reproductive, and sexual health care services, including contraception, are therefore also covered without a co-pay; as part of the mandate, all insurance plans must provide coverage without a co-pay for all methods of contraception approved by the Food and Drug Administration (FDA). Employees *earn* their salaries and their benefits, and many pay for all or a portion of their health care premiums out of their salaries. As such, none of this coverage is "free," but is rather covered by the policies they are earning or for which they are paying.

In January 2013 the Obama administration issued a rule that most employers, including religiously affiliated institutions such as Catholic universities and hospitals, must provide health care coverage that includes contraceptive services for all women employees and their dependents, at no cost to the employee. A narrow exemption exists for some religious employers, limited in most cases to houses of worship. The requirement only affects health care plans created after March 23, 2010. Plans in effect before that date do not have to meet the new rules.

While women's health advocates applauded the new rule, intense pressure from prominent religious organizations, including the U.S. Conference of Catholic Bishops, immediately followed. In response the Obama administration issued a compromise. Objecting nonprofit religious employers will not be required to pay for contraceptive services, instead shifting the cost to the employer's health insurance company. Those opposed to the compromise find the mandate a stark contradiction to the First Amendment to the U.S. Constitution: "Congress shall make no law respecting an establishment of religion." In addition, many Catholic organizations say that shifting the cost of birth control to the insurer does not resolve the moral objection, because they are self-insured, meaning the insurance provider and the organization are one in the same. Opponents also feel the government should not have permission to come in and force an organization to

violate its religious beliefs. While there is religious opposition, there are some strong proponents of the mandate who maintain that no one is denying anybody's religious rights. Religious activists hold that while protecting religious liberties is an important responsibility of government, blocking a plan designed to serve all people based on the values of one faith system becomes a violation of their rights. Those who favor the bill also contend that the bill is about women's right to comprehensive and preventive (as elsewhere) health care with equal access regardless of cost, and it's just good health care.

In the spring of 2013, 18 for-profit companies filed lawsuits to avoid complying with the birth control benefit in the Affordable Care Act (ACA) based on several claims. One is that providing insurance policies that cover birth control violates the religious freedom of the companies' owners. The owners of these companies share the belief that a woman is pregnant as soon as there is a fertilized egg (the medical definition of pregnancy is successful implantation of an embryo in the uterine wall) and that a fertilized egg has the same rights as a born person. They also claim that the ACA forces them to cover "abortifacients," with most pointing to emergency contraception methods such as Plan B to make their case. Emergency contraception, however, prevents ovulation, and therefore fertilization, and does not work after an egg has been fertilized. These lawsuits, now in various phases of litigation, are posing a critical challenge to the Affordable Care Act. Wesley J. Smith believes birth control cases are just the beginning for far more intrusive violation of religious liberty to come and is concerned over a slippery slope where businesses might be required to provide free abortions to their employees. Attorney and editor Aram A. Schvey argues that access to affordable contraception is a cornerstone of women's independence and equality and that the Affordable Care Act does not violate religious freedom.

Does the Affordable Health Care Act Violate Religious Freedom by Requiring Health Care Plans to Cover Birth Control? by Daniel

15

YES ↵

Wesley J. Smith

What About Religious Freedom: The Other Consequences of Obamacare

Obamacare won't just ruin health care. It is also a cultural bulldozer. Before the law is even fully in effect, Health and Human Services bureaucrats have begun wielding their sweeping new powers to assault freedom of religion in the name of their preferred social order.

The promulgation of the free birth control rule indicates the regulatory road ahead. The government now requires every covered employer to provide health insurance that offers birth control and sterilization surgeries free of charge—even if such drugs and procedures violate the religious beliefs of the employer. Only houses of worship and monastic communities are exempt. Religious institutions have until August 1, 2013, to comply.

The lawsuits are flying. In August, the Catholic owners of Hercules Industries, a Colorado air conditioning and heating manufacturer, won a preliminary injunction against enforcement of the free birth control rule against their company (*Newland* v. *Sebelius*). The case hinges on the meaning of the Religious Freedom Restoration Act (RFRA), enacted in 1993 to remedy a Supreme Court decision allowing federal drug laws of "general applicability" to supersede Native American religious ceremonies in which peyote is used. Since many laws not aimed at stifling a specific faith can be construed to do so, the threat to religious liberty was clear. A Democratic Congress passed, and President Clinton signed, RFRA.

RFRA states that the government "shall not substantially burden a person's exercise of religion" unless it can demonstrate that the law "is in furtherance of a compelling governmental interest." The *Newland* trial judge found that forcing Hercules to pay for birth control—the company is self-insured—did indeed constitute a substantial burden on the owners' free exercise of their Catholic faith. Since no compelling government interest was found, the judge protected the company from the rule pending trial. The Department of Justice has appealed.

Alas, in a nearly identical case, *O'Brien* v. *U.S. Department of Health and Human Services*, U.S. District Judge Carol E. Jackson reached the opposite legal conclusion. Frank O'Brien is the Catholic owner of O'Brien Industrial Holdings, LLC, a mining company in St. Louis. Demonstrating the sincerity and depth of O'Brien's faith, a statue of the Sacred Heart of Jesus greets visitors in the company's lobby, and the mission statement on its website affirms the intent "to make our labor pleasing to the Lord."

Despite acknowledging "the sincerity of plaintiff's beliefs" and "the centrality of plaintiff's condemnation of contraception to their exercise of the Catholic religion," Jackson dismissed O'Brien's case on the basis that forcing his company to buy insurance covering contraception was not a "substantial burden" on his religious freedom.

Here is the philosophical core of the ruling:

> The challenged regulations do not demand that plaintiffs alter their behavior in a manner that will directly and inevitably prevent plaintiffs from acting in accordance with their religious beliefs. Frank O'Brien is not prevented from keeping the Sabbath, from providing a religious upbringing for his children, or from participating in a religious ritual such as communion. Instead plaintiffs remain free to exercise their religion, by not using contraceptives and by discouraging employees from using contraceptives.

Excuse me, but that's a lot like a judge telling a Jewish butcher that his freedom of religion is not violated by a regulation requiring him to carry nonkosher wares in his shop. After all, the government wouldn't be requiring *the butcher* to eat nonkosher meat.

More to the point, Jackson embraced the Department of Justice's reasoning. If this view prevails, it will shrivel the "free exercise of religion" guaranteed by the First Amendment into mere "freedom of worship," limiting RFRA's protections to personal morality, domestic activities, and religious rites behind closed doors. Worse, the court ruled that O'Brien is the aggressor in the matter, *that it is he who is seeking to violate the rights of his employees.* "RFRA is a shield, not a sword," Judge Jackson wrote, "it is not a means to force one's religious practices upon others."

How does O'Brien's desire not to involve himself in any way with contraception force Catholicism upon his employees? He hasn't threatened anyone's job for not following Catholic moral teaching. He hasn't tried to prevent any employee from using birth control. He hasn't compelled employees to go to confession or get baptized. He merely chooses not to be complicit in what he considers sinful activities.

But that analysis presupposes that O'Brien's religious freedom extends to his actions as an employer. It doesn't, sayeth the Obama administration: "By definition, a secular employer does not engage in any 'exercise of religion,'" the Department of Justice argued in the *Newland* case. In other words, according to the Obama administration, the realm of commerce is a religion-free zone.

Some might dismiss these employers' concerns because birth control is hardly controversial outside of orthodox religious circles. But these birth control cases are stalking horses for far more intrusive violations of religious liberty to come, e.g., requiring businesses to provide free abortions to their employees. Consider the Democratic party's 2012 platform:

> The Democratic party strongly and unequivocally supports *Roe* v. *Wade* and a woman's right to make decisions regarding her pregnancy, including a safe and legal abortion, *regardless of ability to pay*. [Emphasis added.]

If Democrats regain the control of Congress and the presidency they enjoyed in 2009 and 2010, look for the Affordable Care Act to be amended consistent with their platform. After that, it won't take long for HHS to promulgate a free abortion rule along lines similar to the free birth control mandate.

And what could be done about it? According to Judge Jackson's thinking, ensuring free access to abortion would not prevent employers from "keeping the Sabbath." They would not be prohibited from "providing a religious upbringing" for their children or "participating in a religious ritual such as communion." Rather, they would be barred from "forcing their religious practices" on employees by leaving employees to pay for their own terminations. In time, why shouldn't in-vitro fertilization, assisted suicide, and sex change operations be added to the list?

If higher courts accept this radically antireligious view, the only corrective will be to amend RFRA to spell out that its protections extend to the actions of employers. In fact, why not take that step now and short circuit what could be years of litigation defending religious liberty in the public square?

WESLEY J. SMITH is a senior fellow in the Discovery Institute's Center on Human Exceptionalism and consults for the Patients Rights Council and the Center for Bioethics and Culture.

Does the Affordable Health Care Act Violate Religious Freedom by Requiring Health Care Plans to Cover Birth Control? by Daniel

17

Aram A. Schvey

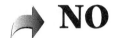 **NO**

Much Ado About Nothing?

Religious Freedom and the Contraceptive-Coverage Benefit

August 1, 2012: A date that will live in infamy. Or so some religious conservatives contend. Matt Smith, president of the Catholic Advocate, solemnly declared that "August first will be remembered as the day our most cherished liberty was thrown in a government dumpster and hauled away." L. Brent Bozell III, president of the conservative Media Research Center, inveighed that "the beginning of the end of freedom as America has known it and loved it" was nigh. And, unsatisfied with even that level of rhetoric, Rep. Mike Kelly (R-PA) went so far as to compare August 1, 2012, to America's darkest hours:

> [Y]ou can think of the times America was attacked. One is December 7, that's Pearl Harbor Day. The other is September 11, and that's the day the terrorists attacked. I want you to remember August 1, 2012, the attack on our religious freedom. That is a day that will live in infamy, along with those other dates.

What event occurred on August 1, 2012, to give rise to such fire-and-brimstone rhetoric? A terrorist attack? A dastardly sneak attack by an enemy nation? A tyrannical military coup d'état?

Hardly. Instead, August 1, 2012, is the day that the 99 percent of American women who have used contraception (including 98 percent of Catholic women) could kiss their copays goodbye and save hundreds of dollars a year on essential reproductive health care. On that date, the contraceptive-coverage benefit of the Affordable Care Act (also known as "Obamacare") went into effect. Under the new policy, most employers' health-insurance plans (other than those for houses of worship) must begin covering FDA-approved contraception (including sterilization and emergency contraception) and associated counseling without cost-sharing—eliminating contraceptive copays.

What to most Americans was a tremendous health care benefit—saving them hundreds of dollars per year in out-of-pocket costs and putting contraception, and, in particular, expensive long-term contraceptive methods, within reach—is to some an affront to and violation of their religious liberty. Critics of the policy who see contraception as sinful are outraged that employees might access contraception through a company-subsidized health-insurance plan despite the company owner's sincerely held belief that contraception is sinful.

This notion—that the contraceptive-coverage benefit runs roughshod over employers' religious liberty—is a claim that has been repeated often and with great fervor. But the dispute cannot be fairly reduced to a conflict between those who support and those who oppose religious liberty. Indeed, all sides agree that religious liberty is a bedrock American value and worthy of protection. What is at issue in the debate is whose religious liberty is at stake: the employers who object to the fact that some employees may access contraception through health-insurance plans, or employees, who risk losing essential health-insurance coverage based on their employer's religious beliefs. Ultimately, this article concludes, religious liberty belongs equally to all Americans. But it is not a sword to be used by those at the top of the employment ladder to hack away at those at lower rungs; rather, it is a shield that protects all individuals' religious beliefs equally.

Background

The contraceptive-coverage policy was recommended as part of a comprehensive set of preventive services for women through the Women's Health Amendment to the Affordable Care Act by a blue-ribbon panel of acclaimed medical experts convened by the Institute of Medicine (other recommendations included improved cancer and sexually transmitted infection (STI) screenings, broadly available lactation counseling, and no-copay annual well-woman preventivecare visits). The purpose of the contraceptive-coverage policy is to promote the health of women and children nationwide by addressing America's sky-high unintended-pregnancy rate: Half of all U.S. pregnancies are unintended, and those unintended pregnancies pose real health risks for women, and, where the pregnancy is taken to term, for newborns. By making contraception—and, in particular, more expensive, but more effective, long-acting contraception (such as intrauterine devices (IUDs) and implants)—more affordable, the policy aims to cut the unintended pregnancy rate, promote health, and save money in the process (because studies demonstrate that a dollar spent on contraception can save more than four dollars in medical costs).

In rolling out the no-copay-contraception policy, the administration recognized that churches and other religious employers might have objections to carrying health insurance that in turn covered contraception. Consequently, the Department of Health and Human Services proposed carving out a special exemption to the policy for houses of worship, as a means of respecting "the unique relationship between a house of worship and its employees in ministerial positions," even though such an exemption was not required as a matter of law. The exemption applies to a nonprofit employer if its purpose is the inculcation of religious values and if it primarily employs and serves those sharing its religious tenets, such as a church or mosque. The exemption does not, however, extend to institutions claiming a religious affiliation that hire and serve nonadherents, such as hospitals and universities; nor does it apply to for-profit companies. The reason is simple: Allowing any corporation or institution to claim exemptions from the law would, in effect, allow the exceptions to swallow the rule, turning the law into Swiss cheese and blunting its purpose of promoting the health of women and infants. It would also have the effect of imposing the employer's religious beliefs on nonbelievers, thus making employees' benefits subject to their employer's religious views.

The exemption did little to quiet critics, and the outcry from religious conservatives and others was quick and vociferous. Despite the fact that most states already mandate coverage for contraceptive drugs and devices, and that many of those states include no exemption whatsoever, the U.S. Conference of Catholic Bishops decried the contraception-coverage benefit as "unprecedented" and numerous institutions claiming a religious affiliation, for-profit companies, and a group of state attorneys general have filed lawsuits to try to halt the implementation of the law. In response, the administration proposed an additional accommodation whereby the cost of the contraception would be explicitly borne by the health-insurance companies, rather than the employer issuing the insurance policy. But neither this second accommodation, nor a one-year safe-harbor provision for groups with religious objections, has quieted the furor.

A number of the suits have been dismissed as premature in light of the safe-harbor provision, but in July 2012 a federal district judge in Colorado granted a preliminary injunction preventing the policy from being enforced against Hercules Industries, a for-profit heating, ventilation, and air-conditioning company, whose owners object to contraception. In late September 2012, however, a federal district judge in Missouri dismissed on the merits a challenge to the contraceptive-coverage benefit brought by a for-profit mining company whose mission includes "mak[ing] our labor a pleasing offering to the Lord."

The current debate surrounding the contraceptive-coverage benefit continues, both in Congress and in the courts. Assuming the Affordable Care Act is not repealed, it may take a Supreme Court decision, in light of the possibility of the circuit courts of appeals splitting on the issue (a likely scenario, given that lawsuits have been filed in numerous circuits). While the claims made in each case differ, the major claims are based on the First Amendment and on the Religious Freedom Restoration Act (RFRA), a 1993 federal statute that applies a strict-scrutiny test to federal actions that substantially burden a person's exercise of **religion.**

Legal Claims

At first blush, one might assume that the First Amendment claims being made by those challenging the contraceptive-coverage benefit are strong. But, in fact, the Supreme Court has roundly rejected the proposition that an otherwise neutral and generally applicable law is unconstitutional simply because it happens to interfere with someone's religious beliefs. Perhaps even more surprising is the fact that this understanding of the First Amendment's intended contours was set forth by the very Supreme Court justice who is commonly thought of as conservative and therefore assumed to be sympathetic to religious-liberty claims—Justice Antonin Scalia.

In *Employment Division v. Smith*, 494 U.S. 872 (1990), the Court confronted a challenge to a statute that denied unemployment benefits to drug users, including Native Americans who consumed sacramental peyote. Justice Scalia, writing for the Court, rejected the claim that the drug-use prohibition violated the Free Exercise Clause as applied to Native Americans who consumed peyote: "The government's ability to carry out aspects of public policy, cannot depend on measuring the effects of a governmental action on a religious objector's spiritual development"; otherwise, every religious objector would "become a law unto himself," a result that Justice Scalia found to be unsupported by both the Constitution and common sense. If a law is neutral and generally applicable, and does not directly target religious activity qua religious activity, it is constitutional. Whether or not an exemption might be desirable, Justice Scalia emphasized, "is not to say that it is constitutionally required."

There is no question that the contraception-coverage benefit is both neutral and generally applicable, and thus accords with the First Amendment. Far from deliberately targeting religious activity, the policy focuses on insurance coverage. And the policy, of course, applies to employers irrespective of their religiosity, or the nature of their religious views. There is simply no support for the claim by the U.S. Conference of Catholic Bishops that the law "targets Catholicism for special disfavor." Indeed, the policy was based on the recommendation of a blue-ribbon panel of medical experts, which in turn was based on substantial scholarship and research.

The stronger claim advanced by opponents of the contraceptive-coverage benefit is that the policy violates the RFRA, a statute designed to overturn legislatively Employment Division and impose a strict-scrutiny test on laws that burden religious exercise. Under RFRA, any federal policy that substantially burdens a person's religious exercise must be justified by a compelling interest, and

Does the Affordable Health Care Act Violate Religious Freedom by Requiring Health Care Plans to Cover Birth Control? by Daniel

19

use the least restrictive means of achieving that interest. Opponents of the contraceptive-coverage benefit argue that a company owner or other employer's religious exercise is substantially burdened by the fact that his or her employees may seek, and access, contraception that the owner/employer finds sinful.

There are numerous problems with this claim—most centrally, the fact that it utterly ignores the religious-liberty interest of the employees, whose health-insurance benefits would be restricted based on their employer's religious beliefs. Indeed, in the Hercules Industries case mentioned above, when the judge sought to balance the harms in deciding whether to grant a preliminary injunction, he weighed the employer's religious-liberty interest against the government's interest in enforcing laws. What is shockingly absent is any consideration of the impact of the decision on the company's 265 employees and their dependents, who have the most to lose in any decision.

This factor—the impact on third parties—is what distinguishes the religious-liberty claims being made here from those made in previous instances where the Supreme Court has permitted a derogation from an otherwise applicable law. For example, in *Wisconsin v. Yoder*, 406 U.S. 205 (1972), the Supreme Court permitted an exemption to school-attendance laws for Amish children. But, in so doing, the Court emphasized that "there is no intimation" that permitting the children to opt out of public schooling "is in any way deleterious to their health."

But with respect to the contraceptive-coverage benefit, there is an obvious impact on employees' well-being—an opt-out for employers would directly harm employees' health. And the Supreme Court has emphasized that one person's sphere of religious liberty only extends to the boundary of another person's sphere of religious liberty. The common thread in the Court's exemptions-related cases is that the religious exercise protected in each instance "did not, or would not, impose substantial burdens on non-beneficiaries while allowing others to act according to their religious beliefs nor [would they] impose monetary costs on [those] who opposed the religious instruction."

In contrast, exempting employers from the contraceptive-coverage benefit would directly impose both a health and a monetary burden on employees. This differentiates the sought exemption from other religious exemptions—for example, allowing Sikh policemen to have beards or allowing a Saturday-Sabbath observer to collect unemployment benefits if the only jobs she can find require Saturday labor.

In addition, it is wholly unclear whether RFRA even applies to corporations and companies, rather than actual flesh-and-blood human beings, or, as the court in the Hercules Industries case posited, "can a corporation exercise religion?" To answer in the affirmative would certainly open the floodgates to substantial mischief, potentially allowing corporations to flout discrimination laws and other worker protections, zoning policies, and safety regulations by claiming a religious posture. And even if RFRA protections were extended to companies and corporations, it is a highly dubious proposition that purchasing insurance coverage constitutes "religious exercise."

To the extent that a corporate employer can invoke RFRA, the burden on religious exercise is minimal. In the cases where the Supreme Court has found a burden on religious exercise, an individual was prohibited by law from actually exercising his or her religion—keeping the Saturday Sabbath, for example, or using prescribed sacramental substances. In contrast, the employers in the various lawsuits are not being prevented from keeping the Sabbath, participating in communion, or providing religious schooling for their children. And they are certainly not being forced to use contraception or encourage its use; indeed, they remain free to speak out against it. Instead, as the federal district judge noted in the case dismissing an employer's lawsuit, the supposed burden complained of is that an employer will contribute to a health care plan that might, after a series of independent decisions by employees and medical professionals, lead some employees to access contraception that is in some way subsidized by the employer. The link between the employer's subsidization of insurance coverage and the ultimate receipt of contraceptives by an individual employee is so remote as to be meaningless. Indeed, it is difficult to distinguish an employer's supposed interest in how employees use their health insurance from an employer's interest in how employees use their salaries (which are, of course, paid by the employer).

Finally, the contraceptive-coverage benefit is consonant with RFRA because it advances a compelling governmental interest and uses the least restrictive means to achieve it. As noted, the policy furthers a compelling interest in women's health and newborn health. It furthers a compelling interest in combating sex-based inequality—in December 2000, the Equal Employment Opportunity Commission held that Title VII of the Civil Rights Act bars employer-sponsored health-insurance plans that provide prescription-drug coverage but fail to cover contraceptives. It also helps remedy the insurance "penalty" women pay by virtue of being female: Senator Barbara Mikulski, the architect of the legislation underlying the contraceptive-coverage benefit, noted that she hoped that the Women's Health Amendment would remedy the sex discrimination women face when purchasing insurance. And, finally, the policy promotes a compelling government interest in women's autonomy. As a society, we recognize that access to affordable contraception is a cornerstone of women's independence and equality. Justice Sandra Day O'Connor, the first female Supreme Court justice, said it best: "The ability of women to participate equally in the economic and social life of the Nation has been facilitated by their ability to control their reproductive lives."

These are powerful and compelling governmental interests. Where such compelling interests are present, the Supreme Court has consistently rejected religious opt-outs. It bears remembering that groups have often sought exemptions from broadly applicable laws based on religious beliefs. Religious groups have, over time, sought to be exempt from laws banning polygamy, from laws banning child labor, from laws banning racial discrimination, and from laws requiring the payment of taxes. In all of these cases, and in many more, the courts roundly rejected such claims. And with respect to the contraceptive-coverage policy, the highest courts of California and New York confronted challenges to their state's contraceptive-coverage laws, in both cases rejecting religious-liberty challenges to the same narrow religious exemption currently at issue in the federal policy. The California Supreme Court's decision is particularly instructive, holding, "We are unaware of any decision in which the United States Supreme Court has exempted a religious objector from the operation of a neutral, generally applicable law despite the recognition that the requested exemption would detrimentally affect the rights of third parties."

Conclusion

Religious liberty is a core American value, and the delicate balance between the First Amendment's Free Exercise and Establishment Clauses is a uniquely American contribution to global jurisprudence. But in a nation blessed with almost endless religious diversity—with those subscribing to all manner of faiths and none, and innumerable interpretations and manifestations of those beliefs—preferencing one person's religious liberty, or one group of people's religious liberty, without regard to others inevitably results in a diminution of rights.

As a nation, we have, and will continue, to struggle to balance laws and policies protecting the individual and those protecting the community. Where religious liberty is used as a shield, the courts have rightly upheld exemptions to protect religious worship and customs from government intrusion. But the courts have rightly rejected—and should continue to reject—claims where religious liberty is used as a sword to subordinate the rights of others. Indeed, the nation was founded on the principle that all Americans, whether corner-office prince or mail-room pauper, have an equal claim to religious liberty.

Aram A. Schvey serves as policy counsel at the Center for Reproductive Rights, a global human rights organization dedicated to promoting reproductive rights in the United States and around the world. He previously served as litigation counsel at Americans United for Separation of Church and State and has served as a fellow at the Georgetown University Law Center and Fordham Law School. He also serves on the editorial board for *Human Rights*.

EXPLORING THE ISSUE

Does the Affordable Health Care Violate Religious Freedom by Requiring Employers' Health Insurance Plans to Cover Birth Control?

Critical Thinking and Reflection

1. Why might affordable birth control be considered the cornerstone of women's independence and equality?
2. Does the Affordable Care Act violate religious freedom?
3. Describe how providing birth control through the Affordable Care Act might be perceived as a violation of religious liberty.

Is There Common Ground?

The government estimated that the Affordable Care Act legislation will lower the number of the uninsured by 32 million, leaving 23 million uninsured residents by 2019 after the bill's mandates have all taken effect. Among the people in this uninsured group will be approximately 8 million illegal immigrants, individuals eligible but not enrolled in Medicare, and mostly the young and single men and women not otherwise covered who choose to pay the annual penalty instead of purchasing insurance.

Early experience under the Act was that, as a result of the tax credit for small businesses, some businesses offered health insurance to their employees for the first time. On September 13, 2011, the Census Bureau released a report showing that the number of uninsured 19- to 25-year-olds (now eligible to stay on their parents' policies) had declined by 393,000, or 1.6 percent. A later report from the Government Accountability Office in 2012 found that of the 4 million small businesses that were offered the tax credit only 170,300 businesses claimed it. Due to the effect of the U.S. Supreme court ruling, states can opt in or out of the expansion of Medicaid.

Also, a component ensuring children could remain included on their parents' plans until age 26 remains a popular, fairly noncontroversial part of the bill. The contraceptive coverage, however, remains contentious. The Affordable Care Act includes a contraceptive coverage mandate that, with the exception of churches and houses of worship, applies to all employers and educational institutions. These regulations made under The Act rely on the recommendations of the Institute of Medicine, which concluded that access to contraception is medically necessary "to ensure women's health and well-being."

The initial regulations proved controversial among Christian hospitals, Christian charities, Catholic universities, and other enterprises owned or controlled by religious organizations that oppose contraception on doctrinal grounds. To accommodate those concerns while still guaranteeing access to contraception, the regulations were adjusted to "allow religious organizations to opt out of the requirement to include birth control coverage in their employee insurance plans. In those instances, the insurers themselves will offer contraception coverage to enrollees directly, at no additional cost." Unfortunately, this didn't entirely satisfy religious organizations who still believe their beliefs are being compromised.

Create Central

www.mhhe.com/createcentral

Additional Resources

Afendulis, C. C., Landrum, M., & Chernew, M. E. (2012). The impact of the Affordable Care Act on Medicare Advantage Plan availability and enrollment. *Health Services Research, 47*(6), 2339–2352.

Burlone, S., Edelman, A. B., Caughey, A. B., Trussell, J., Dantas, S., & Rodriguez, M. I. (2013). Extending contraceptive coverage under the Affordable Care Act saves public funds. *Contraception, 87*(2), 143–148.

Morse, E. A. (2013). Lifting the fog: Navigating penalties in the Affordable Care Act. *Creighton Law Review, 46*(2), 207–257.

Shaffer, E. R. (2013). The Affordable Care Act: The value of systemic disruption. *American Journal of Public Health, 103*(4), 1180-e4.

What are the White House and The Bishops fighting about? (2012). *America, 206*(5), 6–7.

Internet References . . .

Health Care

www.healthcare.gov

Health Care Law and You

www.healthcare.gov/law/

Planned Parenthood

www.plannedparenthood.org

Selected, Edited, and with Issue Framing Material by:
Eileen Daniel, *SUNY College at Brockport*

ISSUE

Should Health Care Be Rationed in the U.S.?

YES: Daniel Callahan, from "Rationing: Theory, Politics, and Passions," *Hastings Center Report* (March/April 2011)

NO: James Ridgeway, from "Meet the Real Death Panels," *Mother Jones* (July/August 2010)

Learning Outcomes
After reading this issue, you should be able to:
• Discuss the different types of health care rationing in the United States.
• Address criteria used to determine who is treated.
• Discuss the justification for rationing health care.

ISSUE SUMMARY

YES: Ethicist and philosopher Daniel Callahan believes that while some individuals may be hurt by health care rationing, these decisions must and will be made eventually.

NO: Author James Ridgeway argues that health care should be treated as a human right instead of a profit-making opportunity.

There are different types of health care rationing in the United States. Rationing is defined as restricting or limiting health care services or supplies to only those individuals who can afford to pay. Currently about one-sixth of the U.S. population is either too poor to pay for health care services or does not qualify for government-supported programs such as Medicaid. Rationing, however, is based not only on ability to pay but also on employment benefits, age, preexisting medical conditions, and even lifestyle. Should health care benefits cover expensive treatments such as liver transplants to chronic alcoholics? Over 40 million Americans have no health insurance while others are denied coverage based on preexisting health problems. Government programs for the poor such as Medicaid also ration coverage by income levels, while Health Maintenance Organizations restrict access and coverage for certain procedures and drugs.

Because of their high health care utilization, there is talk of rationing health care for those over age 65. In 1980, 11 percent of the U.S. population was over age 65, but they utilized about 29 percent ($219 billion) of the total American health care expenditures. By the beginning of the new millennium, the percentage of the population over 65 had risen to 12 percent, which consumed 31 percent of total health care expenditures,

or $450 billion. It has been projected that by the year 2040, people over 65 will represent 21 percent of the population and will consume 45 percent of all health care expenditures.

Medical expenses at the end of life appear to be particularly high in relation to other health care costs. Studies have shown that nearly one-third of annual Medicare costs are for the beneficiaries who die that year. Expenses for dying patients increase significantly as death nears, and payments for health care during the last weeks of life make up 40 percent of the medical costs for the entire last year of life. Some studies have shown that up to 50 percent of the medical costs incurred during a person's entire life are spent during their last year!

Overall as health care costs for Americans of all ages rise, there will be consequences of not controlling these costs. Rationing health care means getting value for the billions we are spending by setting limits on which treatments should be paid for from the public purse. If we ration we won't be writing blank checks to pharmaceutical companies for the patented drugs, nor paying for whatever procedures doctors choose to recommend. When public funds subsidize health care or provide it directly, it is crazy not to try to get value for the money. The debate over health care reform in the United States should start from the promise that some form of health care rationing is both inescapable and desirable. Then we can ask, "What is the best way to follow it?" While Daniel Callahan is an advocate for rational rationing, others such as James Ridgeway believe that we need to make our system more efficient, so we can economically provide health care services to all Americans, not just those who can pay.

In the YES selection, Daniel Callahan argues that it is critical that we adopt some time of systematic rationing as the costs of health care continue to rise. In the NO selection, James Ridgeway maintains that health care must be appropriate, not rationed. He stresses that health care is a basic right of all humans and should not be viewed as an opportunity to make a profit.

YES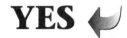

Daniel Callahan

Rationing: Theory, Politics, and Passions

A confession is in order. As did almost everyone else of a certain persuasion, I recoiled when Sarah Palin invoked the notion of a "death panel" to characterize reform efforts to improve end-of-life counseling. That was wrong and unfair. But I was left uneasy by her phrase. Had I not been one of a handful of bioethicists over the years who had pushed to bring the need for rationing of health care to public attention and proposed ways to carry it out? And was not a common thread running through the latter efforts the likely necessity of some kind of committee or other public mechanism to make the hard decisions? Were we not in other words talking about a "death panel," even if none of us has been so imprudent to use such a phrase? And did we not regularly bemoan the fact that politicians, left and right, would not go near the word "rationing"?

My answer to all those questions is yes, but with some important distinctions. One of them bears on the theoretical efforts to make a case for rationing and to propose means to carry it out. Another is the gap between that effort and the political realities of bringing rationing theory before the public eye. Still another is whether it is possible to envision an ethical theory that takes politics fully into account. But there is first a larger background story to be told about all that.

The larger story appropriately begins with the 1960 event that has often been thought of as the birth of bioethics. In that year, the University of Washington nephrologist Belding Scribner devised a shunt that would allow those suffering from kidney failure to be hooked up to a dialysis machine that could keep them alive for many years. But there were few of those machines and many more candidates for their use than could be accommodated. Rationing decisions of the most wrenching kind had to be made.[1]

The solution was a procedural one: the formation of two committees, one of them to determine the medical criteria for selecting candidates. The other was an Admissions and Policy Committee to choose, as the prominent journalist Shana Alexander wrote, "who shall live and who shall die." For four years that committee—whose membership was anonymous—made case-by-case decisions, and its general criterion was a troubling concept, that of the "social worth" of the patients. The committee had a dreadful time making such choices, and the very idea of such a committee was widely assaulted.

Dr. Scribner said later that "we had been naive" not to realize that what seemed to be the "reasonable and simple solution of . . . letting a committee of responsible members of the community choose patients" would evoke "a very serious storm of criticism."[2] Among those in ethics who entered the fray were James Childress and Paul Ramsey, who contended that a random lottery solution would be more fair, and the philosopher Nicholas Rescher, who favored a utilitarian solution that tacitly seemed to accept the "social worth" standard.

The dialysis controversy finally came to an end in 1972, when Congress passed a bill providing Medicare coverage for it. Money, in short, was the way out of the moral dilemmas of committee decisions. But why, many commentators asked, did Congress not do the same with lethal conditions such as cancer and heart disease? That question was answered with silence. Consistency is not one of the behavioral traits of Congress.

So far as I know, no similar effort to have committees make life and death decisions has ever been mounted in this country. Nonetheless, among those in bioethics who have written much on rationing over the years—Norman Daniels, Leonard Fleck, Paul Menzel, Alan Buchanan, Peter Ubel, and myself, for instance—there is a fair degree of consensus. I would sum it up as follows: if not at once, then sooner or later, rationing will be necessary (the steady rise of cost inflation will necessitate it); bedside rationing will not be acceptable (too open to bias and erratic criteria); rationing will have to be done at the policy level (mainly out of the hands of individual doctors and patients); and at that level there will have to be a decision-making procedure (most likely committees of some kind that will, with democratic deliberation, make transparent decisions with "accountability for reasonableness," to use Daniels's standard). The key point is that rationing decisions would be made at the policy level, not case by case.

• • •

I have left out most details with that list, as well as various disagreements among those who have written on rationing. Much of what we have written is theoretical in the sense that it has not been tested by much American experience—little save for Seattle is available—and makes ideal assumptions about ideal behavior in an ideally rational society.

But there is one European model that has been closely watched here, that of the United Kingdom's National Institute for Clinical Excellence (NICE). Technically, NICE was not established as a rationing agency—quality of care is its main emphasis—but it has the option of recommending to the British National Health Service that NHS not provide coverage for treatments thought to be of little medical value or judged to be too costly for their benefits. Most notable is its use of quality-adjusted life years (QALYs), an economics tool, to help it make decisions. The aim of that tool is to find a way around the subjectivity of decisions that will have to encompass individual quality-of-life judgments while at the same time not falling into the "social worth" swamp. The use of this tool is not meant to trump rational deliberation, but to supply it with an economic criterion, recognizing that it would inevitably have some value considerations. It was, not surprisingly, singled out for particular condemnation by opponents of the reform legislation, a this-could-happen-to-us menace if we are not vigilant.

The recent and no doubt endless health care reform debate in the United States was a shock to many of us who have toiled in the neatly tilled vineyard of rationing theory. At first all looked well. Fully recognized was the reality of unsustainable cost escalation with its fallout of a growing number of uninsured, excessive out-of-pocket expenses, Medicaid crises in most states, and a projected insolvency of Medicare in seven to eight years. The Democratic leadership, with at least initial Republican support, made perfectly clear that strong steps to control costs would be necessary.

But as time went on, the expected fast-track drive to manage costs became more a soft, slow, decade-long shuffle. Nervousness about the subject of costs was perfectly exemplified in President Obama's assurance that there would be no reduction of Medicare benefits for seniors. I have seen no serious analysis of Medicare's future that does not include just such a reduction to remain sustainable. "Bending the curve" became the anodyne term of choice in light of the political reality that rapid, fast options would not make it.

Perhaps the reform legislation will make a long-term difference, but even if it does, there is some consensus that it will not do what is necessary: bringing annual cost escalation in line with the annual rise of the gross domestic product, from the present 6 percent to 3 percent. The costs of care for the baby boomers about to enter the Medicare program by the millions will be staggering. Many astute policy analysts have long noted that, for Medicare to survive, either a doubling of the tax rate or a 50 percent cut in benefits will be necessary. No one talks that way in Congress.

Nor does the reform legislation do much to stem the steady stream of expensive biologic drugs for cancer care and costly medical devices for heart disease, many of which cry out for some rationing. How many new cancer drugs costing between fifty and one hundred thousand dollars for just a few extra months of life can be afforded? The stipulation in the reform legislation that comparative effectiveness research could be used neither to fashion practice guidelines nor even to make recommendations

for the use of its findings was as good a sign as any that cost control would not encompass directly saying no to patients, doctors, or industry. Pressures from the drug and device industries and some physician groups were responsible for that crippling provision.

If end-of-life care as legislatively envisioned was the wrong place to affix the label of "death panels," Sarah Palin surely had a good nose for the political unacceptability of any rationing talk. Republicans fastened unrelentingly on any whiff of it (particularly exploiting slippery slope arguments), and Democrats shied away from it no less persistently. What candidate for reelection will go home admitting to his elderly constituents that he favors a cut in their benefits? Far from opening the door for some serious discussion of rationing, it was slammed shut in the reform run-up.

Most of the assumptions about the value and plausibility of deliberative democracy (bringing the public into direct engagement) that have been a key part of the theoretical rationing ensemble have been rendered inoperable. Too many people seem to want no deliberation of any kind. How can we have a sensible public discussion of panels making use of "accountability for reasonableness" if perhaps half of our fellow citizens consider it immoral even to talk about it? Putting aside the often hostile hysteria that marked any efforts to even raise the topic, it is not hard to discern the roots of the opposition. There is the deeply embedded hostility to government interference in the doctor–patient relationship—assumed to be a bulwark against rationing—financially well supported by many medical groups and the drug and device industry. Then there is the popular expectation that in principle the benefits of medical progress and health care should be available to everyone regardless of costs. That view is held by many physicians and encouraged by a research enterprise ever ready to trumpet its benefits, that of the decisive nostrums and cures just over the next hill. That public expectation is not matched by a willingness to pay for the promised benefits, but it is strong enough to stifle any talk of limits to care.

Most important, perhaps, is the belief that, in a rich country like ours, the money is really out there to pay for all we want or need. Liberals can point to the billions spent on unnecessary wars or agricultural subsidies. Conservatives claim that the problem is a failure to let the market, with its potentially rich mix of private choice and insurer competition, be given its unregulated head. Again and again, moreover, I have found it possible with some patience to persuade all but the fanatical in some general fashion that some rationing, in some way, at some time or other, will be necessary, only to be told, "Yes, you're right, but not if it is my spouse, child, or grandparent." For them, the moral bottom line is that rationing life and death is intrinsically wrong, and the test case is someone they cherish.

Nor is that just an American problem. In sketching the earlier cited consensus among the bioethicists who have worked on rationing, I left out the agreement that fair rationing could take place only in a universal health care system, one with equal access to care and (I would add) a fixed annual budget. That would force tradeoffs in the face of scarcity and allow consideration of the opportunity costs of different rationing possibilities.

The United Kingdom has such a health care system, and in NICE it has a way of doing some rationing. But does that combination save it from the kind of politics that stifle debate here? Possibly a little, but not entirely by any means. While there have been critics of NICE's methodology, including its use of QALYs, they have been matched by complaints that its deliberations are not sufficiently transparent, particularly among the subcommittees that carry out most of them. That may well be true about the process, but the recommendations, and the NHS role in responding to them, make their way to the public by means of an ever-alert, aggressive media. The NHS is obliged to cover those treatments and technologies that meet the NICE standards (one reason why these treatments often raise costs), but its conclusions about covering treatments that fall short of the standards can be made only as recommendations.

Recommendations against coverage (or to limit coverage) of some expensive drugs for cancer and dementia on grounds of their high cost per QALY have caught the eye of the media—and the British media is far more unbuttoned than its American counterpart. Its reporters typically fan out to interview those who will be denied a drug. For cancer patients, that drug will often extend their lives, even if not for long. No less typically, those denied the drug or their families believe the drug has desirable benefits (never mind what unseen experts say) and that it would be inhumane to put a price tag on their lives. Why inflict that nastiness on them? This equals a perfect tabloid story. As Robert Steinbrook noted in a paper on NICE, "After all, saying no takes courage—and inevitably provokes outrage."[3]

Ironically, then, transparency can turn out to make rationing decisions all the more difficult to implement. As a result of public outcries, a number of NICE recommendations against coverage have been taken to court, and the NHS has had to back down on some that it initially accepted. Efforts to include more patients in NICE's rationing deliberations may well exacerbate that result. As two advocates for that shift put it, the economic techniques used by NICE "do not measure the quality of someone's life in a way that is sensitive to a variety of conditions or that allows individuals to indicate what is important to them personally and how their illness affects that. . . . Although the direct costs of some treatments may place a huge burden on society, rationing such treatments places even greater (indirect) costs on individuals, their careers, and the wider population."[4]

The logic of that kind of individual patient variation argument is but a short step to a Seattle-type committee, with case-by-case decisions. It also has a more recent familiar ring: U.S. opponents of evidence-based guidelines based on population statistics have said much the same thing. They conclude that it would be better to leave all final decisions in the hands of doctors and their patients, not government panels peopled by faceless bureaucrats. A sick person's notion of "accountability for reasonableness," much less the results of even full democratic deliberation, may offer little solace to someone deprived of a longer (even if not much longer) or in their eyes better life, however awful it might seem in ours.

Yet however much individual patients may be hurt or aggrieved by rationing decisions, they will have to be made eventually. They will have to be a main, if hardly the only, ingredient in any long-term solution to the cost escalation problem—a problem that has the potential to wreak economic and medical havoc if not taken more seriously. It is the classic and always difficult dilemma of individual versus common good. To make matters worse, we do not ordinarily attribute a desire to live rather than die, or to feel less pain rather than more, to gross selfishness. In the case of just wars, we are prepared to sacrifice our children to defend us from societal ruin—but only when there is no other choice. But in the case of health care rationing, it has proved nearly impossible to have a serious debate about something many consider a prima facie evil. As in the United Kingdom, the American media would instantly seize upon the predictable moral outrage.

It is harder still to cut through the plethora of upbeat ideas to avoid rationing, starting with those old nostrums: first, the assertion that we need no rationing until we have eliminated all waste and inefficiency in our health care system or carried out more and better research to rid us of all those expensive diseases; or second—all other ideas failing—the assertion that it does not matter what we spend on health care, held by some economists to be the best possible way to spend money (even in a severe recession, health care remains one of the few economic domains that regularly adds jobs).

Is there some way to develop a theory of rationing that takes full account of the political turbulence of health care reform and the deep repugnance felt by many, maybe even most, at the possibility of rationing? None that I have heard of. If politics has made it hard to manage in the United Kingdom, with its tradition of more readily accepting health care limits than the United States has, it seems almost insurmountable in our hyperindividualistic culture, suffused with skepticism about, or outright hostility to, a strong role for government and an excessively great love of new, always better, technologies.

• • •

I find it plausible to think of rationing in three categories. One of them I call "direct and naked": an unveiled denial of some important health benefit, including life-extending treatment, by either a private or public institution that has the power to do so. To be sure, there is a great difference between rationing in the context of absolute shortages, as with the early dialysis machines, and denying the sick an insurance or Medicare benefit, but leaving them free to buy it for themselves. The latter will be small comfort for anyone other than the very affluent; many families bankrupt themselves these days to cover treatments they cannot otherwise afford.

By "indirect and veiled" rationing, I have in mind the use of copayments and deductibles, particularly when they are set high enough to discourage but not to openly stop people from using expensive services. By "covert" rationing, I mean the kind that existed in the United Kingdom from the 1950s through at least the early 1980s. Restrained by tight budgets, it came to be understood as an unwritten rule that patients over the age of fifty-five would be denied dialysis and some forms of heart surgery. They were to be told by their physicians that nothing could be done for them. That was a flat lie, but it offered cover to physicians who knew their limited budgets could not stand it.

The eminent British policy analyst Rudolf Klein has suggested that a less visible form of that earlier practice still exists in the United Kingdom: "the most pervasive form of rationing is the least explicit and least visible: rationing by dilution . . . not to order an expensive diagnostic test, or to reduce ward staffing levels in order to balance the budget normally attract little attention unless they explode in a scandal . . . such decisions are as much a form of rationing as the refusal to prescribe a drug . . . however, in the times ahead no generally accepted decision-making model is likely to emerge." "The best that ministers can hope for," Klein concludes, "is that most rationing will continue to take the form of dilution rather than excision and that decisions can be taken in the name of clinical discretion and thus be politically invisible."[5]

If present ethical theories—not designed for nasty fights—will not help or be much listened to, just what might otherwise happen? I would bet on a combination of gradually increased taxes, an expanded government role despite conservative hostility, and a steady, even accelerating, rise of copayments, deductibles, and coinsurance—already a pervasive practice. Will there be complaints? Of course. But a long-losing Yale football coach once said that the trick with the alumni was to "keep them sullen, but not mutinous." Copayments and deductibles have managed to walk that fine line. They will surely continue to rise and are steadily doing so across Medicare, Medicaid, and private insurance.

While covert rationing will undoubtedly be condemned, I would not be surprised if it starts happening. For at least some physicians, it will be an enticing way of dealing with cost pressures, a kind of well-meant falsehood to avoid the pain of brutal candor. Available information in the media and on the Internet will make it much harder now to get away with that tactic, but since patients tend to trust their doctors, some doctors may succeed. Rudolf Klein's dour but sober judgment of rationing in the United Kingdom may, and probably will, be applicable here as well.

The rationing problem in the end is that we have a culture and politics that invite evasion of hard ethical dilemmas, outrage and shouting instead of deliberative democracy, and a bad case of what has been called "the California disease"—a limit on taxation combined simultaneously with unlimited demands for ever-more benefits. We want unbounded medical progress, an all-out war on death, lower taxes, and no medical rationing. It is a mix that cannot long be sustained but, like a drug-resistant virus, it continues mutating to keep us sick. It is a chronic economic disease as tenacious as the medical ones. No less pathological is an unwillingness on the part of politicians to talk openly about the need for rationing, not just what's wrong with it. Euphemisms, evasions, and rosy scenarios of bending the curve, or of simultaneously improving quality while lowering costs, make up the rhetoric of choice.

The culture of evasion directly clashes with the necessity of cost control. The same political forces clamoring for deficit reduction are those that have most vehemently condemned any talk of rationing. They cannot have it both ways. Something has to give. But there is little reason to think that what gives will be evasion. I find it hard to imagine that open rationing will be possible other than with the low-hanging fruit—whatever is the least threatening and economically marginal. The really hard choices will be pushed into the territory of indirect and covert rationing. The reigning ethical theory on rationing has it right: only committee decisions with considerable public input ought to be acceptable. But that model has not yet been taken seriously in the world of politics—a failure that simply increases the likelihood that ethically flawed strategies will be embraced. That will be a shame.

Notes

1. A.R. Jonsen, *The Birth of Bioethics* (New York: Oxford University Press, 1998), 211 ff; R.C. Fox and J.P. Swazey, *Courage to Fail: A Social View of Organ Transplants and Dialysis* (Chicago, Ill.: University of Chicago Press, 1974).
2. Quoted in Fox and Swazey, *Courage to Fail*, 76.
3. R. Steinbrook, "Saying No Isn't NICE—The Travails of Britain's Institute for Health and Clinical Excellence," *New England Journal of Medicine* 359 (2008): 1981.
4. J. Speight and M. Reaney, "Wouldn't It Be NICE to Consider Patient's Views When Rationing Health Care," *British Medical Journal* 338 (2009): b85.
5. R. Klein, "Rationing in the Fiscal Ice Age," *Health Economics, Policy and Law* 5, no. 4 (2010): 389–96, at 389–90 and 394.

DANIEL CALLAHAN is a senior research scholar and President Emeritus of the Hastings Center. He holds a PhD in philosophy from Harvard University.

James Ridgeway

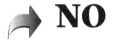 **NO**

Meet the Real Death Panels

*H*ealth care reform is done, but the battle over "entitlement reform" is just beginning—and already, deficit hawks are suggesting that geezers like me need to pull the plug on ourselves for the good of society. Are they looking out for future generations—or just the bonuses of *health care* execs?

There's a certain age at which you cease to regard your own death as a distant hypothetical and start to view it as a coming event. For me, it was 67—the age at which my father died. For many Americans, I suspect it's 70—the age that puts you within striking distance of our average national life expectancy of 78.1 years. Even if you still feel pretty spry, you suddenly find that your roster of doctor's appointments has expanded, along with your collection of daily medications. You grow accustomed to hearing that yet another person you once knew has dropped off the twig. And you feel more and more like a walking ghost yourself, invisible to the younger people who push past you on the subway escalator. Like it or not, death becomes something you think about, often on a daily basis.

Actually, you don't think about death, per se, as much as you do about dying—about when and where and especially how you're going to die. Will you have to deal with a long illness? With pain, immobility, or dementia? Will you be able to get the *care* you need, and will you have enough money to pay for it? Most of all, will you lose control over what life you have left, as well as over the circumstances of your death?

These are precisely the preoccupations that the right so cynically exploited in the debate over *health care* reform, with that ominous talk of Washington bean counters deciding who lives and dies. It was all nonsense, of course—the worst kind of political scare tactic. But at the same time, supporters of *health care* reform seemed to me too quick to dismiss old people's fears as just so much paranoid foolishness. There are reasons why the death-panel myth found fertile ground—and those reasons go beyond the gullibility of half-senile old farts.

While politicians of all stripes shun the idea of *health care rationing* as the political third rail that it is, most of them accept a premise that leads, one way or another, to that end. Here's what I mean: Nearly every other industrialized country recognizes *health care* as a human right, whose costs and benefits are shared among all citizens. But in the United States, the leaders of both political parties along with most of the "experts" persist in treating *health care* as a commodity

that is purchased, in one way or another, by those who can afford it. Conservatives embrace this notion as the perfect expression of the all-powerful market; though they make a great show of recoiling from the term, in practice they are endorsing *rationing* on the basis of wealth. Liberals, including supporters of President Obama's *health care* reform, advocate subsidies, regulation, and other modest measures to give the less fortunate a little more buying power. But as long as *health care* is viewed as a product to be bought and sold, even the most well-intentioned reformers will someday soon have to come to grips with *health care rationing*, if not by wealth then by some other criteria.

In a country that already spends more than 16 percent of each GDP dollar on *health care*, it's easy to see why so many people believe there's simply not enough of it to go around. But keep in mind that the rest of the industrialized world manages to spend between 20 and 90 percent less per capita and still rank higher than the US in overall *health care* performance. In 2004, a team of researchers including Princeton's Uwe Reinhardt, one of the nation's best known experts on *health* economics, found that while the US spends 134 percent more than the median of the world's most developed nations, we get less for our money—fewer physician visits and hospital days per capita, for example—than our counterparts in countries like Germany, Canada, and Australia. (We do, however, have more MRI machines and more cesarean sections.)

Where does the money go instead? By some estimates, administration and insurance profits alone eat up at least 30 percent of our total *health care* bill (and most of that is in the private sector—Medicare's overhead is around 2 percent). In other words, we don't have too little to go around—we overpay for what we get, and we don't allocate our spending where it does us the most good. "In most [medical] resources we have a surplus," says Dr. David Himmelstein, cofounder of Physicians for a National *Health* Program. "People get large amounts of *care* that don't do them any good and might cause them harm [while] others don't get the necessary amount."

Looking at the numbers, it's pretty safe to say that with an efficient *health care* system, we could spend a little less than we do now and provide all Americans with the most spectacular *care* the world has ever known. But in the absence of any serious challenge to the *health-care-as-commodity* system, we are doomed to a battlefield scenario where Americans must fight to secure their share of a "scarce" resource in a life-and-death struggle that pits the rich against the poor, the insured against the uninsured—and increasingly, the old against the young.

For years, any push to improve the nation's finances—balance the budget, pay for the bailout, or help stimulate the economy—has been accompanied by rumblings about the greedy geezers who resist entitlement "reforms" (read: cuts) with their unconscionable demands for basic *health care* and a hedge against destitution. So, too, today: Already, President Obama's newly convened deficit commission looks to be blaming the nation's fiscal woes not on tax cuts, wars, or bank bailouts, but on the burden of Social Security and Medicare. (The commission's co-chair, former Republican senator Alan Simpson, has declared, "This country is gonna go to the bow-wows unless we deal with entitlements.")

Old people's anxiety in the face of such hostile attitudes has provided fertile ground for Republican disinformation and fearmongering. But so has the vacuum left by Democratic reformers. Too often, in their zeal to prove themselves tough on "waste," they've allowed connections to be drawn between two things that, to my mind, should never be spoken of in the same breath: death and cost.

Dying Wishes

The death-panel myth started with a harmless minor provision in the *health* reform bill that required Medicare to pay in case enrollees wanted to have conversations with their own doctors about "advance directives" like *health care* proxies and living wills. The controversy that ensued, thanks to a host of right-wing commentators and Sarah Palin's Facebook page, ensured that the advance-planning measure was expunged from the bill. But the underlying debate didn't end with the passage of *health care* reform, any more than it began there. For if *rationing* is inevitable once you've ruled out reining in private profits, the question is who should be denied *care,* and at what point. And given that no one will publicly argue for withholding cancer treatment from a seven-year-old, the answer almost inevitably seems to come down to what we spend on people—old people—in their final years.

As far back as 1983, in a speech to the *Health* Insurance Association of America, a then-57-year-old Alan Greenspan suggested that we consider "whether it is worth it" to spend so much of Medicare's outlays on people who would die within the year. (Appropriately, Ayn Rand called her acolyte "the undertaker"—though she chose the nickname because of his dark suits and austere demeanor.)

Not everyone puts the issue in such nakedly pecuniary terms, but in an April 2009 interview with *The New York Times Magazine,* Obama made a similar point in speaking of end-of-life *care* as a "huge driver of cost." He said, "The chronically ill and those toward the end of their lives are accounting for potentially 80 percent of the total *health care* bill out here."

The president was being a bit imprecise. Those figures are actually for Medicare expenditures, not the total *health*

care tab, and more important, lumping the dying together with the "chronically ill"—who often will live for years or decades—makes little sense. But there is no denying that end-of-life *care* is expensive. Hard numbers are not easy to come by, but studies from the 1990s suggest that between a quarter and a third of annual Medicare expenditures go to patients in their last year of life, and 30 to 40 percent of those costs accrue in the final month. What this means is that around one in ten Medicare dollars—some $50 billion a year—are spent on patients with fewer than 30 days to live.

Pronouncements on these data usually come coated with a veneer of compassion and concern: How terrible it is that all those poor dying old folks have to endure aggressive treatments that only delay the inevitable; all we want to do is bring peace and dignity to their final days! But I wonder: If that's really what they're worried about, how come they keep talking about money?

At this point, I ought to make something clear: I am a big fan of what's sometimes called the "right to die" or "death with dignity" movement. I support everything from advance directives to assisted suicide. You could say I believe in one form of *health care rationing*: the kind you choose for yourself. I can't stand the idea of anyone—whether it's the government or some hospital administrator or doctor or Nurse Jackie—telling me that I must have some treatment I don't want, any more than I want them telling me that I can't have a treatment I do want. My final wish is to be my own one-member death panel.

A physician friend recently told me about a relative of hers, a frail 90-year-old woman suffering from cancer. Her doctors urged her to have surgery, followed by treatment with a recently approved cancer medicine that cost $5,000 a month. As is often the case, my friend said, the doctors told their patient about the benefits of the treatment, but not about all the risks—that she might die during the surgery or not long afterward. They also prescribed a month's supply of the new medication, even though, my friend says, they must have known the woman was unlikely to live that long. She died within a week. "Now," my friend said, "I'm carrying around a $4,000 bottle of pills."

Perhaps reflecting what economists call "supplier-induced demand," costs generally tend to go up when the dying have too little control over their *care,* rather than too much. When geezers are empowered to make decisions, most of us will choose less aggressive—and less costly—treatments. If we don't do so more often, it's usually because of an overbearing and money-hungry *health care* system, as well as a culture that disrespects the will of its elders and resists confronting death.

Once, when I was in the hospital for outpatient surgery, I woke up in the recovery area next to a man named George, who was talking loudly to his wife, telling her he wanted to leave. She soothingly reminded him that they had to wait for the doctors to learn the results of the surgery, apparently some sort of exploratory thing. Just then, two doctors appeared. In a stiff, flat voice, one of them told George that he had six months to live. When his wife's shrieking had subsided, I heard George say, "I'm getting the fuck out of this place." The doctors sternly advised him that they had more tests to run and "treatment options" to discuss. "Fuck that," said George, yanking the IV out of his arm and getting to his feet. "If I've got six months to live, do you think I want to spend another minute of it here? I'm going to the Alps to go skiing."

I don't know whether George was true to his word. But not long ago I had a friend, a scientist, who was true to his. Suffering from cancer, he anticipated a time when more chemotherapy or procedures could only prolong a deepening misery, to the point where he could no longer recognize himself. He prepared for that time, hoarding his pain meds, taking *care* to protect his doctor and pharmacist from any possibility of legal retribution. He saw some friends he wanted to see, and spoke to others. Then he died at a time and place of his choosing, with his family around him. Some would call this euthanasia, others a sacrilege. To me, it seemed like a noble end to a fine life. If freedom of choice is what makes us human, then my friend managed to make his death a final expression of his humanity.

My friend chose to forgo medical treatments that would have added many thousands of dollars to his *health care* costs—and, since he was on Medicare, to the public expense. If George really did spend his final months in the Alps, instead of undergoing expensive surgeries or sitting around hooked up to machines, he surely saved the *health care* system a bundle as well. They did it because it was what they wanted, not because it would save money. But there is a growing body of evidence that the former can lead to the latter—without any *rationing* or coercion.

One model that gets cited a lot these days is La Crosse, Wisconsin, where Gundersen Lutheran hospital launched an initiative to ensure that the town's older residents had advance directives and to make hospice and palliative *care* widely available. A 2008 study found that 90 percent of those who died in La Crosse under a physician's *care* did so with advance directives in place. At Gundersen Lutheran, less is spent on patients in their last two years of life than nearly any other place in the US, with per capita Medicare costs 30 percent below the national average. In a similar vein, Oregon, in 1995, instituted a two-page form called Physician Orders for Life-Sustaining Treatment; it functions as doctor's orders and is less likely to be misinterpreted or disregarded than a living will. According to the Dartmouth Atlas of *Health Care,* a 20-year study of the nation's medical costs and resources, people in Oregon are less likely to die in a hospital than people in most other states, and in their last six months, they spend less time in the hospital. They also run up about 50 percent less in medical expenditures.

It's possible that attitudes have begun to change. Three states now allow what advocates like to call "aid-in-dying" (rather than assisted suicide) for the terminally ill. More Americans than ever have living wills and other advance directives, and that can only be a good thing:

One recent study showed that more than 70 percent of patients who needed to make end-of-life decisions at some point lost the capacity to make these choices, yet among those who had prepared living wills, nearly all had their instructions carried out.

Here is the ultimate irony of the deathpanel meme: In attacking measures designed to Promote advance directives, conservatives were attacking what they claim is their core value—the individual right to free choice.

The QALY of Mercy

A wonkier version of the reform-equals-*rationing* argument is based less on panic mongering about Obama's secret euthanasia schemes and more on the implications of something called "comparative effectiveness research." The practice got a jump start in last year's stimulus bill, which included $1.1 billion for the Federal Coordinating Council for Comparative Effectiveness Research. This is money to study what treatments work best for which patients. The most obvious use of such data would be to apply the findings to Medicare, and the effort has already been attacked as the first step toward the government deciding when it's time to kick granny to the curb. Senate minority leader Mitch McConnell (R-Ky.) has said that Obama's support for comparative effectiveness research means he is seeking "a national *rationing* board."

Evidence-based medicine, in itself, has absolutely nothing to do with age. In theory, it also has nothing to do with money—though it might, as a byproduct, reduce costs (for example, by giving doctors the information they need to resist pressure from drug companies). Yet the desire for cost savings often seems to drive comparative effectiveness research, rather than the other way around. In his *Time Magazine* interview last year, Obama said, "It is an attempt to say to patients, you know what, we've looked at some objective studies concluding that the blue pill, which costs half as much as the red pill, is just as effective, and you might want to go ahead and get the blue one."

Personally, I don't mind the idea of the government promoting the blue pill over the red pill, as long as it really is "just as effective." I certainly trust the government to make these distinctions more than I trust the insurance companies or pharma reps. But I want to know that the only target is genuine waste, and the only possible casualty is profits.

There's nothing to give me pause in the *health care* law's comparative effectiveness provision, which includes $500 million a year for comparative effectiveness research. The work is to be overseen by the nonprofit Patient-Centered Outcomes Research Institute, whose 21-member board of governors will include doctors, patient advocates, and only three representatives of drug and medical-device companies.

Still, there's a difference between comparative effectiveness and comparative cost effectiveness—and from the latter, it's a short skip to outright cost-benefit analysis. In other words, the argument sometimes slides almost imperceptibly from comparing how well the blue pill and the red pill work to examining whether some people should be denied the red pill, even if it demonstrably works better.

The calculations driving such cost-benefit analyses are often based on something called QALYs—quality-adjusted life years. If a certain cancer drug would extend life by two years, say, but with such onerous side effects that those years were judged to be only half as worth living as those of a healthy person, the QALY is 1.

In Britain, the National *Health* Service has come close to setting a maximum price beyond which extra QALYs are not deemed worthwhile. In assessing drugs and treatments, the NHS's National Institute for *Health* and Clinical Excellence usually approves those that cost less than 20,000 pounds per QALY (about $28,500), and most frequently rejects those costing more than 30,000 pounds (about $43,000).

It's not hard to find examples of comparative effectiveness research—complete with QALYs—that hit quite close to home for almost anyone. Last year I was diagnosed with atrial fibrillation, a disturbance in the heart rhythm that sometimes leads to blood clots, which can travel to the brain and cause a stroke. My doctor put me on warfarin (brand name Coumadin), a blood-thinning drug that reduces the chances of forming blood clots but can also cause internal bleeding. It's risky enough that when I go to the dentist or cut myself shaving, I have to watch to make sure it doesn't turn into a torrent of blood. The levels of warfarin in my bloodstream have to be frequently checked, so I have to be ever mindful of the whereabouts of a hospital with a blood lab. It is a pain in the neck, and it makes me feel vulnerable. I sometimes wonder if it's worth it.

It turns out that several comparative effectiveness studies have looked at the efficacy of warfarin for patients with my heart condition. One of them simply weighed the drug's potential benefits against its dangerous side effects, without consideration of cost. It concluded that for a patient with my risk factors, warfarin reduced the chance of stroke a lot more than it increased the chance that I'd be seriously harmed by bleeding. Another study concluded that for a patient like me, the cost per QALY of taking warfarin is $8,000—cheap, by most standards.

Prescription drug prices have more than doubled since the study was done in 1995. But warfarin is a relatively cheap generic drug, and even if my cost per QALY was $15,000 or $20,000, I'd still pass muster with the NHS. But if I were younger and had fewer risk factors, I'd be less prone to stroke to begin with, so the reduction in risk would not be as large, and the cost per QALY would be correspondingly higher, about $370,000. Would I still want to take the drug if I were, say, under 60 and free of risk factors? Considering the side effects, probably not. But would I want someone else to make that decision for me?

Critics of the British system say, among other things, that the NHS's cost-per-QALY limit is far too low. But raising it wouldn't resolve the deeper ethical question: Should anyone but the patient get to decide when life is not worth living? The Los Angeles Times' Michael Hiltzik, one of the few reporters to critically examine this issue, has noted that "healthy people tend to overestimate the effect of some medical conditions on their sufferers' quality of life. The hale and hearty, for example, will generally rate life in a wheelchair lower than will the wheelchair-bound, who often find fulfillment in ways 'healthier' persons couldn't imagine."

Simone de Beauvoir wrote that fear of aging and death drives young people to view their elders as a separate species, rather than as their future selves: "Until the moment it is upon us old age is something that only affects other people." And the more I think about the subject, the more I am sure of one thing: It's not a good idea to have a 30-year-old place a value on my life.

Whose Death Is It Anyway?

Probably the most prominent advocate of age-based *rationing* is Daniel Callahan, cofounder of a bioethics think tank called the Hastings Center. Callahan's 1987 book, *Setting Limits: Medical Goals in an Aging Society,* depicted old people as "a new social threat," a demographic, economic, and medical "avalanche" waiting to happen. In a 2008 article, Callahan said that in evaluating Medicare's expenditures, we should consider that "there is a duty to help young people to become old people, but not to help the old become still older indefinitely . . . One may well ask what counts as 'old' and what is a decently long lifespan? As I have listened to people speak of a 'full life,' often heard at funerals, I would say that by 75–80 most people have lived a full life, and most of us do not feel it a tragedy that someone in that age group has died (as we do with the death of a child)." He has proposed using "age as a specific criterion for the allocation and limitation of *care*," and argues that after a certain point, people could justifiably be denied Medicare coverage for life-extending treatments.

You can see why talk like this might make some old folks start boarding up their doors. (It apparently, however, does not concern Callahan, who last year at age 79 told *The New York Times* that he had just had a life-saving seven-hour heart procedure.) It certainly made me wonder how I would measure up.

So far, I haven't cost the system all that much. I take several different meds every day, which are mostly generics. I go to the doctor pretty often, but I haven't been in the hospital overnight for at least 20 years, and my one walk-in operation took place before I was on Medicare. And I am still working, so I'm paying in as well as taking out.

But things could change, perhaps precipitously. Since I have problems with both eyesight and balance, I could easily fall and break a bone, maybe a hip. This could mean a hip replacement, months of therapy, or even long-term immobility. My glaucoma could take a turn for the worse, and I would face a future of near blindness, with all the associated costs. Or I could have that stroke, in spite of my drug regimen.

I decided to take the issue up with the Australian philosopher Peter Singer, who made some waves on this issue with a *New York Times* op-ed published last year, titled "Why We Must Ration *Health Care*." Singer believes that *health care* is a scarce resource that will inevitably be limited. Better to do it through a public system like the British NHS, he told me, than covertly and inequitably on the private US model. "What you are trying to do is to get the most value for the money from the resources you have," he told me.

In the world he imagines, I asked Singer over coffee in a Manhattan café, what should happen if I broke a hip? He paused to think, and I hoped he wouldn't worry about hurting my feelings. "If there is a good chance of restoring mobility," he said after a moment, "and you have at least five years of mobility, that's significant benefit." He added, "Hip operations are not expensive." A new hip or knee runs between $30,000 and $40,000, most of it covered by Medicare. So for five years of mobility, that comes out to about $7,000 a year—less than the cost of a home-*care* aide, and exponentially less than a nursing home.

But then Singer turned to a more sobering thought: If the hip operation did not lead to recovery of mobility, then it might not be such a bargain. In a much-cited piece of personal revelation, Obama in 2009 talked about his grandmother's decision to have a hip replacement after she had been diagnosed with terminal cancer. She died just a few weeks later. "I don't know how much that hip replacement cost," Obama told the *Times Magazine*. "I would have paid out of pocket for that hip replacement just because she's my grandmother." But the president said that in considering whether "to give my grandmother, or everybody else's aging grandparents or parents, a hip replacement when they're terminally ill . . . you just get into some very difficult moral issues."

Singer and I talked about what choices we ourselves might make at the end of our lives. Singer, who is 63, said that he and his wife "know neither of us wants to go on living under certain conditions. Particularly if we get demented. I would draw the line if I could not recognize my wife or my children. My wife has a higher standard—when she couldn't read a novel. Yes, I wouldn't want to live beyond a certain point. It's not me anymore." I'm 10 years older than Singer, and my own advance directives reflect similar choices. So it seems like neither one of us is likely to strain the public purse with our demands for expensive and futile life-prolonging *care*.

You can say this is all a Debbie Downer, but people my age know perfectly well that these questions are not at all theoretical. We worry about the time when we will no longer be able to contribute anything useful to society and will be completely dependent on others. And we worry about the day when life will no longer seem worth living,

and whether we will have the courage—and the ability—to choose a dignified death. We worry about these things all by ourselves we don't need anyone else to do it for us. And we certainly don't need anyone tallying up QALYs while our overpriced, underperforming private *health care* system adds a few more points to its profit margin.

Let It Bleed

What happened during the recent *health care* wars is what military strategists might call a "bait-and-bleed" operation: Two rival parties are drawn into a protracted conflict that depletes both their forces, while a third stands on the sidelines, its strength undiminished. In this case, Republicans and Democrats alike have shed plenty of blood, while the clever combatant on the sidelines is, of course, the *health care* industry.

In the process, *health care* reform set some unsettling precedents that could fuel the phony intergenerational conflict over *health care* resources. The final reform bill will help provide coverage to some of the estimated 46 million Americans under 65 who live without it. It finances these efforts in part by cutting Medicare costs—some $500 billion over 10 years. Contrary to Republican hysteria, the cuts so far come from all the right places—primarily from ending the tip-offs by insurers who sell government-financed "Medicare Advantage" plans. The reform law even manages to make some meaningful improvements to the flawed Medicare prescription drug program and preventive *care*. The legislation also explicitly bans age-based *health care rationing*.

Still, there are plenty of signs that the issue is far from being put to rest. Congress and the White House wrote into the law something called the Independent Payment Advisory Board, a presidentially appointed panel that is tasked with keeping Medicare's growth rate below a certain ceiling. Office of Management and Budget director Peter Orszag, the economics wunderkind who has made Medicare's finances something of a personal project, has called it potentially the most important aspect of the legislation: Medicare and Medicaid, he has said, "are at the heart of our long-term fiscal imbalance, which is the motivation for moving to a different structure in those programs." And then, of course, there's Obama's deficit commission: While the president says he is keeping an open mind when it comes to solving the deficit "crisis," no one is trying very hard to pretend that the commission has any purpose other than cutting Social Security, Medicare, and probably Medicaid as well.

Already, the commission is working closely with the Peter G. Peterson Foundation, headed by the billionaire businessman and former Nixon administration official who has emerged as one of the nation's leading "granny bashers"—deficit hawks who accuse old people of bankrupting the country.

In the end, of course, many conservatives are motivated less by deficits and more by free-market ideology:

Many of them want to replace Medicare as it now exists today with a system of vouchers, and place the emphasis on individual savings and tax breaks. Barring that, Republicans have proposed a long string of cuts to Medicaid and Medicare, sometimes defying logic—by, for example, advocating reductions in in-home *care,* which can keep people out of far more expensive nursing homes.

The common means of justifying these cuts is to attack Medicare "waste." But remember that not only are Medicare's administrative costs less than one-sixth of those of private insurers, Medicare pays doctors and hospitals less (20 and 30 percent, respectively) than private payment rates; overall, Medicare pays out less in annual per capita benefits than the average large employer *health* plan, even though it serves an older, sicker population.

That basic fact is fully understood by the *health care* industry. Back in January 2009, as the nation suited up for the health care wars, the Lewin Group—a subsidiary of the *health* insurance giant United *Health*—produced an analysis of various reform proposals being floated and found that the only one to immediately reduce overall *health care* costs (by $58 billion) was one that would have dramatically expanded Medicare.

Facts like these, however, have not slowed down the granny bashers. In a February op-ed called "The Geezers' Crusade," commentator David Brooks urged old people to willingly submit to entitlement cuts in service to future generations. Via Social Security and Medicare, he argued, old folks are stealing from their own grandkids.

I'm as public spirited as the next person, and I have a Gen X son. I'd be willing to give up some expensive, life-prolonging medical treatment for him, and maybe even for the good of humanity. But I'm certainly not going to do it so some WellPoint executive can take another vacation, so Pfizer can book $3 billion in annual profits instead of $2 billion, or so private hospitals can make another campaign contribution to some gutless politician.

Here, then, is my advice to anyone who suggests that we geezers should do the right thing and pull the plug on ourselves: Start treating *health care* as a human right instead of a profit-making opportunity, and see how much money you save. Then, by all means, get back to me.

JAMES RIDGEWAY is a senior Washington correspondent for *Mother Jones.*

EXPLORING THE ISSUE

Should Health Care Be Rationed in the U.S.?

Critical Thinking and Reflection

1. What are the primary reasons we should consider health care rationing?
2. Is health care a basic right or a luxury?
3. If health care was rationed, what criteria should be used to determine who is treated and who is not?

Is There Common Ground?

In October 1986 Dr. Thomas Starzl of Pittsburgh, Pennsylvania, transplanted a liver into a 76-year-old woman at a cost of over $200,000. Soon after that, Congress ordered organ transplantation to be covered under Medicare, which ensured that more older persons would receive this benefit. At the same time these events were taking place, a government campaign to contain medical costs was under way, with health care for the elderly targeted.

Not everyone agrees with this means of cost cutting. In "Public Attitudes About the Use of Chronological Age as a Criterion for Allocating Health Care Resources," *The Gerontologist* (February 1993), the authors report that the majority of older people surveyed accept the withholding of life-prolonging medical care from the hopelessly ill but that few would deny treatment on the basis of age alone. Two publications that express opposition to age-based health care rationing are "Health Care Rationing: Goodwill to All?" *Social Research* (vol. 64, spring 2007) and "Who Should We Treat: Rights, Rationing and Resources in the NHS," *Journal of Medical Ethics* (vol. 33, March 2007).

Currently, about 40 million Americans have no medical insurance and are at risk of being denied basic health care services. At the same time, the federal government pays most of the health care costs of the elderly. While it may not meet the needs of all older people, the amount of medical aid that goes to the elderly is greater than that goes to any other demographic group, and the elderly have the highest disposable income.

Most Americans have access to the best and most expensive medical care in the world. As these costs rise, some difficult decisions may have to be made regarding the allocation of these resources. As the population ages and more health care dollars are spent on care during the last years of life, medical services for the elderly or the dying may become a natural target for reduction in order to balance the health care budget. Other population groups may also be affected including the disabled, substance abusers, and others.

Create Central

www.mhhe.com/createcentral

Additional Resources

Callahan, D. (2012). Must we ration health care for the elderly? *Journal of Law, Medicine & Ethics*, *40*(1), 10–16.

Coleman, R. (2011). The independent Medicare advisory committee: Death panel or smart governing? *Issues in Law & Medicine*, *27*(2), 121–177.

Gruenewald, D. A. (2012). Can health care rationing ever be rational? *Journal of Law, Medicine & Ethics*, *40*(1), 17–25.

Priaulx, N. & Wrigley, A. (2013). *Ethics, law & society.* Farnham: Ashgate Publishing Ltd.

Rubenfeld, G. D. (2012). Cost-effective critical care: Cost containment and rationing. *Seminars in Respiratory & Critical Care Medicine, 4,* 413–420.

Internet References . . .

U.S. Department of Health and Human Services

www.os.dhhs.gov

U.S. National Institutes of Health (NIH)

www.nih.gov

American Medical Association (AMA)

www.ama-assn.org

MedScape: The Online Resource for Better Patient Care

www.medscape.com

Selected, Edited, and with Issue Framing Material by:
Eileen Daniel, *SUNY College at Brockport*

ISSUE

Should Prescription Drugs Be Advertised Directly to Consumers?

YES: Paul Antony, from "PhRMA Chief Medical Officer Testifies on DTC Advertising," www.phrma.org/

NO: Marc-André Gagnon and Joel Lexchin, from "The Cost of Pushing Pills: A New Estimate of Pharmaceutical Promotion Expenditures in the United States," *PLoS Medicine* (January 2008)

Learning Outcomes

After reading this issue, you should be able to:

- Discuss the advantages to consumers from direct advertised prescription drugs.
- Assess the risks associated with direct advertised prescription drugs.
- Discuss direct marketing of prescription drugs from a historical perspective.
- Assess the reasons why drug prices have soared in recent years.

ISSUE SUMMARY

YES: Paul Antony, chief medical officer at the Pharmaceutical Research and Manufacturers of America (PhRMA), claims that direct-to-consumer advertising of prescription medications has been beneficial to American patients and is a powerful tool in educating consumers and improving their health.

NO: Professors Marc-André Gagnon and Joel Lexchin argue that drug companies spend almost twice as much on advertising to consumers as they do on research and product development.

Prescription drug spending continues to grow at a faster pace than any other component of health care in the United States, and it is expected to continue for at least the next several years. The nation's prescription drug bill has been rising 14–18 percent a year and exceeded $168 billion in 2012. About 50 percent of Americans have no prescription drug coverage and government programs such as Medicare lack a comprehensive pharmacy benefit. Unfortunately, some people solve the problem of high drug costs by cutting back on other life necessities such as food or utility payments. Others simply go without some or all of their medications. A survey conducted recently by the American Association of Retired Persons (AARP) found that one in five older Americans didn't fill one or more prescriptions for financial reasons.

There are two primary reasons drug spending has increased: higher use and a higher average cost per prescription. Research indicates that each year, drug spending will account for 18–25 percent of overall health care spending. Prescription drug costs have increased from less than 10 percent of total health care costs to 15 percent plus of the total health care bill—and could approach 20 percent of total health care costs in the future. There are several key drivers of these cost increases, which include the significant increase in the elderly population over the next decade. People tend to use more drugs as they grow older to treat chronic conditions and, on average, tend to use drugs that cost more. Also, interestingly, the thresholds for determining diabetes and high cholesterol were recently lowered. As a result, more than 38 million additional people fell under the guidelines for prescription drug treatment. While this should have a long-term, positive impact on patients' health, the short-term impact on drug spending is significant.

Costs for prescription drugs continue to escalate to allow pharmaceutical companies to recoup costs for advertising and research and development. Drug companies have invested heavily in advertising directly to consumers for the latest heartburn, allergy, arthritis, erectile dysfunction, or pain medication, to name a few. This has led to a nation of consumers entering their doctors' offices with a particular brand name drug in mind that they think will cure their ailment.

In 1977, regulations were liberalized by the Food and Drug Administration allowing direct-to-consumer advertising of prescription drugs. Though legal, the practice remains controversial and may influence the way doctors prescribe drugs. At an estimated annual cost of $2.5 billion, pharmaceutical advertising on television and in the popular press has made drug companies and their brands household names. Recent analysis from the managed care industry has shown that prescriptions written for the top 50 most heavily advertised drugs rose nearly 25 percent, compared to 4.3 percent for all other drugs combined. Drug manufacturing, a $122 billion industry, is becoming more dependent on advertising to sell their products.

In addition to advertising expenditures, the drug companies claim they must heavily spend on research and development to bring new, better drugs to market. More new drugs are being released, with additional drugs in clinical trials. In 2000, the Food and Drug Administration approved 27 new drugs plus many improved or enhanced versions of existing drugs. Currently, more than 1,000 drugs are in the pipeline. The pharmaceutical companies claim that it costs an average of $800 million to bring a new drug to market. Critics claim that much of the research and development needed to bring a drug to market is supported by taxpayers via support by the federal government. A study by the National Institute for Health Care Management Foundation found, however, that two-thirds of the prescription drugs recently approved by the Food and Drug Administration were modified or enhanced versions of existing drugs. Only 15 percent of the approved drugs were both new and improved over existing medications.

While it is clear that drug prices have risen dramatically, there are some positive effects to this trend to consider as many key drugs will lose their patent protection in the next couple of years, providing an opportunity to switch to generics. While the initial cost of the generic alternatives for some of these drugs may be high, it does provide for a more competitive environment. In addition, some of the drugs being introduced will significantly improve the health of patients. Patients who continue to comply with drug therapies may improve their health for the long term. However, the role of direct advertising costs remains an issue from both an economic and a moral perspective.

In the YES and NO selections, Paul Antony claims direct-to-consumer advertising has been a benefit to American patients and has had a powerful impact on the education of consumers and their health improvement. Marc-André Gagnon and Joel Lexchin argue that the pharmaceutical industry continues to spend an inordinate amount of money on direct patient advertising and that this money should be earmarked toward research and development of better, more effective medications.

YES ⤹

Paul Antony

PhRMA Chief Medical Officer
Testifies on DTC Advertising

Washington, D.C. (September 29, 2005)—PhRMA Chief Medical Officer Paul Antony testified before Congress today at a hearing held by the U.S. Senate Special Committee on Aging on direct-to-consumer advertising and submitted the following written statement:

Mr. Chairman, Ranking Member Kohl and Members of the Committee, on behalf of the Pharmaceutical Research and Manufacturers of America (PhRMA), I am pleased to appear at this hearing today on direct-to-consumer (DTC) advertising. I am Paul Antony, M.D., Chief Medical Officer at PhRMA.

DTC advertising has been proven to be beneficial to American patients. And, continuing regulatory oversight by the FDA helps ensure that the content of DTC advertising informs and educates consumers about medical conditions and treatment options. PhRMA and its member companies have a responsibility to ensure that ads comply with FDA regulations. We take that job seriously. We want to continue to be a valuable contributor to improving public health.

DTC Advertising can be a powerful tool in educating millions of people and improving health. Because of DTC advertising, large numbers of Americans are prompted to discuss illnesses with their doctors for the first time. Because of DTC advertising, patients become more involved in their own health care decisions, and are proactive in their patient–doctor dialogue. Because of DTC advertising, patients are more likely to take their prescribed medicines.

PhRMA's Guiding Principles on Direct-to-Consumer Advertisements About Prescription Medicines

PhRMA and its member companies have long understood the special relationship we have with the patients [who] use our innovative medicines. Despite the very positive role DTC advertising plays in educating patients about health issues and options, over the years, we have heard the concerns expressed about DTC advertising—that some ads may oversell benefits and undersell risks; that some ads may lead to inappropriate prescribing; that some patients may not be able to afford the advertised medicines; and

that some ads may not be appropriate for some audiences. Some doctors have also complained that drug companies launch advertising campaigns without helping to educate doctors in advance. Although actual practice and data on the effects of DTC advertising differ from these concerns, PhRMA recognized our obligation to act. On July 29, 2005, PhRMA's Board of Directors unanimously approved Guiding Principles on Direct-to-Consumer Advertisements About Prescription Medicines. These principles help ensure that DTC advertising remains an important and powerful tool to educate patients while at the same time addressing many of the concerns expressed about DTC advertising over the past few years.

First, PhRMA member companies take their responsibility to fully comply with FDA advertising regulations very seriously. Our advertising is already required to be accurate and not misleading; it can only make claims supported by substantial evidence; it must reflect the balance between risks and benefits; and it must be consistent with FDA-approved labeling. However, patients, health care providers, and the general public expect us to do more than just meet our exacting legal obligations, and our Guiding Principles do go further.

Our principles recognize that at the heart of our companies' DTC communications efforts is patient education. This means that DTC communications designed to market a medicine should responsibly educate patients about a medicine, including the conditions for which it may be prescribed. DTC advertising should also foster responsible communications between patients and health care professionals to help the patient achieve better health and a better appreciation of a medicine's known benefits and risks. Specifically, the Principles state that risk and safety information should be designed to achieve a balanced presentation of both risks and benefits associated with the advertised medicines.

Our Guiding Principles recognize that companies should spend appropriate time educating health care professionals about a new medicine before it is advertised to patients. That way, providers will be prepared to discuss the appropriateness of a given medication with a patient.

Current law provides that companies must submit their DTC television advertisements to FDA upon first use for FDA's review at its discretion. Companies that sign onto these Guiding Principles agree to submit all new

Antony, Paul. Testimony at hearing of U.S. Senate Special Committee on Aging, September 29, 2005. Reprinted from PhRMA.org, Pharmaceutical Research and Manufacturers of America (PhRMA).

DTC television ads to the FDA before releasing these ads for broadcast, giving the Agency an opportunity to review consistent with its priorities and resources. Companies also commit to informing FDA of the earliest date the advertisement is set to air. Should new information concerning a previously unknown safety risk be discovered, companies commit to work with FDA to "responsibly alter or discontinue a DTC advertising campaign."

In addition, the Principles encourage companies to include, where feasible, information about help for the uninsured and underinsured in their DTC communications. Our member companies offer a host of programs that can assist needy patients with their medicines.

The Principles also recognize that ads should respect the seriousness of the health condition and medicine being advertised and that ads employing humor or entertainment may not be appropriate in all instances.

As a result of concerns that certain prescription drug ads may not be suitable for all viewing audiences, the Guiding Principles state that, "DTC television and print advertisements should be targeted to avoid audiences that are not age appropriate for the messages involved."

Signatory companies are committed to establishing their own internal processes to ensure compliance with the Guiding Principles and to broadly disseminate them internally and to advertisers. In addition, PhRMA's Board unanimously approved the creation of an office of accountability to ensure the public has an opportunity to comment on companies' compliance with these Principles. The office of accountability will be responsible for receiving comments from the general public and from health care professionals regarding DTC ads by any company that publicly states it will follow the principles. The PhRMA office of accountability will provide to these companies any comment that is reasonably related to compliance with the Principles. Periodic reports will be issued by the PhRMA office of accountability to the public regarding the nature of the comments. Each report will also be submitted to the FDA.

PhRMA's Board also agreed to select an independent panel of outside experts and individuals to review reports from the office of accountability after one year and evaluate overall trends in the industry as they relate to the Principles. The panel will be empowered to make recommendations in accordance with the Principles. The Principles will go into effect in January 2006.

We believe these Principles will help patients and health care professionals get the information they need to make informed health care decisions.

The Value of DTC Advertising

Informing and Empowering Consumers

Surveys indicate that DTC advertising makes consumers aware of new drugs and their benefits, as well as risks and side effects with the drugs advertised. They help consumers recognize symptoms and seek appropriate care. According to an article in the New England Journal of Medicine, DTC

advertising is concentrated among a few therapeutic categories. These are therapeutic categories in which consumers can recognize their own symptoms, such as arthritis, seasonal allergies, and obesity; or for pharmaceuticals that treat chronic diseases with many undiagnosed sufferers, such as high cholesterol, osteoporosis, and depression.

DTC advertising gets patients talking to their doctors about conditions that may otherwise have gone undiagnosed or undertreated. For example, a study conducted by RAND Health and published in the New England Journal of Medicine found that nearly half of all adults in the United States fail to receive recommended health care. According to researchers on the RAND study, "the deficiencies in care . . . pose serious threats to the health of the American public that could contribute to thousands of preventable deaths in the United States each year." The study found underuse of prescription medications in seven of the nine conditions for which prescription medicines were the recommended treatment. Conditions for which underuse was found include asthma, cerebrovascular disease, congestive heart failure, diabetes, hip fracture, hyperlipidemia, and hypertension. Of those seven conditions for which RAND found underuse of recommended prescription medicines, five are DTC advertised.

The Rand study, as well as other studies, highlight the underuse of needed medications and other healthcare services in the U.S.

- According to a nationally representative study of 9,090 people aged 18 and up, published in JAMA, about 43 percent of participants with recent major depression are getting inadequate therapy.
- A 2004 study published in the Archives of Internal Medicine, found that, "In older patients, failures to prescribe indicated medications, monitor medications appropriately, document necessary information, educate patients, and maintain continuity are more common prescribing problems than is use of inappropriate drugs."
- A May/June 2003 study published in the Journal of Managed Care Pharmacy, which examined claims data from 3 of the 10 largest health plans in California to determine the appropriateness of prescription medication use based upon widely accepted treatment guidelines, found that "effective medication appears to be underused." Of the four therapeutic areas of study—asthma, CHF, depression, and common cold or upper respiratory tract infections—asthma, CHF, and depression were undertreated. The researchers concluded that "the results are particularly surprising and disturbing when we take into account the fact that three of the conditions studied (asthma, CHF, and depression) are known to produce high costs to the healthcare system."
- According to a study released in May 2005 by the Stanford University School of Medicine, among patients with high cholesterol in moderate and high-risk groups, researchers found fewer than half of patient visits ended with a statin

recommendation. Based on the findings, the researchers say physicians should be more aggressive in investigating statin therapy for patients with a high or moderate risk of heart disease, and that patients should ask for their cholesterol levels to be checked regularly.

Increasing Communication Between the Doctor and Patient

A vast majority of patients (93 percent) who asked about a drug reported that their doctor "welcomed the questions." Of patients who asked about a drug, 77 percent reported that their relationship with their doctor remained unchanged as a result of the office visit, and 20 percent reported that their relationship improved. In addition, both an FDA survey of physicians (from a random sample of 500 physicians from the American Medical Association's database) and a survey by the nation's oldest and largest African-American medical association, found that DTC advertisements raise disease awareness and bolster doctor-patient ties.

The doctor-patient relationship is enhanced if DTC advertising prompts a patient to talk to his doctor for the first time about a previously undiscussed condition, to comply with a prescribed treatment regimen, or to become aware of a risk or side effect that was otherwise unknown. A 2002 Prevention Magazine survey found that 24.8 million Americans spoke with their doctor about a medical condition for the first time as a result of seeing a DTC advertisement. Similarly, the FDA patient survey on DTC advertising found that nearly one in five patients reported speaking to a physician about a condition for the first time because of a DTC ad.

PhRMA and its member companies believe it is vital that patients, in consultation with their doctors, make decisions about treatments and medicines. Prescribing decisions should be dominated by the doctor's advice. While our member companies direct a large majority of their promotional activities toward physicians, such promotion in no way guarantees medicines will be prescribed.

According to a General Accounting Office report, of the 61.1 million people (33 percent of adults) who had discussions with their physician as a result of a DTC advertisement in 2001, only 8.5 million (5 percent of adults) actually received a prescription for the product, a small percentage of the total volume of prescriptions dispensed. Indeed, an FDA survey of physicians revealed that the vast majority of physicians do not feel pressure to prescribe. According to the survey, 91 percent of physicians said that their patients did not try to influence treatment courses in a way that would have been harmful and 72 percent of physicians, when asked for prescription for a specific brand name drug, felt little or no pressure to prescribe a medicine.

De-Stigmatizing Disease

DTC advertising also encourages patients to discuss medical problems that otherwise may not have been discussed because it was either thought to be too personal or that there was a stigma attached to the disease. For example, a Health Affairs article examined the value of innovation and noted that depression medications, known as selective serotonin reuptake inhibitors (SSRIs), that have been DTC advertised, have led to significant treatment expansion. Prior to the 1990's, it was estimated that about half of those persons who met a clinical definition of depression were not appropriately diagnosed, and many of those diagnosed did not receive clinically appropriate treatment. However, in the 1990's with the advent of SSRIs, treatment has been expanded. According to the article, "Manufacturers of SSRIs encouraged doctors to watch for depression and the reduced stigma afforded by the new medications induced patients to seek help." As a result, diagnosis and treatment for depression doubled over the 1990's.

Utilization and DTC Advertising

According to reports and studies, there is no direct relationship between DTC advertising and the price growth of drugs. For example, in comments to the FDA in December 2003, the FTC stated, "[DTC advertising] can empower consumers to manage their own health care by providing information that will help them, with the assistance of their doctors, to make better informed decisions about their treatment options. . . . Consumer[s] receive these benefits from DTC advertising with little, if any, evidence that such advertising increases prescription drug prices." Notably, since January 2000, the CPI component that tracks prescription medicines [has] been in line with overall medical inflation.

The FTC comments referenced above also note, "DTC advertising accounts for a relatively small proportion of the total cost of drugs, which reinforces the view that such advertising would have a limited, if any, effect on price." Likewise, a study by Harvard University and the Massachusetts Institute of Technology and published by the Kaiser Family Foundation found that DTC advertising accounts for less than 2 percent of the total U.S. spending for prescription medicines.

One study in the American Journal of Managed Care looked at whether pharmaceutical marketing has led to an increase in the use of medications by patients with marginal indications. The study found that high-risk individuals were receiving lipid-lowering treatment "consistent with evidence-based practice guidelines" despite the fact that "a substantial portion of patients continue to remain untreated and undertreated. . . ." The study concluded that "greater overall use did not appear to be associated with a shift towards patients with less CV [cardiovascular] risk."

Pharmaceutical utilization is increasing for reasons other than DTC advertising. As the June 2003 study of DTC advertising commissioned by the Kaiser Family Foundation found, "[O]ur estimates indicate that DTCA is important, but not the primary driver of recent growth [in prescription drug spending]."

Other reasons pharmaceutical utilization is increasing include:

- Improved Medicines—Many new medicines replace higher-cost surgeries and hospital care. In 2004 alone, pharmaceutical companies added 38 new medicines and over the last decade, over 300 new medicines have become available for treating patients. These include important new medicines for some of the most devastating and costly diseases, including: AIDS, cancer, heart disease, Alzheimer's, and diabetes. According to a study prepared for the Department of Health and Human Services, "[n]ew medications are not simply more costly than older ones. They may be more effective or have fewer side effects; some may treat conditions for which no treatment was available."
- New Standards of Medical Practice Encouraging Greater Use of Pharmaceuticals—Clinical standards are changing to emphasize earlier and tighter control of a range of conditions, such as diabetes, hypertension and cardiovascular disease. For example, new recommendations from the two provider groups suggest that early treatment, including lifestyle changes and treatment with two or more types of medications, can significantly reduce the risk of later complications and improve the quality of life for people with type 2 diabetes.
- Greater Treatment of Previously Undiagnosed and Untreated Conditions—According to guidelines developed by the National Heart, Lung, and Blood Institute's National Cholesterol Education Program (NCEP) Adult Treatment Panel (ATP), approximately 36 million adults should be taking medicines to lower their cholesterol, a number that has grown from 13 million just 8 years ago.
- Aging of America—The aging of American translates into greater reliance on pharmaceuticals. For example, congestive heart failure affects an estimated 2 percent of Americans age[d] 40 to 59, more than 5 percent of those aged 60 to 69, and 10 percent of those [aged] 70 or more.

While some assume that DTC advertising leads to increased use of newer medicines rather than generic medicines, generics represent just over 50 percent of all prescriptions (generics are historically not DTC advertised). In contrast, in Europe, where DTC advertising is prohibited, the percentage of prescriptions that are generic is significantly lower. Likewise, it is worth noting that while broadcast DTC has been in place since 1997, the rate of growth in drug cost increases has declined in each of the last 5 years and in 2004 was below the rate of growth in overall health care costs.

Economic Value of DTC Advertising

Increased spending on pharmaceuticals often leads to lower spending on other forms of more costly health care. New drugs are the most heavily advertised drugs, a point critics often emphasize. However, the use of newer drugs tends to lower all types of non-drug medical spending, resulting in a net reduction in the total cost of treating a condition. For example, on average replacing an older drug with a drug 15 years newer increases spending on drugs by $18, but reduces overall costs by $111.

The Tufts Center for the Study of Drug Development reports that disease management organizations surveyed believe that increased spending on prescription drugs reduces hospital inpatient costs. "Since prescription drugs account for less than 10 percent of total current U.S. health care spending, while inpatient care accounts for 32 percent, the increased use of appropriate pharmaceutical therapies may help moderate or reduce growth in the costliest component of the U.S. health care system," according to Tufts Center Director Kenneth I. Kaitin.

Opponents also compare the amount of money spent by drug companies on marketing and advertising to the amount they spend on research and development of new drugs. However, in 2004, pharmaceutical manufacturers spent an estimated $4.15 billion on DTC advertising, according to IMS Health, compared to $49.3 billion in total R&D spending by the biopharmaceutical industry, according to Burrill & Company. PhRMA members alone spent $38.8 billion on R&D in 2004.

Conclusion

DTC advertising provides value to patients by making them aware of risks and benefits of new drugs; it empowers patients and enhances the public health; it plays a vital role in addressing a major problem in this country of undertreatment and underdiagnosis of disease; encourages patients to discuss medical problems with their health care provider that may otherwise not be discussed due to a stigma being attached to the disease; and encourages patient compliance with physician-directed treatment regimens.

Given the progress that continues to be made in society's battle against disease, patients are seeking more information about medical problems and potential treatments. The purpose of DTC advertising is to foster an informed conversation about health, disease and treatments between patients and their health care practitioners. Our Guiding Principles are an important step in ensuring patients and health care professionals get the information they need to make informed health care decisions.

This concludes my written testimony. I would be happy to answer any questions or to supply any additional material by Members or Committee Staff on this or any other issue.

PAUL ANTONY is the chief medical officer at the Pharmaceutical Research and Manufacturers of America.

Gagnon and Lexchin

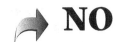 **NO**

The Cost of Pushing Pills: A New Estimate of Pharmaceutical Promotion Expenditures in the United States

In the late 1950s, the late Democratic Senator Estes Kefauver, Chairman of the United States Senate's Anti-Trust and Monopoly Subcommittee, put together the first extensive indictment against the business workings of the pharmaceutical industry. He laid three charges at the door of the industry: (1) Patents sustained predatory prices and excessive margins; (2) Costs and prices were extravagantly increased by large expenditures in marketing; and (3) Most of the industry's new products were no more effective than established drugs on the market. Kefauver's indictment against a marketing-driven industry created a representation of the pharmaceutical industry far different than the one offered by the industry itself. As Froud and colleagues put it, the image of life-saving "researchers in white coats" was now contested by the one of greedy "reps in cars." The outcome of the struggle over the image of the industry is crucial because of its potential to influence the regulatory environment in which the industry operates.

Fifty years later, the debate still continues between these two depictions of the industry. The absence of reliable data on the industry's cost structures allows partisans on both sides of the debate to cite figures favorable to their own positions. The amount of money spent by pharmaceutical companies on promotion compared to the amount spent on research and development is at the heart of the debate, especially in the United States. A reliable estimate of the former is needed to bridge the divide between the industry's vision of research-driven, innovative, and life-saving pharmaceutical companies and the critics' portrayal of an industry based on marketing-driven profiteering.

IMS, a firm specializing in pharmaceutical market intelligence, is usually considered to be the authority for assessing pharmaceutical promotion expenditures. The US General Accounting Office, for example, refers to IMS numbers in concluding that "pharmaceutical companies spend more on research and development initiatives than on all drug promotional activities." Based on the data provided by IMS, the Pharmaceutical Research and Manufacturers of America (PhRMA), an American industrial lobby group for research-based pharmaceutical companies, also contends that pharmaceutical firms spend more

on research and development (R&D) than on marketing: US$29.6 billion on R&D in 2004 in the US as compared to US$27.7 billion for all promotional activities.

In this paper, we make the case for the need for a new estimate of promotional expenditures. We then explain how we used proprietary databases to construct a revised estimate and finally, we compare our results with those from other data sources to argue in favor of changing the priorities of the industry.

The Case for a New Estimate of Pharmaceutical Promotion

There are many concerns about the accuracy of the IMS data. First, IMS compiles its information through surveys of firms, creating the possibility that companies may systematically underestimate some of their promotional costs to enhance their public image. Second, IMS does not include the cost of meetings and talks sponsored by pharmaceutical companies featuring either doctors or sales representatives as speakers.

The number of promotional meetings has increased dramatically in recent years, going from 120,000 in 1998 to 371,000 in 2004. In 2000, the top ten pharmaceutical companies were spending just under US$1.9 billion on 314,000 such events. Third, IMS does not include the amount spent on phase IV "seeding" trials, trials designed to promote the prescription of new drugs rather than to generate scientific data. In 2004, 13.2% (US$4.9 billion) of R&D expenditures by American pharmaceutical firms was spent on phase IV trials. Almost 75% of these trials are managed solely by the commercial, as opposed to the clinical, division of biopharmaceutical companies, strongly suggesting that the vast majority of these trials are done just for their promotional value.

Finally, IMS data seem inconsistent with estimates based on the information in the annual reports of pharmaceutical companies. For example, in an accounting study based on the annual reports of ten of the largest global pharmaceutical firms, Lauzon and Hasbani showed that between 1996 and 2005, these firms globally spent a total of US$739 billion on "marketing and administration."

Gagnon, Marc-André and Lexchin, Joel. From *PLoS Medicine,* January 2008, Public Library of Science.

In comparison, these same firms spent US$699 billion in manufacturing costs, US$288 billion in R&D, and had a net investment in property and equipment of US$43 billion, while receiving US$558 billion in profits.

Annual reports, however, have their own limitations. First, pharmaceutical firms are multinational and diversified; their annual reports provide no information on how much they spend on pharmaceutical marketing, as compared to the marketing of their non-pharmaceutical products, and they do not provide information about how much is spent on marketing specifically in the US. Second, annual reports merge the categories of "marketing" and "administration," without delineating the relative importance of each. Finally, "marketing" is a category that includes more than just promotion; it also includes the costs of packaging and distribution. In terms of offering a more precise estimate of overall expenditures on pharmaceutical promotion in the US, annual reports are thus far from satisfactory.

In the absence of any collection of information on promotional spending by government or any other noncommercial source, the market research company IMS has long been the only source of such information, which it gains by surveying pharmaceutical firms. Since 2003, however, the market research company CAM has been providing comprehensive information on promotion expenditures by surveying doctors instead of firms. (In July 2005, CAM was merged into the Cegedim Group, another market research company.) We chose to compare IMS data to those produced by CAM in order to provide a more accurate estimate of promotional spending in the US. Other proprietary sources of data do not break down promotional expenditures into different categories and therefore were not used in our comparison.

Methods

According to its Web site (http://www.imshealth.com/), IMS provides business intelligence and strategic consulting services for the pharmaceutical and health care industries. It is a global company established in more than 100 countries. IMS gathers data from 29,000 data suppliers at 225,000 supplier sites worldwide. It monitors 75% of prescription drug sales in over 100 countries, and 90% of US prescription drug sales. It tracks more than 1 million products from more than 3,000 active drug manufacturers. IMS data for 2004 were obtained from its Web site for the amount spent on: visits by sales representatives (detailing), samples, direct-to-consumer advertising, and journal advertising.

The Cegedim Web site (http://www.cegedim-crm.com/index.php?id=12) describes CAM as a global company dedicated to auditing promotional activities of the pharmaceutical industry, established in 36 countries worldwide. CAM annually surveys a representative sample of 2,000 primary care physicians and 4,800 specialists in a variety of specialties in selected locations in the US. From CAM's newsletter,

we obtained access to data from CAM for the same promotion categories as from IMS. In addition, CAM provided figures for the amount of spending on company-sponsored meetings, e-promotion, mailings, and clinical trials.

We used 2004 as the comparison year because it was the latest year for which information was available from both organizations. We focused on the US because it is the only country for which information is available for all important promotional categories. The US is also, by far, the largest market for pharmaceuticals in the world, representing around 43% of global sales and global promotion expenditures.

We asked both CAM and IMS about the procedures that they used to collect information on different aspects of promotion. Based on the answers we received, we determined the relevant figures for expenditures for samples and detailing. Each author independently decided on which values should be used, based on an understanding of the methods that the companies used to collect the information and the limitations of those methods. Differences were resolved by consensus.

We queried CAM and IMS about the estimated value of unmonitored promotional expenditures. IMS did not provide an answer to this question. In order to validate its estimates, CAM relies on a validation committee that includes representatives from various pharmaceutical firms, including Merck, Pfizer, Bristol-Myers Squibb, Eli Lilly, Aventis, Sanofi-Synthelabo, AstraZeneca, and Wyeth. Under a confidentiality agreement, the firms supply CAM with internal data related to their detailing activity and promotional costs in the US. Through the validation committee, CAM can thus compare totals obtained through its own audits with the firms' internal data about their promotional budgets in order to evaluate if all promotion has been properly audited through its physician surveys. As a result of this comparison, CAM's validation committee considers that about 30% of promotional spending is not accounted for in its figures. CAM is unable to provide an exact breakdown of unmonitored promotion, but it believes that around 10% is due to incomplete disclosure and omissions by surveyed physicians and the remaining 20% comes from a combination of promotion directed at categories of physicians that are not surveyed, unmonitored journals in which pharmaceutical promotion appears, and possibly unethical forms of promotion. We adjusted total expenditures to account for this unreported 30%.

Results

For 2004, CAM reported total promotional spending in the US of US$33.5 billion, while IMS gave the figure of US$27.7 billion for the same year. Both CAM and IMS cited the media intelligence company CMR as the source for the amount spent on direct-to-consumer advertising (US$4 billion), and they also gave the same figure for journal advertising (US$0.5 billion).

There were two major differences between the two sets of figures: the amounts spent on detailing and the amounts spent on samples. IMS estimated the amount spent on detailing at US$7.3 billion versus US$20.4 billion for CAM, and while IMS gave a retail value of US$15.9 billion for samples, CAM estimated a wholesale value of US$6.3 billion.

Using the IMS figure of US$15.9 billion for the retail value of samples, and adding the CAM figures for detailing and other marketing expenses after correcting for the 30% estimate of unaccounted promotion, we arrived at US$57.5 billion for the total amount spent in the US in 2004, more than twice what IMS reported (see Table 1).

Discussion

Our revised estimate for promotional spending in the US is more than twice that from IMS. This number compares to US$31.5 billion for domestic industrial pharmaceutical R&D (including public funds for industrial R&D) in 2004 as reported by the National Science Foundation.

However, even our revised figure is likely to be incomplete. There are other avenues for promotion that would not be captured by either IMS or CAM, such as ghostwriting and illegal off-label promotion. Furthermore, items with promotional potential such as "seeding trials" or educational grants might be included in other budgets and would not be seen in the confidential material provided to CAM's validation committee.

IMS and CAM data were used for comparison purposes for a number of reasons: data from both were publicly available, both operate on a global scale and are well regarded by the pharmaceutical industry, both break down their information by different categories of promotion, and, most importantly, they use different methods for gathering their data, thereby allowing us to triangulate on a more accurate figure for each category.

Methodological differences between the ways that IMS and CAM collect data will affect the values for promotional spending depending on the category being considered. Because of the problematic nature of some data from each firm, we believe that the most precise picture of industry spending can be obtained by selectively using both sets of figures.

CAM compiles its data on the value of detailing and samples through systematic surveys of primary care providers and specialists and by estimating an average cost for each visit by a sales representative according to the type of physician. By contrast, IMS compiles its data on the value of detailing through surveys of firms, while its data on samples are obtained by monitoring products directly from manufacturers.

There is a significant discrepancy between the two sets of data in the cost of detailing: US$7.3 billion for IMS and US$20.4 billion for CAM. This difference can be explained by the fact that CAM offers a more complete data set since it includes in the average cost of a call (a sales representative's visit to a physician) not only the "cost to field the rep" (salary and benefits of the representative and the transportation cost) but also the costs for the area and regional managers, the cost of the training, and the cost of detail aids such as brochures and advertising material. By contrast, in reporting the cost of detailing IMS only considers the "cost to field the rep." Furthermore, relying on physician-generated data to estimate the amount spent on detailing is likely to give a more accurate figure than using figures generated by surveying firms. Companies may not report some types of detailing, for example, the use of sales representatives for illegal off-label promotion, whereas doctors are not likely to distinguish between on- and off-label promotion and would report all encounters with sales representatives.

In the case of samples, there is also a large difference between the IMS (US$15.9 billion) and CAM (US$6.3 billion)

Table 1

Pharmaceutical Marketing Expenditures in the United States in 2004: Data from IMS, CAM, and Our New Estimate

Type of Promotion	IMS (US$ Billions)	CAM (US$ Billions)	New Estimate (US$ Billions)	Percent of Total of New Estimate
Samples	15.9	6.3	15.9 (IMS)	27.7
Detailing	7.3	20.4	20.4 (CAM)	35.5
DTCA (data provided by CMR)	4	4	4 (CMR)	7
Meetings	nd	2	2 (CAM)	3.5
E-promotion, mailing, clinical trials	nd	0.3	0.3 (CAM)	0.5
Journal advertising	0.5	0.5	0.5 (CAM/IMS)	0.9
Unmonitored promotion (estimate[a])	nd	14.4	14.4 (CAM)	25
Total	27.7	47.9	57.5	100

[a]Includes incomplete disclosure and omissions by surveyed physicians, promotion to unaudited physician categories, promotion in unmonitored journals, and could possibly include unethical forms of promotion funded out of the firms' marketing budget. See text for details about this category.
DTCA, direct-to-consumer advertising; nd, no data
doi:10.1371/journal.pmed.0050001.t001

estimates. CAM estimates the amount spent on samples by multiplying the number of samples declared by physicians with their wholesale value. The latter is determined by using the average wholesale price (AWP), which is the amount set by manufacturers and used by Medicare in the US to determine reimbursement. CAM then divides that amount in half to account for the fact that samples are frequently given out in small dosage forms. CAM admits, however, that the amount for samples is understated because, when physicians fill out their survey, any quantity of samples of the same product left during a call is considered to be only one sample unit. CAM's calculations also rely on the AWP, which has been criticized for not taking into account the various discounts and rebates that are negotiated between manufacturers and purchasers.

IMS provides exact figures for the retail value for samples by monitoring 90% of all pharmaceutical transactions and by tracking products directly from manufacturers. This method for calculating the value of samples is much more direct than CAM's and therefore is likely to be subject to less error.

Using the wholesale value for samples, the CAM figure would be appropriate if we were arguing that the money spent on samples should go to another activity such as R&D. However, we have used the retail value of samples because this is consistent with companies' reporting of drugs they donate. As these are both categories of products that are being distributed without a charge to the user, it is inconsistent for donations to be reported in terms of retail value and samples in terms of wholesale value.

We believe that it is appropriate to correct for unmonitored promotion and that the figure we used is a reliable estimate. The 30% correction factor is based on a direct comparison that CAM is able to make between the data it collects through its surveys and the amount reported by companies.

There are other ways of combining the data that we have presented, but with the exception of choosing the lower amounts for detailing and samples and ignoring the 30% for unmonitored promotion, all of them yield a higher figure than the one from IMS. Some examples of alternative estimates follow: using the CAM estimate for the wholesale value of samples and the 30% adjustment, the total amount would be US$47.9 billion; without the 30% adjustment CAM's estimate is US$33.5 billion. Adding the figures for the categories that IMS does not cover (meetings, e-promotion, mailing, clinical trials) boosts its estimate to US$31 billion; using the lower figures for detailing and samples plus the CAM amounts for the other categories and applying the 30% adjustment gives an amount of US$29.1 billion. Therefore, the actual amount could range from a low of US$27.7 billion to a high of US$57.5 billion. Our analysis shows, however, that the figure of US$57.5 billion is the most appropriate one when using the most relevant figures for each category of promotional spending.

Excluding direct-to-consumer advertising, CAM considers that around 80% of the remaining promotion is directed towards physicians, with 20% of this figure going to pharmacists. (IMS does not provide any comparable values.) With about 700,000 practicing physicians in the US in 2004, we estimate that with a total expenditure of US$57.5 billion, the industry spent around US$61,000 in promotion per physician. As a percentage of US domestic sales of US$235.4 billion, promotion consumes 24.4% of the sales dollar versus 13.4% for R&D.

Our new estimate of total promotion costs and promotion as a percentage of sales is broadly in line with estimates of promotional or marketing spending from other sources. The annual reports of Novartis distinguish "marketing" from "administration." Marcia Angell extrapolates from this annual report to the entire industry and calculates a figure of US$54 billion spent on pharmaceutical promotion in the US in 2001. As a proportion of sales, she estimates 33% is spent on marketing. Using similar methodology, the Office of Technology Assessment derived an estimate for marketing costs in the US by extrapolating from the cost structure of Eli Lilly. The Office of Technology Assessment considers that firms spend around 22.5% of their sales on marketing. Based on United Nations Industrial Development Organization estimates, a report from the Organization for Economic Cooperation and Development estimated that, in 1989, pharmaceutical firms globally spent 24% of their sales on marketing, but few details of the methodology used were provided, making it impossible to verify the accuracy of the estimate. Finally, in 2006 Consumers International surveyed 20 European pharmaceutical firms to obtain more information about their exact expenditures on drug promotion. Among the 20 firms contacted, only five agreed to provide separate figures for marketing, which ranged from 31% to 50% of sales depending on the firm.

The results are also consistent with data on the share of revenue allocated to "marketing and administration" according to annual reports of large pharmaceutical companies, if we consider that the largest part of "marketing and administration" is devoted to promotion. Lauzon and Hasbani found that 33.1% of revenues was allocated to "marketing and administration," similar to the 31% reported by the Centers for Medicare and Medicaid Services and the 27% from Families USA.

The value of our estimate over these others is that it is not based on extrapolating from annual reports of firms that are both diversified and multinational. Our estimate is driven by quantifiable data from highly reliable sources and concerns only the promotion of pharmaceutical products in the US. The derivation of our figure is thus transparent and can form the basis for a vigorous debate.

Conclusion

From this new estimate, it appears that pharmaceutical companies spend almost twice as much on promotion as they do on R&D. These numbers clearly show how promotion predominates over R&D in the pharmaceutical industry, contrary to the industry's claim. While the amount spent on promotion is not in itself a confirmation of Kefauver's depiction of the pharmaceutical industry, it confirms the public image of a marketing-driven industry and provides an important argument to petition in favor of transforming the workings of the industry in the direction of more research and less promotion.

MARC-ANDRÉ GAGNON is an assistant professor in the School of Public Policy and Administration at Carlton University, Ottawa, Ontario, Canada.

JOEL LEXCHIN is a physician and professor in the School of Health Policy and Management at York University and an associate professor in the Department of Family and Community Medicine at the University of Toronto.

EXPLORING THE ISSUE

Should Prescription Drugs Be Advertised Directly to Consumers?

Critical Thinking and Reflection

1. What are the advantages of patent protection to consumers?
2. Describe the justification the drug companies use to directly market prescription drugs to consumers.
3. What are the primary reasons drug costs continue to spiral?

Is There Common Ground?

While new prescription drugs may save lives, it can also be argued that the pharmaceutical industry, via advertising to consumers and physicians, has increased the demand for their products and the costs of drugs. Television advertisements for heartburn medicine imply that overeating is not a problem if one takes the right pill. Shifting to a healthier lifestyle may help many Americans avoid and reduce their need for costly prescription medications. Also, advertising may divert money away from research, and may influence physicians' prescribing practices. "Who Are the Opinion Leaders? The Physicians, Pharmacists, Patients, and Direct-to-Consumer Prescription Drug Advertising," *Journal of Health Communication* (September 2010) discusses the popular perception that physicians prescribe requested drugs to patients influenced by prescription drug advertising seen on television or in magazines. In "Consumer Responses to Coupons in Direct-to-Consumer Advertising of Prescription Drugs," *Health Marketing Quarterly* (December 2009), the authors determined that coupons for prescription drugs in newspapers, magazines, or online had an impact on drugs requested by patients when visiting their physicians.

There appears to be a drug war in America. Rapidly escalating prescription costs from advertising and other issues are affecting the most vulnerable among us—the elderly. The lack of a pharmacy benefit in Medicare coverage plus the rising costs of medications causes too many seniors to make tough choices: their prescription drugs or other necessities such as food. Some states including Maine, Florida, and Michigan have taken on the drug companies to lower the cost of prescription medications. The industry has vowed to fight the states on every front. More states are ready to address the problem of rising drug prices under the Medicaid program and a battle may be looming.

Some American consumers are also fighting back. They're traveling to Mexico and Canada in search of lower prices. Others are asking for generic versions of their medications and also requesting double dosage pills and splitting them. Often the larger dose pills have a lower unit cost. Still others are shopping online, by mail, or through prescription drug groups. While all these techniques may save money, critics of the pharmaceutical industry assert the real problem is that the drug companies' rising profits, monopolies on patented drugs, high advertising costs, and political contributions all play a role in high prescription costs.

Create Central

www.mhhe.com/createcentral

Additional Resources

An, S. & Muturi, N. (2011). Subjective health literacy and older adults' assessment of direct-to-consumer prescription drug ads. *Journal of Health Communication, 16,* 242–255.

Boltz, K. (2012). Advertising and promoting prescription drugs: The FDA speaks. *AMWA Journal: American Medical Writers Association Journal, 27*(4), 161–162.

Frosch, D. L., Grande, D., Tarn, D. M., & Kravitz, R. L. (2010). A decade of controversy: Balancing policy with evidence in the regulation of prescription drug advertising. *American Journal of Public Health, 100*(1), 24–32.

La Barbera, C. P. (2012). Irresponsible reminders: Ethical aspects of direct-to-consumer drug advertising. *Ethics & Medicine: An International Journal of Bioethics, 28*(3), 95–112.

Mintzes, B. (2012). Advertising of prescription-only medicines to the public: Does evidence of benefit counterbalance harm? *Annual Review of Public Health, 33,* 259–277.

Internet References . . .

Food and Drug Administration (FDA)

This site includes FDA news, information on drugs, and drug toxicology facts.

www.fda.gov

National Institute on Drug Abuse (NIDA)

www.nida.nih.gov

Pharmaceutical Research and Manufacturers of America (PhRMA)

www.phrma.org/

Prescription Drugs: The Issue

www.opensecrets.org/news/drug/

Selected, Edited, and with Issue Framing Material by:
Eileen Daniel, *SUNY College at Brockport*

ISSUE

Are We Winning the War on Cancer?

YES: John R. Seffrin, from "Winning the War on Cancer: Public Health or Public Policy Challenge?" *Vital Speeches of the Day* (September 2006)

NO: Reynold Spector, from "The War on Cancer: A Progress Report for Skeptics," *Skeptical Inquirer* (January/February 2010)

Learning Outcomes
After reading this issue, you should be able to:
• Understand the complex nature of cancer.
• Discuss the reasons why the disease has been so difficult to eradicate.
• Assess why Reynold Spector believes so little progress has been made.
• Discuss cancer treatments and their side effects.
• Discuss the causes of various types of cancer.

ISSUE SUMMARY

YES: American Cancer Society President John R. Seffrin claims we are winning the war against cancer and that it is possible to eliminate the disease as a major public health problem.

NO: Physician and professor of medicine Reynold Spector argues that the gains made against cancer have been limited and that overall there has been very little progress in the war on cancer.

Cancer is a group of diseases characterized by uncontrolled cellular growth, invasion that intrudes on and destroys nearby tissues, and may metastasize or spread to other locations in the body via blood or lymph. The malignant characteristics of cancers differentiate them from benign growths or tumors, which do not invade or metastasize. Fortunately, most cancers can be treated with drugs or chemotherapy, surgery, and/or radiation. The outcome of the disease is based on the type of cancer, for example, lung or breast, and the extent of disease. Although cancer affects people of all ages, and a few types of cancer are actually more common in children, most cancer risks increase with age. Cancer rates are increasing as more people live longer and lifestyles change such as increased smoking occur in the developing world.

Most cancers have an environmental link, with 90–95 percent of cases attributed to environmental factors and 5–10 percent due to heredity. Typical environmental factors that contribute to cancer deaths include diet and obesity (30–35 percent), smoking and tobacco use (25–30 percent), infectious agents (15–20 percent), and ionizing and non-ionizing radiation (up to 10 percent). The remaining may be caused by stress, lack of exercise, and some environmental pollutants. Cancer prevention is related to those active measures that decrease the incidence of the disease. Since the vast majority of cancer risk factors are environmental or lifestyle-related, cancer is largely a preventable disease. Individuals who avoid tobacco, maintain a healthy weight, eat a diet rich in fruits and vegetables, exercise, use alcohol in moderation, take measures to prevent the transmission of sexually transmitted diseases, and avoid exposure to air pollution are likely to significantly reduce their risks of the disease.

Cancer's reputation is a deadly one. In reality, about half of the patients receiving treatment for invasive cancer will not survive the disease or the treatment. The survival rate, however, can vary significantly by the type of cancer, ranging from basically all patients surviving to almost no patients surviving. Predicting either short-term or long-term survival is challenging and depends on a variety of factors. The most important factors are the type of cancer and the patient's age and overall health. Medically frail patients suffering simultaneously from other illnesses have lower survival rates than otherwise healthy patients. Despite strong social pressure to maintain an upbeat, optimistic attitude or act like a determined "fighter" to "win the battle," research has not shown that personality traits have a connection to survival.

In 1971, the then president Richard Nixon signed the National Cancer Act of 1971. The goal of the act was to find a cure for cancer by increased research to improve the understanding of cancer biology and the development of more effective treatments such as targeted drug therapies. The act is also viewed as the beginning of the war on cancer and the vow to end the disease for good. Despite significant progress in the treatment of certain forms of cancer, the disease in general remains a major cause of death 40 years after this effort began, leading to a perceived lack of progress and to new legislation aimed at augmenting the original National Cancer Act of 1971. New research directions, in part based on the results of the Human Genome Project, hold promise for a better understanding of the hereditary factors underlying cancer and the development of new diagnostics, treatments, preventive measures, and early detection ability.

In the YES and NO selections, American Cancer Society President John R. Seffrin claims we are winning the war against cancer and that it is possible to eliminate the disease as a major public health problem. Physician and professor of medicine Reynold Spector argues that the gains made against cancer have been limited and that overall there has been very little progress in the war on cancer.

YES ←

John R. Seffrin

Winning the War on Cancer: Public Health or Public Policy Challenge?

Ladies and gentlemen—we are winning!

For the first time—we can today state that we are winning the war on cancer.

What is even more—we now know essentially what it will take to finish the job—that is eliminating cancer as a major public health problem—first here in the US and then worldwide. Indeed, the progress made in our understanding of the cancer problem is so great—so substantial—that we find ourselves in a very different place—and in a very different situation—than when the American Cancer Society was founded in 1913 or even when the National Cancer Act was passed in 1971.

Today, we know more about cancer than ever before. We understand many of its causes. We know how to prevent it, and, we increasingly know how to cure it, especially in its early stages. Despite this significant growth in the knowledge base, we have not succeeded in stemming the growing burden of cancer. The gap between what is and what could be in cancer control and cancer care is the single most important issue facing the cancer community in the world today.

So it is in this context that I would like to share with you these four facts of life or new realities which form the core of my message today.

1. For the first time, we know what it will take to win the war on cancer, based on evidence.
2. We can eliminate cancer as a major health problem in the US in this century, if we do the right things.
3. However, if we fail to intervene—if we fail to do the right things, cancer will become the leading cause of death in the US by 2018 and eventually, likely, the leading cause of death in the world.
4. So the conquest of the world's most feared disease is a question of choice, priority, resources, and resolve, not luck or a magic bullet or a single miracle cure.

While the hopeful side of cancer has never been more hopeful—and the prospects for saving and improving lives are truly extraordinary—we do have our work cut out for us.

Science alone, public health alone, or public policy alone cannot get us to where we need to be to realize this very possible dream. It will take all three and a lot of commitment and collaboration to make it happen. And as I speak, the cancer burden is actually getting worse—not better—and cancer will kill more people in the world this year than HIV/AIDS, tuberculosis, and malaria combined.

Perhaps ironically, in the last 60 years, science has made remarkable progress toward unraveling the mystery of cancer. But so much of what we know about cancer is not being adequately translated into what we do about cancer.

As a result, if current trends persist, by 2020, the number of new cancer cases worldwide will grow to 15 million and the number of deaths will double to as many as 12 million. An estimated 70 percent of these deaths will occur in developing countries, which are least prepared to address their growing cancer burdens.

With recent advances in our understanding of cancer, these are people whose lives need not be lost. They continue to experience unnecessary suffering and death not because we don't know how to prevent it or detect it early or treat it, but because we refuse to ensure that all people in all nations—including our own—have equal access to lifesaving cancer advances.

That's why this July the American Cancer Society is doing something that hasn't been done before—bringing together two world conferences that have rarely been held in the same year, and never in the same country—the World Cancer Congress and the 13th World Conference on Tobacco OR Health.

These two conferences will bring together over 5,500 participants from more than 130 countries: oncologists, public health leaders, tobacco control advocates, cancer association leaders, health ministries, and journalists. These meetings will reach across the entire breadth of cancer control and cancer care to focus energy and attention not just on talking about the cancer problem, but on identifying and sharing practical solutions that can make a lifesaving difference in communities around the world now.

Why is it so critical to unite the global cancer and tobacco control communities? Because, if your aim is to solve the cancer problem, the two are inseparable. The world is on a collision course if we fail to take action against the scourge of tobacco. Indeed, it's a train wreck not waiting to happen! Indeed, it's already happening and its repercussions will have a public health and economic impact unlike any we have ever experienced before.

As the only consumer product proven to kill more than half of its regular users, tobacco will be responsible

Seffrin, John R. From address delivered to the National Press Club, Washington, D.C., June 26, 2006.

for 4.9 million deaths worldwide this year alone. Today, that burden is almost evenly shared by industrialized and developing nations, but the trend is rapidly changing to the developing countries of the world.

If we fail to act to prevent this tragedy in the making, the consequences will most certainly be dire and destabilizing. As a direct result of tobacco use, at current rates, 650 million people alive today will eventually die, half of whom are now children. Half of these people will die in middle age—when they are most productive for their economies, their communities, and their families. In the last century, tobacco use killed 100 million people. If left unchecked, tobacco use will kill more than one billion people in this century, and if we let it happen, it will be the worst case of avoidable loss of life in world history. Yet, we know with comprehensive, concerted action, we can eliminate the global scourge of tobacco and save hundreds of millions of lives within the next few decades, if we do the right things.

Let's take the United States as an example. We have enjoyed many resounding victories against Big Tobacco that are making a real difference toward the ultimate bottom line—lives saved. More than 2,200 communities nationwide have enacted smoke-free laws that are protecting the health of millions of Americans. In fact, tomorrow the Surgeon General will release the first report in 20 years focusing on secondhand smoke, and we expect it to confirm the public health and economic benefits of clean indoor air laws.

However, as smoking rates decline in the US and many other industrialized nations, the tobacco industry has dramatically stepped up its efforts in emerging markets. Because tobacco kills the majority of its customer base, the industry must persuade millions of people to become new smokers each year just to break even. In the largely unrestricted markets of the developing world, that means that no one is immune to the industry's tactics, especially the most vulnerable people of all—children.

Fortunately, thanks to the rigorous educational, scientific, and advocacy efforts of dedicated tobacco control activists worldwide, many nations are taking a stand against tobacco by supporting the world's first global public health treaty—the World Health Organization Framework Convention on Tobacco Control (FCTC). This treaty's evidence-based interventions have been proven to work in diverse cultures around the world.

The treaty hits the tobacco companies where they live by restricting their insidious and immoral marketing tactics. It gives nations—particularly the low-income nations the tobacco companies have targeted as their most promising markets—powerful new tools to protect their citizens from the tobacco industry's deception.

The US is to be commended for supporting adoption of the treaty, but our nation's role in this arena has been halted because we have so far refused to ratify it. As of June 20, 2006, 131 countries already have ratified the treaty, making it the most rapidly embraced treaty in UN history.

Why are we lagging behind? The United States ratification and effective implementation of the treaty is essential to turning the tide of the global tobacco pandemic. To that end, I have urged President Bush to send the treaty to the Senate for ratification. And since many of the ratifying countries will be represented at the upcoming conferences, we will use that opportunity to bring pressure to bear on the administration and the US Senate to promptly join the rest of the world in ratifying the treaty. When ratified and implemented, we know from experience and evidence that human suffering will be reduced and lives will be saved.

In addition to taking immediate action against tobacco, there are three actions I believe it will take to eliminate cancer as a major public health problem at the earliest possible time.

First, we must accelerate discovery by redoubling and balancing our cancer research portfolio. Thanks to decades of well-funded, peer-reviewed research, cancer research has gone from a good bet to a sure bet. Remarkable achievements such as the mapping of the human genome make new cancer cures virtually inevitable, if we do the right things—and that is fully fund NIH and its National Cancer Institute. Further progress is guaranteed if research funding keeps pace. Landmark discoveries such as cancer vaccines and better and more targeted therapies are inevitable (assumed), but only if we fuel the engines of discovery. And we know that's what the American tax-payer and voter wants us to do!

And we must, at the same time, balance our research portfolio to include applied behavioral research, psychosocial and translational research, and evidence-based prevention interventions. If we redouble and balance cancer research efforts, the number of lives we could improve and save is unlimited over time. Unfortunately, funding for the NIH—the worldwide leader among cancer research institutions—is in jeopardy. If we fail to continue stoking the engines of research, we will effectively renege on our nation's commitment to the American people. And that's wrong!

Second, we must promote and elevate prevention into public policy and standard practice nationwide. One example of the enormous potential of prevention is cervical cancer. In nations like ours, where screening tests are available and early detection is standard practice, screening and follow-up treatment has reduced cervical cancer deaths by as much as 80 percent. And yet, despite these advances in prevention, in many parts of the world, cervical cancer is still a leading cause of cancer death in women.

As you know, recent FDA approval of the HPV vaccine, the first vaccine targeted specifically to preventing cancer, is one of the most important advances in women's health in recent decades. Successful global implementation of an effective HPV vaccine offers a truly unprecedented opportunity to prevent millions of deaths and dramatically reduce the world's cancer burden. The challenge is to make such advances available to every woman who needs them.

This is typical of the challenge facing cancer control advocates worldwide. Science has given us the tools to save lives, but our medical care and political systems are not equipped to deliver on those advances, which brings me to the third action.

Thirdly, we must drive delivery of state-of-the-art cancer care and control at the community level. In places where public health organizations, governments, and the private sector have worked together to drive delivery at the community level, there have been impressive results. With state-of-the-art cancer care, as many as 75 percent of cancer patients could survive long-term. Today, tragically, nowhere near this many will receive treatment that fully takes advantage of what science has taught us.

Access to the means for the attainment and preservation of health is a basic human need and right and should not be thought of as a privilege for just the few.

If we fail to do the right things, it will not only result in an otherwise avoidable public health catastrophe, but also an economic missed opportunity. For example, here in the US, a 20% reduction in cancer mortality will yield a 10 trillion dollar value to the American people, according to a study done by Kevin M. Murphy and Robert H. Topel entitled The Economic Value of Medical Research.

Because cancer tends to strike and kill in the prime of one's life, its human and economic impact is difficult to exaggerate. Truly, a nation's very competitiveness in the future will be tied to how healthy its citizens are.

So the underlying key to achieving each of these goals is advocacy. Cancer is as much a political and public policy issue as it is a medical and public health issue. Remarkable advances in prevention, early detection, and treatment virtually guarantee lower incidence and mortality rates—if they are available to everyone who needs them.

That means our most pressing challenge is to make cancer a policy priority—to educate lawmakers, governments, and civic leaders about the urgency of cancer control and inspire their commitment to enact public policies that will make cancer advances available to all people everywhere.

Obviously, this is an enormously complicated task, but we need only look to advocacy successes here in the United States to see the remarkable, lifesaving potential of public policy solutions to the world's public health problems.

Let me cite one contemporary example. Recently, the American Cancer Society Cancer Action Network (ACS CAN)—the Society's sister 501(c)4 advocacy organization—took action against the small business health care legislation known as "Health Insurance Marketplace Modernization and Affordability Act," or S. 1955, which would have effectively gutted state laws that require health insurers to cover lifesaving cancer screenings and treatments.

Working with our partners—AARP and the American Diabetes Association—ACS CAN launched a multi-media advertising campaign that received an immediate, strong response from grassroots volunteers. More than 170,000 emails poured into US Senate offices and nearly 10,000 calls came in from constituents requesting to be connected to the target Senate offices. I'm proud to report that our collaborative efforts were successful. On May 12, the bill was stopped in the US Senate.

But, although we've made extraordinary progress, we still have a long way to go.

That's why ACS CAN is planning to bring 10,000 energetic advocates representing every congressional district in the country to Capitol Hill this September 19 and 20 for Celebration on the Hill to meet with their elected officials and participate in activities on the National Mall with an important message: "We care about cancer, and we will be heard. We will do our part, but you must do yours. And we will not take 'no' for an answer." Cancer survivors don't take life and health for granted—and they vote with their feet and voices as well as their ballots.

Our ability to make a difference in the lives of people touched by cancer increases exponentially when we help pass laws and establish public policies that secure investments in research and prevention, and access to quality health care.

Ultimately, the challenge for all of us will be to do what we can to redouble our efforts in pursuit of our common cancer-fighting agenda. This means we must have the courage to share, the courage to take responsible, bold risks, and the courage to persevere. In other words, we must have the courage to transform what is into what could be.

In conclusion, I leave you with the following truth: When the American Cancer Society was founded in 1913, a diagnosis of cancer was a virtual death sentence only to be preceded by an often protracted period of pain and suffering. Due to an indefatigable commitment to research and intervention at the community level, cancer has been transformed and is today potentially the most preventable and most curable of the major life-threatening diseases facing humankind.

We now have the knowledge and know-how to turn that potentiality into reality, if we do the right things. And may God speed that day.

Thank you.

John R. Seffrin is the president of the American Cancer Society.

Reynold Spector

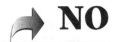

The War on Cancer: A Progress Report for Skeptics

In 1971, President Nixon and Congress declared war on cancer. Since then, the federal government has spent well over $105 billion on the effort. What have we gained from that huge investment? David Nathan, a well-known professor and administrator, maintains in his book *The Cancer Treatment Revolution* (Wiley, 2007) that we have made substantial progress. However, he greatly overestimates the potential of the newer so-called "smart drugs." Researchers Psyrri and De Vita (2008) also claim important progress. However, they cherry-pick the cancers with which there has been some progress and do not discuss the failures. Moreover, they only discuss the last decade rather than a more balanced view of 1950 or 1975 to the present.

On the other hand, Gina Kolata pointed out in *The New York Times* that the cancer death rate, adjusted for the size and age of the population, has decreased by only 5 percent since 1950. She argues that there has been very little overall progress in the war on cancer.

In this article, I will focus on adult cancer, since child cancer makes up less than 1 percent of all cancer diagnosed. I will then place the facts in proper perspective after an overview of the epidemiology, diagnosis, and treatment (especially with smart drugs) of adult cancer in the United States.

The Cancer Facts

Summary statistics show that the war on cancer has not gone well. This is in marked contrast to death rates from stroke and cardiovascular disease (adjusted for the age and size of the population), which have fallen by 74 percent and 64 percent, respectively, from 1950 through 2006; and by 60 percent and 52 percent, respectively, from 1975 through 2006. These excellent results against stroke and heart disease are mainly due to improvements in drug therapy, especially the control of high blood pressure to prevent stroke and the use of statins, aspirin, beta blockers, calcium channel blockers, and ACE inhibitors (now all generic) to prevent and treat heart disease. Cancer therapy is clearly decades behind. However, these data conceal a great deal of useful information and do not provide guidance on how to make progress against cancer.

Methodological Issues

To understand the issues, we must describe a few statistical traps and define our terms (see table 1). For example, there are several types of detection bias. First, if one discovers a malignant tumor very early and starts therapy immediately, even if the therapy is worthless, it will appear that the patient lives longer than a second patient (with an identical tumor) treated with another worthless drug if the cancer in the second patient was detected later. Second, detection bias can also occur with small tumors, especially of the breast and prostate, that would not harm the patient if left untreated but can lead to unnecessary and sometimes mutilating

Figure 1

U.S. Mortality, 2006

Rank	Cause of Death	No. of Deaths	% of All Deaths
1.	Heart Diseases	631,636	26.0
2.	Cancer	559,888	23.1
3.	Cerebrovascular Diseases	137,119	5.7
4.	Chronic Lower Respiratory Diseases	124,583	5.1
5.	Accidents (unintentional injuries)	121,599	5.0
6.	Diabetes Mellitus	72,449	3.0
7.	Alzheimer Disease	72,432	3.0
8.	Influenza & Pneumonia	56,326	2.3
9.	Nephritis*	45,344	1.9
10.	Septicemia	34,234	1.4

*Includes nephrotic syndrome and nephrosis.

Sources: U.S. Mortality Data 2006, National Health and Statistics, Centers for Disease Control and Prevention, 2009

Table 1

Critical Terms Defined in the Text

1. Cancer—three kinds: local, regional, distant (metastatic)
2. Carcinoma (cancer) in situ—e.g., ductal carcinoma of the breast (DCIS)
3. Slow cancers—e.g., prostate, breast
4. Cancer treatments: surgery, chemotherapy, radiation therapy
5. Partial response
6. Complete response
7. Cure
8. Median survival, one/five-year survival

Figure 2

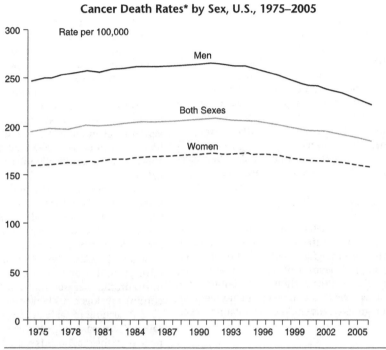

Cancer Death Rates* by Sex, U.S., 1975–2005

*Age-adjusted to the U.S. 2000 standard population.

Sources: U.S. Mortality Data 2006, National Health and Statistics, Centers for Disease Control and Prevention, 2008

therapy. Another type is publication bias, whereby positive studies (especially those funded by the pharmaceutical industry) tend to be published while negative studies do not.

What is cancer? Cancer is a large group of diseases characterized by the uncontrolled growth and spread of abnormal cells locally, regionally, and/or distantly (metastatically). A carcinoma (cancer) in situ is a small cancer that has not invaded the local tissue. Some cancers grow very slowly, and the patient may survive for ten years or more with minimal treatment. Other cancers (e.g., lung and pancreas) grow quickly and, even today, kill more than half of the patients in less than one year (see table 2). The therapy for cancer is generally surgery, if possible, and/or chemotherapy and/or radiation therapy. Chemotherapy aims to kill the cancer cells, but most chemotherapeutic drugs are nonspecific and also kill sensitive normal cells, especially in the intestine and bone marrow. Radiation therapy is also nonspecific. In chemotherapy and radiation therapy, a partial response is defined as shrinkage of the tumor in each dimension by 50 percent; a complete response means no detectable tumor, but this does not necessarily mean a "cure." Many complete responses are only transitory. Median survival is the length of time in which one-half of the patients in a cohort die.

Table 2

Common Cancers Current Death and Survival Statistics (American Cancer Society 2009)

Cancer Origin	Percent of Cancer Deaths	One-Year Survival (%)	Five-Year Survival (%)
Lung	28	41	15
Colon/Rectum	9	83	64
Breast	8	>95	89
Pancreas	6	24	5
Prostate	5	*	*
Leukemia	4	**	51
Lymphoma	4	82	68
Liver	3	†	<10
Other	33	‡	‡

*Survival statistics for prostate cancer are very misleading since they include many treated cancers that would not have harmed (or killed) the patient (see test).

**Leukemia is a heterogenous group of diseases. The five-year survival figure is an average of all types.

†Liver cancer is a rapidly fatal disease in which treatment is ineffective.

‡Other cancers are so heterogenous that the reader should consult the American Cancer Society (2009) for specific data.

What Do We Know About Cancer?

The "causes" of cancer are shown in table 3, though there is still much we don't know. For example, we do not know exactly how smoking causes cancer; in most cases, we do not know how "acquired" mutations cause cancer. In some cancers, there are more than five hundred identifiable genetic abnormalities—no one knows which one(s), if any, is "causative." The importance of epigenetic changes is currently speculative. It is quite possible that there is a completely unknown causal mechanism in many cancers.

The diagnosis of cancer today is relatively straightforward with imaging techniques (x-ray, CAT, MRI, PET) and biopsies that are subjected to routine histology, electron microscopy, and immunological techniques.

Cancer Therapy

To have a reasonable discussion of cancer therapy, we need to agree on the objectives of therapy, as shown in table 4. Everyone agrees that meaningful prolongation of life, preferably complete surgical removal of the tumor and cure, is a high priority. The treatment should also improve the quality of life. But, as is well known, many chemotherapeutic and radiation regimens cause mild to devastating—even

Table 3

Examples of Probable or Definite Causes of Cancer (American Cancer Society 2009)

---

1. External Factors
   a. Tobacco
   b. Chemicals (e.g., asbestos, benzene, alcohol)
   c. Radiation
   d. Infections, organisms (e.g., hepatitis B, papilloma virus, *Helicobacter*)
   e. Hormone replacement therapy with estrogen
2. Inernal Factors
   a. Genetic mutations
      1) inherited
      2) acquired
   b. Hormones (e.g., estrogen)
   c. Immune disorders (e.g., AIDS)
   d. Epigenetic changes
   e. Obesity

Table 4

Criteria for Utility of Cancer Therapy (Fojo and Grady 2009)

---

1. Meaningful prolongation of life or cure (mortality)
2. Improvement of quality of life (symptoms)
3. Value of treatment (compared to cost)

---

fatal—side effects. Nathan (2007) compares conventional chemotherapy to "carpet-bombing," an extreme but realistic metaphor. Finally, the results of a cost-benefit analysis must be reasonable. (In some cases, justifiably and importantly, chemotherapy and/or radiation and/or other drugs are used as palliative measures exclusively to counter symptoms from the disease [e.g., pleural effusions in the chest cavity or bone pain] or from the treatments [e.g., vomiting, mucositis, low white blood counts, heart failure, nerve damage, diarrhea, and/or inflammation of the bladder]). In the final analysis, what counts are the criteria in table 4. Partial or even complete remissions, unless they prolong life and/or improve the overall quality of life at a reasonable cost, are scientifically interesting but of little use to the patient.

Currently there are a few metastatic cancers that can sometimes be cured with chemotherapy and/or radiation therapy, but unfortunately these cures make up a very small percentage of the whole cancer problem. These cancers include testicular cancer, choriocarcinoma, Hodgkin's and non-Hodgkin's lymphoma, leukemia, and rare cases of breast and ovarian cancer. A few cancers can be made into chronic diseases that require daily treatment, e.g., chronic myelogenous leukemia.

Returning to table 2, lung cancer, the most common cancer, is a devastating disease; if the surgeon cannot totally remove it, the diagnosis is grim. In fact, about 60 percent of lung cancer patients are dead within one year of diagnosis with the best available therapy, and only 15 percent survive five years.

There has been some progress in the death rate from colorectal cancer, especially in women. This is mainly due to earlier diagnosis and surgical therapy.

Cancer of the breast is often a slow cancer and has a five- to ten-year median survival rate with just surgical therapy. There has been a modest decline in death rates from breast cancer since 1975. It is worth noting that currently, if the breast cancer is metastatic, five-year survival is only 27 percent. However, breast cancer presents a serious dilemma. Early detection of invasive breast cancer by screening is good; however, about 62,000 cases of ductal carcinoma in situ (DCIS) are also discovered every year. In greater than 50 percent of these women, especially older women, these lesions will not progress and do not need treatment. However, it is difficult to predict who will not need therapy, so the American Cancer Society (2009) recommends all patients with DCIS undergo therapy—generally breast surgery. Thus, more than thirty thousand patents annually are unnecessarily treated. We need to figure out which DCIS are harmless in order to avoid unnecessary treatment. On balance, I feel that breast cancer screening has a small but positive net benefit.

Pancreatic cancer is devastating (see table 2), and little progress has been made against it since 1975. Pancreatic cancer is very challenging because the tumors are surrounded by dense fibrous connective tissue with few blood vessels. Because of this, it is difficult to deliver drugs to pancreatic tumors. Moreover, this explains in part why chemotherapy is so ineffective for pancreatic cancer (see table 2). Better animal models are needed.

Prostate cancer mortality has declined slightly since 1975 with an unexplained increase in the mid-1990s. But prostate cancer therapy also presents a serious quandary. At autopsy, approximately 30 percent (or more) of men have cancer foci in their prostate glands, yet only 1 to 2 percent of men die of prostate cancer. Thus less than 10 percent of prostate cancer patients require treatment. This presents a serious dilemma: whom should the physician treat? Moreover, recently, two large studies of prostate cancer screening with prostate specific antigen (PSA) have seriously questioned the utility of screening. In one study, the investigators had to screen over a thousand men before they saved one life. This led to about fifty "false positive" patients who often underwent surgery and/or radiation therapy unnecessarily. The second study, conducted in the United States, was negative, i.e., no lives were saved due to the screening, but many of the screening-positive patients with prostate cancer were treated. Welch and Albertson (2009) and Brawley (2009) estimate that more than a million men in the U.S. have been unnecessarily treated for prostate cancer between 1986 and 2005, due to over-diagnostic PSA screening tests. In the end, screening for prostate cancer will not be useful until methods are developed to determine which prostate cancers detected by screening will harm the patient. Many men—especially elderly ones—with a histological diagnosis of prostate cancer elect "watchful waiting" with no therapy, a rational strategy.

There are many other things we do not understand about cancer—even on a phenomenological level. For example, in the United States, the incidence and death rates from cancer of the stomach have fallen dramatically since 1930. The reason for this is unknown but may be due to changes in food preservation; it is not due to treatment.

Smart Drugs

David Nathan (2007) extols the virtues and potential of the new "smart drugs." Smart drugs are defined as drugs that focus on a particular vulnerability of the cancer; they are not generalized but rather specific toxins. But the *Journal of the American Medical Association* reports that 90 percent of the drugs or biologics approved by the FDA in the past four years for cancer (many of them smart drugs) cost more than $20,000 for twelve weeks of therapy, and many offer a survival benefit of only two months or less. Let us take bevacizumab (Avastin), the ninth largest selling drug in America ($4.8 billion in 2008), costing about $8,000 per month per patient. Bevacizumab, a putative smart drug, is an intravenous man-made antibody that blocks the action of vascular endothelial growth factor (VEFG). It sometimes works because tumors (and normal tissues) release VEFG to facilitate small blood vessel ingrowth into the tumor. These small blood vessels "nourish" the tumor (or normal tissue). The idea is to "starve" the growing tumor with once or twice monthly intravenous injections of bevacizumab.

The FDA has approved bevacizumab for the cancers listed in table 5. Since the median survival of colorectal cancer is eighteen months, bevacizumab therapy would cost about $144,000 (in such a patient) for four months prolongation of survival. In the other cancers in table 4, there is no prolongation of survival. Moreover, bevacizumab can have terrible side effects, including gastrointestinal perforations, serious bleeding, severe hypertension, clot formation, and delayed wound healing. By the criteria in table 4, bevacizumab is at best a marginal drug. It only slightly prolongs life, demonstrable only in colorectal cancer, has serious side effects, and is very expensive.

Bevacizumab is frequently cited as an example of the so-called newer smart drugs. But by interfering with small blood vessel growth throughout the body, it is a nonspecific toxin—and hence has serious side effects. It is not so different from the older non-specific chemotherapy.

The use of bevacizumab and similar drugs raises another issue. According to Gina Kolata, 60 to 80 percent of oncologists' revenue comes from infusion of anti-cancer drugs in their offices. Many believe that such economic incentives are the reason for the substantial overuse of expensive chemotherapeutic drugs. However, it is very difficult to document the extent of the overuse of cancer chemotherapy. Does it make sense to employ such expensive drugs that do not prolong life (see table 5) and have such serious side effects? Moreover, although VEGF and bevacizumab are interesting science, there has been gross exaggeration of bevacizumab's clinical utility in the press (see tables 4 and 5).

So why does the U.S. Food and Drug Administration (FDA) approve bevacizumab (and other drugs) that do not improve longevity and/or the quality of life (see table 5)? The answer is that bevacizumab coupled with other drugs can cause partial remissions, "stabilization" of the cancer, or "lack of progression" for several months. However, this often does not lead to prolongation of life in most of the cancers in table 5. Moreover, many patients pay a heavy price in terms of side effects and cost. It is also worth noting

Table 5

Bevacizumab (Avastin)—Utility

Cancer	Evidence for Prolongation of Life; time*
Bowel/Rectum	Yes, four months (median survival) with other drugs
Lung	No +
Breast	No
Kidney	No
Glioblastoma (Brain)	No

*Compared to randomized control (if available).

+"No" means a lack of a statistically significant prolongation.

that several European national regulatory authorities do not accept the utility of some of these smart drugs and do not license them for sale in their countries. In agreement with the Europeans, scientists at the U.S. National Cancer Institute are urging the oncology community, regulators, and the public to set limits on the use and pricing of such marginal drugs. They view the current situation as unsustainable.

Why Has the War on Cancer Failed?

As documented above, unlike the successes against heart disease and stroke, the war on cancer, after almost forty years, must be deemed a failure with a few notable exceptions. Why? Is it because cancer is an incredibly tough problem, or are there other explanations? In table 6, I have listed six reasons for the failure, although there is little doubt that effective, safe therapy of the various cancers is a difficult problem.

Where Should We Go from Here?

In my view the principal problem is that we just do not understand the causes of most cancers. We don't even know if the problem is genetic or epigenetic or something totally unknown. In theory, problems 2 through 6 in table 6 are all correctable with political and scientific will and more knowledge. Even though we know cancer of the lung is caused by cigarette smoking, we do not know the mechanism, and (except for surgery) we do not know how to meaningfully intervene (see table 2). The pharmaceutical industry cannot make real progress until we understand the mechanisms and molecular causes of cancer so that industrial, academic, and governmental scientists have rational targets for intervention. We will make no progress if there are five hundred or more genetic abnormalities in a single cancer cell. Where would one begin?

What Should We Do Now?

We can still do a lot even today (see table 7). Smoking and hormone replacement therapy are a cause of lung and breast cancer, respectively, and should be stopped or minimized. For hepatitis B (which causes over 50 percent of liver

Table 6

Why Has the War on Cancer Failed?

1. We don't understand the cause/pathogenesis in most case of cancer—smoking is an obvious phenomenological exception.
2. Most treatments (except surgery) are nonspecific cell killers and not "smart."
3. Clinical trials and the grant system don't foster innovation—need reform.
4. Screening for useful drugs against cancer cells has not worked.
5. Animal models of cancer are often inadequate—e.g., pancreatic cancer as described in this article.
6. Unproductive "facts" in research come and go.

Table 7

The Way Forward

1. Prevention (cancer prevented)
   a. Stop smoking (lung; others)
   b. Minimize hormone replacement therapy (breast)
   c. Vaccines
      1) Hepatitis B (liver)
      2) Papilloma virus (cervical, anal, penis)
   d. Eliminate *Helicobacter* with antibiotics (stomach)
   e. Prevent contracting AIDS (sarcoma)
   f. Chemoprophylaxis
      3) finasteride (prostate)
      4) tamoxifen (high risk breast)
   g. Decrease alcohol (liver, esophagus)
   h. Decrease obesity (many types)
2. Screening for
   a. Cervical cancer
   b. Colorectal cancer
   c. Breast cancer
3. More knowledge of cancers' causes and better animal models
4. Better drugs—once appropriate targets identified

cancer) and papilloma virus (which causes almost all cervical cancer and some anal and mouth cancers), we can vaccinate with vaccines that are essentially 100 percent effective. *Helicobacter* (the probable cause of some stomach cancer) can be easily eliminated with antibiotics. Prophylactic finasteride and tamoxifen (both generic) can decrease prostate and breast cancer, respectively (in high risk patients). We must also decrease alcohol intake (liver and esophageal cancer) and obesity. Obesity is associated with increased cancer risk but the mechanism, if causal, is obscure.

We can screen for cervical, colorectal, and breast cancer, although the value of breast cancer screening is not clear (due to overdiagnosis), as I discussed above. However, in my view, the benefit of breast cancer screening slightly outweighs the harm. For example, if DCIS treatment could be rationalized and provided only to those who need it, breast cancer screening would then be unarguably useful. All attempts to screen for lung cancer, even in smokers, have so far been futile.

If all these recommendations were followed, we could cut cancer deaths in half. Moreover, with better mechanistic understanding of cancer, we could make truly "smart" drugs, as has been done in recent years for atherosclerosis (heart attacks), hypertension (strokes), gastrointestinal diseases (ulcers), and AIDS—with truly remarkable results. Let us hope cancer is next.

Reynold Spector is a physician and clinical professor of medicine at the Robert Wood Johnson Medical School in New Jersey.

EXPLORING THE ISSUE

Are We Winning the War on Cancer?

Critical Thinking and Reflection

1. Why are some cancers so difficult to successfully treat?
2. What are effective ways to reduce the risk of developing cancer?
3. Describe what factors are involved in predicting short- and long-term cancer survival rates.

Is There Common Ground?

While many diseases have similar or worse outcomes, cancer is generally more feared than heart disease or diabetes. Cancer is regarded as a disease that must be "battled" and a "war" on cancer has been declared. Fighting or military-like descriptions are often used to address cancer's human effects, and they emphasize the need for the patient to take immediate, decisive actions him or herself, rather than to delay, to ignore, or to rely on others caring for him or her.

Forty years ago, talk therapy to change a patient's outlook on life was a relatively popular alternative cancer treatment. It was based on the idea that cancer was caused by a negative personality or attitude. People with a "cancer personality"—depressed, repressed, self-hating, and unable to express their emotions—were believed to have developed cancer through their personality and/or their attitudes. This theory allowed society to blame the victim for having developed cancer or having prevented its cure by their negative attitude and personality. It also increased patients' anxieties as they incorrectly believed that natural emotions of sadness, anger, or fear either gave them the disease or prevented them from being cured. The author Susan Sontag helped promote this idea in her book *Illness as a Metaphor* written in 1978 while recovering from treatment for breast cancer. While the idea of personality causing cancer has not been supported by research, the belief that thinking positively will increase survival especially among breast cancer patients is common. An article titled "Invited Commentary: Personality as a Causal Factor in Cancer Risk and Mortality—Time to Retire a Hypothesis?" *American Journal of Epidemiology* (2010) reports findings from a large-scale study of the value of two *personality* dimensions: neuroticism and extraversion, for *cancer* risk and life expectancy. Overall, no relationship was found between personality and cancer onset or survival. The authors question whether it is time for the field to move on from considering a role for *personality* in *cancer* to more promising and modifiable factors.

For further information on the progress of the war on cancer see "Declining Death Rates Reflect Progress against Cancer," *PLoS ONE* (2010). The article discusses the success of the "war on cancer" initiated in 1971. The authors found that death rate for all cancers combined in men showed a net decline of 21 percent and 11 percent from the 1990 and 1970 rates, respectively. Similarly, the all-cancer death rate in women showed a net decline of 12 percent and 6 percent from the 1991 and 1970 rates, respectively. These decreases since 1990/1991 translate to prevention of 561,400 cancer deaths in men and 205,700 deaths in women. The decrease in death rates from all-cancers involved all ages and racial/ethnic groups. The positive change in cancer death rates since 1990 resulted mostly from reductions in smoking, increased screening allowing early detection of several cancers, and improvements in treatment for specific cancers. While much overall progress has been made in cancer treatment and prevention, lung cancer remains a difficult disease to treat, with generally poor prognoses. In "Lung Cancer: Progress in Diagnosis, Staging and Therapy," *Respirology* (January 2010), the authors indicate that lung cancer remains one of the greatest medical challenges with nearly 1.5 million new cases worldwide each year and a growing tobacco epidemic in the developing world. The value of screening for early disease is not yet established and trials to see if mortality can be improved as a result are in progress. For further reading see "Two Decades of Declining Cancer Mortality: Progress with Disparity," *Annual Review of Public Health* (2010). In this article, the authors claim that despite considerable progress in preventing and treating cancer, disparities in cancer mortality persist across different races and social classes. Because all the factors that account for declining cancer trends are related to social class, and because of large social class disparities in cancer risk factors, there will likely be a widening gap in cancer deaths among those in lower socioeconomic groups in the future.

Create Central

www.mhhe.com/createcentral

Additional Resources

Duncan, D. E. (2012). Your cancer, your cure. *Discover, 33*(9), 56–61.

Garnick, M. B. (2012). The great prostate cancer debate. *Scientific American, 306*(2), 38–46.

Sulik, G. A. (2011). *Pink ribbon blues: How breast cancer culture undermines women's health.* New York, NY: Oxford University Press.

Welch, H. G., Schwartz, L. M., & Woloshin, S. (2011). *Overdiagnosed: Making people sick in the pursuit of health.* Boston, MA: Beacon Press.

Internet References . . .

American Cancer Society

This site offers tips on staying healthy and preventing cancer, a resource for support and treatment, and research into cancer prevention and treatment.

www.cancer.org

American Medical Association (AMA)

The AMA offers this site to find up-to-date medical information, peer-review resources, discussions of such topics as HIV/AIDS and women's health, examination of issues related to managed care, and important publications.

www.ama-assn.org

Centers for Disease Control and Prevention

This CDC site provides updates, information, key facts, questions and answers, and ways to prevent and treat illnesses.

www.cdc.gov/

MedScape: The Online Resource for Better Patient Care

For health professionals and interested consumers, this site offers peer-reviewed articles, self-assessment features, medical news, and annotated links to Internet resources. It also contains the *Morbidity & Mortality Weekly Report*, which is a publication of Centers for Disease Control and Prevention.

www.medscape.com

U.S. National Institutes of Health (NIH)

Consult this site for links to extensive health information and scientific resources. Comprising 24 separate institutes, centers, and divisions, the NIH is one of eight health agencies of the Public Health Service, which, in turn, is part of the U.S. Department of Health and Human Services.

www.nih.gov

Selected, Edited, and with Issue Framing Material by:
Eileen Daniel, *SUNY College at Brockport*

ISSUE

Should Marijuana Be Legalized for Medicinal Purposes?

YES: Kevin Drum, from "The Patriot's Guide to Legalization," *Mother Jones* (July/August 2009)

NO: Christian Science Monitor Editorial Board, from "Legalize Marijuana? Not So Fast," *The Christian Science Monitor* (May 22, 2009)

Learning Outcomes
After reading this issue, you should be able to: • Discuss the physical risks associated with marijuana use. • Assess the cognitive, social, behavioral, and legal issues associated with the use of marijuana. • Assess the viability of legalization of marijuana. • Discuss marijuana's medicinal purposes.

ISSUE SUMMARY

YES: Political columnist and blogger Kevin Drum contends that medical marijuana is now legal in more than a dozen states without any serious problems or increased usage.

NO: The editorial board of *The Christian Science Monitor* maintains that the drug can lead to dependence and can cause lung damage and other health concerns.

At one time, there were no laws in the United States regulating the use or sale of drugs, including marijuana. Rather than by legislation, their use was regulated by religious teaching and social custom. As society grew more complex and more heterogeneous, the need for more formal regulation of drug sales, production, and use developed.

Attempts at regulating patent medications through legislation began in the early 1900s. In 1920, Congress, under pressure from temperance organizations, passed an amendment prohibiting the manufacture and sale of all alcoholic beverages. From 1920 until 1933, the demand for alcohol was met by organized crime, who either manufactured it illicitly or smuggled it into the United States. The government's inability to enforce the law, as well as increasing violence, finally led to the repeal of prohibition in 1933.

Many years later, in the 1960s, drug usage again began to worry many Americans. Heroin abuse had become epidemic in urban areas, and many middle-class young adults had begun to experiment with marijuana and LSD by the end of the decade. Cocaine also became popular first among the middle class and later among inner-city residents. More recently, crack houses, babies born with drug addictions, and drug-related crimes and shootings are the images of a new epidemic of drug abuse.

Many of those who believe illicit drugs are a major problem in America, however, are usually referring to hard drugs, such as cocaine and heroin. Soft drugs like marijuana, though not legal, are not often perceived as a major threat to the safety and well-being of citizens. Millions of Americans have tried marijuana and did not become addicted. The drug has also been used illegally by those suffering from AIDS, glaucoma, and cancer to alleviate their symptoms and to stimulate their appetites. Should marijuana be legalized as a medicine, or is it too addictive and dangerous? In California, Proposition 215 was passed in the November 1996 ballot. A similar measure was passed in Arizona. These initiatives convinced voters to relax current laws against marijuana use for medical and humane reasons. Several other states followed and legalized marijuana for medicinal purposes.

Opponents of these recent measures argue that marijuana use has been steadily rising among teenagers and that this may lead to experimentation with hard drugs. There is concern that if marijuana is legal via a doctor's prescription, the drug will be more readily available. There is also concern that the health benefits of smoking marijuana are overrated. For instance, among glaucoma sufferers, in order to achieve benefits from the drug, patients would literally have to be stoned all the time. Unfortunately, the efficacy of marijuana is unclear because, as an illicit drug, studies to adequately test it have been thwarted by drug control agencies.

Although marijuana's effectiveness in treating the symptoms of disease is unclear, is it actually dangerous and addictive? Scientists contend that the drug can negatively affect cognition and motor function. It can also have an impact on short-term memory and can interfere with perception and learning. Physical health effects include lung damage. Until recently, scientists had little evidence that marijuana was actually addictive. Although heavy users did not seem to experience actual withdrawal symptoms, studies with laboratory animals given large doses of THC, the active ingredient in marijuana, suffered withdrawal symptoms similar to those of rodents withdrawing from opiates.

Not all researchers agree, however, that marijuana is dangerous and addictive. The absence of well-designed, long-term studies on the effects of marijuana use further complicates the issue, as does the current potency of the drug. Growers have become more skilled about developing strains of marijuana with high concentrations of THC. Today's varieties may be three to five times more potent than the pot used in the 1960s. Much of the data are unclear, but what is known is that young users of the drug are likely to have problems learning. In addition, some users are at risk for developing dependence.

In the YES and NO selections, Kevin Drum states that there are no proven studies to support the view that marijuana prohibition is justified. The editors of *The Christian Science Monitor* argue that marijuana causes many physical and psychological effects, particularly to adolescents.

YES ↵

Kevin Drum

The Patriot's Guide to Legalization

Have you ever looked at our marijuana policy? I mean really looked at it?

When we think of the drug war, it's the heavy-duty narcotics like heroin and cocaine that get most of the attention. And why not? That's where the action is. It's not marijuana that is sustaining the Taliban in Afghanistan, after all. When Crips and Bloods descend into gun battles in the streets of Los Angeles, they're not usually fighting over pot. The junkie who breaks into your house and steals your Blu-ray player isn't doing it so he can score a couple of spliffs.

No, the marijuana trade is more genteel than that. At least, I used to think it was. Then, like a lot of people, I started reading about the open warfare that has erupted among the narcotraffickers in Mexico and is now spilling across the American border. Stories of drugs coming north and arsenals of guns going south. Thousands of people brutally murdered. Entire towns terrorized. And this was a war not just over cocaine and meth, but marijuana as well.

And I began to wonder: Maybe the war against pot is about to get a lot uglier. After all, in the 1920s, Prohibition gave us Al Capone and the St. Valentine's Day Massacre, and that was over plain old whiskey and rum. Are we about to start paying the same price for marijuana?

If so, it might eventually start to affect me, too. Indirectly, sure, but that's more than it ever has before. I've never smoked a joint in my life. I've only seen one once, and that was 30 years ago. I barely drink, I don't smoke, and I don't like coffee. When it comes to mood altering substances, I live the life of a monk. I never really cared much if marijuana was legal or not.

But if a war is breaking out over the stuff, I figured maybe I should start looking at the evidence on whether marijuana prohibition is worth it. Not the spin from the drug czar at one end or the hemp hucksters at the other. Just the facts, as best as I could figure them out. So I did. Here's what I found.

In 1972, the report of the National Commission on Marihuana and Drug Abuse urged that possession of marijuana for personal use be decriminalized. A small wave of states followed this recommendation, but most refused; in Washington, President Carter called for eliminating penalties for small-time possession, but Congress stonewalled. And that's the way things have stayed since the late '70s. Some states have decriminalized, most haven't, and possession is still a criminal offense under federal law. So how has that worked out?

I won't give away the ending just yet, but one thing to know is this: On virtually every subject related to cannabis (an inclusive term that refers to both the sativa and indica varieties of the marijuana plant, as well as hashish, bhang, and other derivatives), the evidence is ambiguous. Sometimes even mysterious. So let's start with the obvious question.

Does decriminalizing cannabis have any effect at all? It's remarkably hard to tell—in part because drug use is faddish. Cannabis use among teens in the United States, for example, went down sharply in the '80s, bounced back in the early '90s, and has declined moderately since. Nobody really knows why.

We do, however, have studies that compare rates of cannabis use in states that have decriminalized vs. states that haven't. And the somewhat surprising conclusion, in the words of Robert MacCoun, a professor of law and public policy at the University of California-Berkeley, is simple: "Most of the evidence suggests that decriminalization has no effect."

But decriminalization is not legalization. In places that have decriminalized, simple possession is still illegal; it's just treated as an administrative offense, like a traffic ticket. And production and distribution remain felonies. What would happen if cannabis use were fully legalized?

No country has ever done this, so we don't know. The closest example is the Netherlands, where possession and sale of small amounts of marijuana is de facto legal in the famous coffeehouses. MacCoun and a colleague, Peter Reuter of the University of Maryland, have studied the Dutch experience and concluded that while legalization at first had little effect, once the coffeehouses began advertising and promoting themselves more aggressively in the 1980s, cannabis use more than doubled in a decade. Then again, cannabis use in Europe has gone up and down in waves, and some of the Dutch increase (as well as a later decrease, which followed a tightening of the coffeehouse laws in the mid-'90s) may have simply been part of those larger waves.

The most likely conclusion from the overall data is that if you fully legalized cannabis, use would almost certainly go up, but probably not enormously. MacCoun guesses that it might rise by half—say, from around 15 percent of the population to a little more than 20 percent. "It's not going to triple," he says. "Most people who want to use marijuana are already finding a way to use marijuana."

Still, there would be a cost. For one thing, a much higher increase isn't out of the question if companies like Philip Morris or R.J. Reynolds set their finest minds on the promotion of dope. And much of the increase would likely come among the heaviest users. "One person smoking eight joints a day is worth more to the industry than fifty people each smoking a joint a week," says Mark Kleiman, a drug policy expert at UCLA. "If the cannabis industry were to expand greatly, it couldn't do so by increasing the number of casual users. It would have to create and maintain more chronic zonkers." And that's a problem. Chronic use can lead to dependence and even long-term cognitive impairment. Heavy cannabis users are more likely to be in auto accidents. There have been scattered reports of respiratory and fetal development problems. Still, sensible regulation can limit the commercialization of pot, and compared to other illicit drugs (and alcohol), its health effects are fairly mild. Even a 50 percent increase in cannabis use might be a net benefit if it led to lower rates of use of other drugs.

So would people just smoke more and drink less? Maybe. The generic term for this effect in the economics literature is "substitute goods," and it simply means that some things replace other things. If the total demand for transportation is generally steady, an increase in sales of SUVs will lead to a decrease in the sales of sedans. Likewise, if the total demand for intoxicants is steady, an increase in the use of one drug should lead to a decrease in others.

Several years ago, John DiNardo, an economist now at the University of Michigan, found a clever way to test this via a natural experiment. Back in the 1980s, the Reagan administration pushed states to raise the drinking age to 21. Some states did this early in the decade, some later, and this gave DiNardo the idea of comparing data from the various states to see if the Reagan policy worked.

He found that raising the drinking age did lead to lower alcohol consumption; the effect was modest but real. But then DiNardo hit on another analysis—comparing cannabis use in states that raised the drinking age early with those that did it later. And he found that indeed, there seemed to be a substitution effect. On average, among high school seniors, a 4.5 percent decrease in drinking produced a 2.4 percent increase in getting high.

But what we really want to know is whether the effect works in the other direction: Would increased marijuana use lead to less drinking? "What goes up should go down," DiNardo told me cheerfully, but he admits that in the absence of empirical evidence this hypothesis depends on your faith in basic economic models.

Some other studies are less encouraging than DiNardo's, but even if the substitute goods effect is smaller than his research suggests—if, say, a 30 percent increase in cannabis use led to a 5 or 10 percent drop in drinking—it would still be a strong argument in favor of legalization. After all, excessive drinking causes nearly 80,000 deaths per year in the United States, compared to virtually none for pot. Trading alcohol consumption for cannabis rise might be a pretty attractive deal.

But what about the gateway effect? This has been a perennial bogeyman of the drug warriors. Kids who use pot, the TV ads tell us, will graduate to ecstasy, then coke, then meth, and then—who knows? Maybe even talk radio.

Is there anything to this? There are two plausible pathways for the gateway theory. The first is that drug use of any kind creates an affinity for increasingly intense narcotic experiences. The second is that when cannabis is illegal, the only place to get it is from dealers who also sell other stuff.

The evidence for the first pathway is mixed. Research in New Zealand, for example, suggests that regular cannabis use is correlated with higher rates of other illicit drug use, especially in teenagers. A Norwegian study comes to similar conclusions, but only for a small segment of "troubled" teenagers. Other research, however, suggests that these correlations aren't caused by gateway effects at all, but by the simple fact that kids who like drugs do drugs. All kinds of drugs.

The second pathway was deliberately targeted by the Dutch when they began their coffeehouse experiment in the '70s in part to sever the connection of cannabis with the illicit drug market. The evidence suggests that it worked: Even with cannabis freely available, Dutch cannabis use is currently about average among developed countries and use of other illicit drugs is about average, too. Easy access to marijuana, outside the dealer network for harder drugs, doesn't seem to have led to greater use of cocaine or heroin.

So, to recap: Decriminalization of simple possession appears to have little effect on cannabis consumption. Full legalization would likely increase use only moderately as long as heavy commercialization is prohibited, although the effect on chronic users might be more substantial. It would increase heroin and cocaine use only slightly if at all, and it might decrease alcohol consumption by a small amount. Which leads to the question:

Can we still afford prohibition? The consequences of legalization, after all, must be compared to the cost of the status quo. Unsurprisingly, this too is hard to quantify. The worst effects of the drug war, including property crime and gang warfare, are mostly associated with cocaine, heroin, and meth. Likewise, most drug-law enforcement is aimed at harder drugs, not cannabis; contrary to conventional wisdom, only about 44,000 people are currently serving prison time on cannabis charges—and most of those are there for dealing and distribution, not possession.

Still, the University of Maryland's Reuter points out that about 800,000 people are arrested for cannabis possession every year in the United States. And even though very few end up being sentenced to prison, a study of three counties in Maryland following a recent marijuana crackdown suggests that a third spend at least one pretrial night in jail and a sixth spend more than ten days. That takes a substantial human toll. Overall, Harvard economist Jeffrey

Miron estimates the cost of cannabis prohibition in the United States at $13 billion annually and the lost tax revenue at nearly $7 billion.

So what are the odds of legalization? Slim. For starters, the United States, along with virtually every other country in the world, is a signatory to the 1961 Single Convention on Narcotic Drugs (and its 1988 successor), which flatly prohibits legalization of cannabis. The only way around this is to unilaterally withdraw from the treaties or to withdraw and then reenter with reservations. That's not going to happen.

At the federal level, there's virtually no appetite for legalizing cannabis either. Though public opinion has made steady strides, increasing from around 20 percent favoring marijuana legalization in the Reagan era to nearly 40 percent favoring it today, the only policy change in Washington has been Attorney General Eric Holder's announcement in March that the Obama administration planned to end raids on distributors of medical marijuana. (Applications for pot dispensaries promptly surged in Los Angeles County.)

The real action in cannabis legalization is at the state level. More than a dozen states now have effective medical marijuana laws, most notably California. Medical marijuana dispensaries are dotted all over the state, and it's common knowledge that the "medical" part is in many cases a thin fiction. Like the Dutch coffeehouses, California's dispensaries are now a de facto legal distribution network that severs the link between cannabis and other illicit drugs for a significant number of adults (albeit still only a fraction of total users). And the result? Nothing. "We've had this experiment for a decade and the sky hasn't fallen," says Paul Armentano, deputy director of the National Organization for the Reform of Marijuana Laws. California Assemblyman Tom Ammiano has even introduced a bill that would legalize, tax, and regulate marijuana; it has gained the endorsement of the head of the state's tax collection agency, which informally estimates it could collect $1.3 billion a year from cannabis sales. Still, the legislation hasn't found a single cosponsor, and isn't scheduled for so much as a hearing.

Which is too bad. Going into this assignment, I didn't care much personally about cannabis legalization. I just had a vague sense that if other people wanted to do it, why not let them? But the evidence suggests pretty clearly that we ought to significantly soften our laws on marijuana. Too many lives have been mined and too much money spent for a social benefit that, if not zero, certainly isn't very high.

And it may actually happen. If attitudes continue to soften; if the Obama administration turns down the volume on anti-pot propaganda; if medical dispensaries avoid heavy commercialization; if drug use remains stable; and if emergency rooms don't start filling up with drug-related traumas while all this is happening, California's experience could go a long way toward destigmatizing cannabis use. That's a lot of ifs.

Still, things are changing. Even GOV icon Arnold Schwarzenegger now says, "I think it's time for a debate." That doesn't mean he's in favor of legalizing pot fight this minute, but it might mean we're getting close to a tipping point. Ten years from now, as the flower power generation enters its 70s, you might finally be able to smoke a fully legal, taxed, and regulated joint.

Kevin Drum is a political columnist and blogger.

**Christian Science Monitor
Editorial Board**

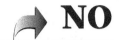 **NO**

Legalize Marijuana? Not So Fast

Backers serve up a timely batch of arguments, but their latest reasons are half-baked.

The American movement to legalize marijuana for regular use is on a roll. Or at least its backers say it is.

They point to California Gov. Arnold Schwarzenegger, who said in early May that it's now time to debate legalizing marijuana—though he's personally against it. Indeed, a legislative push is on in his state (and several others, such as Massachusetts and Nevada) to treat this "soft" drug like alcohol—to tax and regulate its sale, and set an age restriction on buyers.

Several recent polls show stepped-up public support for legalization. This means not only lifting restrictions on use ("decriminalization"), but also on supply—production and sales. The Obama administration, meanwhile, says the US Drug Enforcement Agency will no longer raid dispensaries of medical marijuana—which is illegal under federal law—in states where it is legal.

The push toward full legalization is a well-organized, Internet-savvy campaign, generously funded by a few billionaires, including George Soros. It's built on a decades-long, step-by-step effort in the states. Thirteen states have so far decriminalized marijuana use (generally, the punishment covers small amounts and involves a fine). And 13 states now allow for medical marijuana.

Paul Armentano, deputy director of the National Organization for the Reform of Marijuana Laws (NORML), recently told a Monitor reporter that three reasons account for the fresh momentum toward legalization: 1) the weak economy, which is forcing states to look for new revenue; 2) public concern over the violent drug war in Mexico; and 3) more experience with marijuana itself.

If there is to be a debate, let's look at these reasons, starting with experience with marijuana.

A Harmless Drug?

Supporters of legalization often claim that no one has died of a pot overdose, and that it has beneficial effects in alleviating suffering from certain diseases.

True, marijuana cannot directly kill its user in the way that alcohol or a drug like heroin can. And activists claim that it may ease symptoms for certain patients—though it has not been endorsed by the major medical associations representing those patients, and the Food and Drug Administration disputes its value.

Rosalie Pacula, codirector of the Rand Drug Policy Research Center, poses this question: "If pot is relatively harmless, why are we seeing more than 100,000 hospitalizations a year" for marijuana use?

Emergency-room admissions where marijuana is the primary substance involved increased by 164 percent from 1995 to 2002—faster than for other drugs, according to the Drug Abuse Warning Network.

Research results over the past decade link frequent marijuana use to several serious mental health problems, with youth particularly at risk. And the British Lung Foundation finds that smoking three to four joints is the equivalent of 20 tobacco cigarettes.

While marijuana is not addictive in the way that a drug like crack-cocaine is, heavy use can lead to dependence—defined by the same criteria as for other drugs. About half of those who use pot daily become dependent for some period of time, writes Kevin Sabet, in the 2006 book, "Pot Politics"—and 1 in 10 people in the US who have ever used marijuana become dependent at some time (about the same rate as alcohol). Dr. Sabet was a drug policy adviser in the past two presidential administrations.

He adds that physicians in Britain and the Netherlands—both countries that have experience with relaxed marijuana laws—are seeing withdrawal symptoms among heavy marijuana users that are similar to those of cocaine and heroin addicts. This has been confirmed in the lab with monkeys.

Today's marijuana is also much more potent than in the hippie days of yesteryear. But that doesn't change what's always been known about even casual use of this drug: It distorts perception, reduces motor skills, and affects alertness. When combined with alcohol (not unusual), or even alone, it worsens the risk of traffic accidents.

Would Legalization Take the Violence Out of the Mexican Drug War?

NORML likes to point out that marijuana accounts for the majority of illicit drug traffic from Mexico. End the illicit trafficking, and you end the violence. But that volume gives a false impression of marijuana's role in crime and violence, says Jonathan Caulkins, a professor at Carnegie Mellon and a drug-policy adviser in the US and Australia.

It's the dollars that count, and the big earners—cocaine, methamphetamine, heroin—play a much larger role in crime and violence. In recent years, Mexico has become a major cocaine route to the US. That's what's fanning the violence, according to Dr. Caulkins, so legalizing marijuana is unlikely to quiet Mexico's drug war.

Neither are America's prisons stuffed with users who happened to get caught with a few joints (if that were the case, a huge percentage of America's college students—an easy target—would be behind bars). Yes, there are upward of 700,000 arrests on marijuana charges each year, but that includes repeat arrests, and most of those apprehended don't go to jail. Those who do are usually large-scale offenders.

Only 0.7 percent of inmates in state and federal prisons are in for marijuana possession (0.3 percent counting first-time offenders only, according to a 2002 US Justice Department survey). In federal prisons, the median amount of marijuana for those convicted of possession is 115 pounds—156,000 marijuana cigarettes.

Can Marijuana Rescue State Coffers?

The California legalization bill proposes a $50/ounce tax on marijuana. The aim is to keep pot as close to the black-market price as possible while still generating an estimated $1.3 billion in income for this deficit-challenged state.

But the black market can easily undercut a $50 tax and shrink that expected revenue stream. Just look at the huge trade in illegal cigarettes in Canada to see how taxing can spur a black market (about 30 percent of tobacco bought in Canada is illegal).

A government could attempt to eliminate the black market altogether by making marijuana incredibly cheap (Dr. Pacula at the RAND Organization says today's black market price is about four times what it would be if pot were completely legalized). But then use would skyrocket and teens (though barred) could buy it with their lunch money.

Indeed, legalizing marijuana is bound to increase use simply because of availability. Legalization advocates say "not so" and point to the Netherlands and its legal marijuana "coffee shops." Indeed, after the Dutch de facto legalized the drug in 1976, use stayed about the same for adults and youth. But it took off after 1984, growing by 300 percent over the next decade or so. Experts attribute this to commercialization (sound like alcohol?), and also society's view of the drug as normal—which took a while to set in.

Now the Dutch are finding that normalization has its costs—increased dependence, more dealers of harder drugs, and a flood of rowdy "drug tourists" from other countries. The Dutch "example" should be renamed the Dutch "warning."

As America has learned with alcohol, taxes don't begin to cover the costs to society of destroyed families, lost productivity, and ruined lives—and regulators still have not succeeded in keeping alcohol from underage drinkers.

No one has figured out what the exact social costs of legalizing marijuana would be. But ephemeral taxes won't cover them—nor should society want to encourage easier access to a drug that can lead to dependency, has health risks, and reduces alertness, to name just a few of its negative outcomes.

Why legalize a third substance that produces ill effects, when the US has such a poor record in dealing with the two big "licits"—alcohol and tobacco?

Parents Need to Resist Peer Pressure Too

Legalization backers say the country is at a tipping point, ready to make the final big leap. They hope that a new generation of politicians that has had experience with marijuana will be friendly to their cause.

But this new generation is also made up of parents. Do parents really want marijuana to become a normal part of society—and an expectation for their children?

Maybe parents thought they left peer pressure behind when they graduated from high school. But the push to legalize marijuana is like the peer pressure of the schoolyard. The arguments are perhaps timely, but they don't stand up, and parents must now stand up to them.

They must let lawmakers know that legalization is not OK, and they must carry this message to their children, too. Disapproval, along with information on risk, are the most important factors in discouraging marijuana and cocaine use among high school seniors, according to the University of Michigan's "Monitoring the Future" project on substance abuse.

Parents must make clear that marijuana is not a harmless drug—even if they personally may have emerged unscathed.

And they need to teach the life lesson that marijuana does not really solve personal challenges, be they stress, relationships, or discouragement.

In the same way, a search for joy and satisfaction in a drug is misplaced.

The far greater and lasting attraction is in a life rooted in moral and spiritual values—not in a haze, a daze, or a munchie-craze.

Today's youth are tomorrow's world problem solvers—and the ones most likely to be affected if marijuana is legalized. Future generations need to be clear thinkers. For their sakes, those who oppose legalizing marijuana must become vocal, well-funded, and mainstream—before it's too late.

EXPLORING THE ISSUE

Should Marijuana Be Legalized for Medicinal Purposes?

Critical Thinking and Reflection

1. What are the pros and cons of legalization of marijuana for medicinal purposes?
2. Would legalization of marijuana offer a major benefit to individuals with cancer and other diseases?
3. Describe the impact legalization would have on marijuana usage.
4. Why is marijuana particularly harmful to adolescents?

Is There Common Ground?

Recent laws in several states legalizing marijuana for medicinal purposes make many people nervous. The majority of Americans are against making marijuana completely legal even if prescribed to individuals who have legitimate medicinal need for the drug. A compromise might be to decriminalize marijuana, making it neither strictly legal nor illegal. If decriminalized, there would be no penalty for personal or medical use or possession, although there would continue to be criminal penalties for sale and distribution to minors. Marijuana has been decriminalized in a few states, but it is illegal in most of the country.

While decriminalization appeals to many, in early 1992 the Drug Enforcement Administration published a document stating that the federal government was justified in its continued prohibition of marijuana for medicinal purposes. The report indicated that too many questions surrounded the effectiveness of medicinal marijuana. See "Medical Marijuana on Trial," *The New York Times* (March 29, 2005), and "The Right Not to Be in Pain: Using Marijuana for Pain Management," *The Nation* (February 3, 2003). The effectiveness of marijuana as therapy for cancer patients and AIDS patients continues to be debated, but the Center on Addiction and Substance Abuse of Columbia University maintains that recent research suggests that the drug is addictive and can wreck the lives of users, particularly teenagers.

They argue that legalizing marijuana would undermine the impact of drug education and increase usage.

Create Central

www.mhhe.com/createcentral

Additional Resources

Barbour, S. (2012). *Should marijuana be legalized?* San Diego, CA: ReferencePoint Press.

Borgelt, L. M., Franson, K. L., Nussbaum, A. M., & Wang, G. S (2013). The pharmacologic and clinical effects of medical cannabis. *Pharmacotherapy, 33,* 195–209.

Caulkins, J. P., Hawken, A., Kilmer, B., & Kleiman, M. A. (2012). *Marijuana legalization: What everyone needs to know.* New York, NY: Oxford University Press.

Cerdá, M., Wall, M., Keyes, K. M., Galea, S., & Hasin, D. (2012). Medical marijuana laws in 50 states: Investigating the relationship between state legalization of medical marijuana and marijuana use, abuse and dependence. *Drug & Alcohol Dependence, 120*(1/3), 22–27.

Friese, B. & Grube, J. W. (2013). Legalization of medical marijuana and marijuana use among youths. *Drugs: Education, Prevention & Policy, 20*(1), 33–39.

Internet References . . .

Food and Drug Administration (FDA)

www.fda.gov

National Organization for the Reform of Marijuana Laws (norml)

http://norml.org/

National Institutes on Health: National Institute on Drug Abuse

www.drugabuse.gov/nidahome.html

Web of Addictions

www.well.com/user/woa

National Institute on Drug Abuse (NIDA)

www.nida.nih.gov

Unit 2

UNIT

Health and Society

*H*uman health is complex, influenced not only by the biology and chemistry of the body but also by societal structures, culture, and politics and economics. Interestingly, public policy and medical ethics have not always kept pace with rapidly growing technology and scientific advances, especially if we consider the impact of recent biomedical research. Some developments, for example, those associated with reproductive technologies such as in vitro fertilization and cloning, seem to present us with ethical problems and the need for public policy that are unprecedented. More often, however, the advance of biomedical research has simply added complexity to old problems and created a sense of urgency with regard to their solution. Euthanasia and health care rationing are not new problems, but our ability to save the lives of individuals who would have died in the past has certainly added new dimensions.

Selected, Edited, and with Issue Framing Material by:
Eileen Daniel, *SUNY College at Brockport*

ISSUE

Is the Use of "Smart" Pills for Cognitive Enhancement Dangerous?

YES: **Alan Schwarz**, from "Drowned in a Stream of Prescriptions," *The New York Times* (February 2, 2013)

NO: **Joshua Gowin**, from "How 'Smart Drugs' Enhance Us," *Psychology Today* (September 29, 2009)

Learning Outcomes

After reading this issue, you should be able to:

- Discuss the legitimate uses for drugs such as Ritalin and Adderall.
- Understand the addictive qualities of these drugs.
- Understand how people without ADHD are able to acquire prescriptions for the drugs.
- Understand the consequences of abusing these drugs.
- Assess why illicit use of stimulant drugs has increased dramatically over the past 10 years.

ISSUE SUMMARY

YES: Pulitzer Prize-nominated reporter Alan Schwarz maintains that "smart pills" such as Adderall can significantly improve the lives of children and others with ADHD but that too many young adults who do not have the condition fake the symptoms and get prescriptions for the highly addictive and dangerous drugs.

NO: Psychologist Joshua Gowin argues that these drugs aren't much different from a cup of coffee and should be treated accordingly.

Medication therapy is a major part of treating attention deficit hyperactive disorder (ADHD), a common condition that affects children and adolescents and can continue into adulthood for some. Individuals with ADHD generally have difficulty paying attention, focusing, or concentrating. They seem to be unable to follow directions and are easily bored or frustrated with tasks. They also are likely to continuously move and tend to display impulsive behaviors. Overall, these behaviors are generally common in children without ADHD, but they occur more frequently than usual and are more severe in a child with ADHD.

For the past several decades, multiple types of stimulant drugs have been prescribed to treat the symptoms of ADHD. These medications enable individuals with ADHD to better focus their thoughts and overlook distractions and are effective for the majority of patients who take them.

Stimulant medications used to treat ADHD can have side effects, but these tend to happen early in treatment and are usually mild and short-lived, especially when monitored by a physician. The most common side effects include insomnia, weight loss and decreased appetite, and jitteriness. Occasionally, drugs to treat ADHD can cause more serious side effects such as an increased risk of cardiovascular problems. They may also exacerbate psychiatric conditions like depression, psychosis, or anxiety. ADHD medications are illegal to take without a prescription as they can produce serious side effects and are potentially addictive.

Despite the potential for addiction, prescription stimulant abuse has dramatically increased over the past decade. About 30 percent of stimulant drug use may be diverted to nonmedical usage. College students and young adults take them with the belief that these medications help with mental abilities including studying, memorizing, and test taking. Most people think of ADHD as a difficulty with controlling thought, hence the belief that ADHD medications help with thought control. Interestingly, evidence suggests that when people are given rote learning tasks such as memorizing items on a list, their performance *is* improved by ADHD stimulants. These effects are strongest when people learn the items on the list and have to remember them at least a day after learning. This effect does seem to come from the learning process, because the participants do not need to be on the medication during the test in order to see the effect.

Few research studies, however, have studied memory for complex kinds of information that demand genuine in-depth understanding of the material. So it is not possible to determine whether ADHD stimulants are simply assisting with learning the kinds of random items that typically appear on memory tests or whether they would also help with the types of complex knowledge important in high school and college classes.

Another area where ADHD stimulants seem to have impact is with *working memory*, the amount of information that people can hold in their mind at the same time. Many research investigations suggest that these medications have limited or no effect on working memory but a few studies show otherwise. Improvement is most likely to be seen in individuals whose normal working memory capacity is the smallest. While the research is inconclusive on the overall advantages of taking stimulant drugs on cognitive enhancement, the risks are clear. Over time, continued use of ADHD medications can make users less effec-tive intellectually due to poor mental functioning mostly caused by insomnia, addiction, or malnutrition. Other side effects that can impair performance include paranoia, aggression, and irritability that can accompany these drugs. Individuals taking the drugs prescribed by physicians are regularly monitored for these side effects as well as disturbances in heart rate, sleep, mood, and appetite.

In the YES and NO selections, Pulitzer Prize-nominated reporter Alan Schwarz maintains that "smart pills" such as Adderall can significantly improve the lives of children and others with ADHD but that too many young adults who do not have the condition fake the symptoms and get prescriptions for the highly addictive and dangerous drugs. They take the drugs with the belief that their ability to study, learn, and take tests will be enhanced, though the research is mostly not supportive. Psychologist Joshua Gowin argues that these drugs aren't much different from a cup of coffee and should be treated accordingly.

YES ↵

Alan Schwarz

Drowned in a Stream of Prescriptions

Before his addiction, Richard Fee was a popular college class president and aspiring medical student. "You keep giving Adderall to my son, you're going to kill him," said Rick Fee, Richard's father, to one of his son's doctors.

Virginia Beach—Every morning on her way to work, Kathy Fee holds her breath as she drives past the squat brick building that houses Dominion Psychiatric Associates.

It was there that her son, Richard, visited a doctor and received prescriptions for Adderall, an amphetamine-based medication for attention deficit hyperactivity disorder. It was in the parking lot that she insisted to Richard that he did not have A.D.H.D., not as a child and not now as a 24-year-old college graduate, and that he was getting dangerously addicted to the medication. It was inside the building that her husband, Rick, implored Richard's doctor to stop prescribing him Adderall, warning, "You're going to kill him."

It was where, after becoming violently delusional and spending a week in a psychiatric hospital in 2011, Richard met with his doctor and received prescriptions for 90 more days of Adderall. He hanged himself in his bedroom closet two weeks after they expired.

The story of Richard Fee, an athletic, personable college class president and aspiring medical student, highlights widespread failings in the system through which five million Americans take medication for A.D.H.D., doctors and other experts said.

Medications like Adderall can markedly improve the lives of children and others with the disorder. But the tunnel-like focus the medicines provide has led growing numbers of teenagers and young adults to fake symptoms to obtain steady prescriptions for highly addictive medications that carry serious psychological dangers. These efforts are facilitated by a segment of doctors who skip established diagnostic procedures, renew prescriptions reflexively and spend too little time with patients to accurately monitor side effects.

Richard Fee's experience included it all. Conversations with friends and family members and a review of detailed medical records depict an intelligent and articulate young man lying to doctor after doctor, physicians issuing hasty diagnoses, and psychiatrists continuing to prescribe medication—even increasing dosages—despite evidence of his growing addiction and psychiatric breakdown.

Very few people who misuse stimulants devolve into psychotic or suicidal addicts. But even one of Richard's own physicians, Dr. Charles Parker, characterized his case as a virtual textbook for ways that A.D.H.D. practices can fail patients, particularly young adults. "We have a significant travesty being done in this country with how the diagnosis is being made and the meds are being administered," said Dr. Parker, a psychiatrist in Virginia Beach. "I think it's an abnegation of trust. The public needs to say this is totally unacceptable and walk out."

Young adults are by far the fastest-growing segment of people taking A.D.H.D. medications. Nearly 14 million monthly prescriptions for the condition were written for Americans ages 20 to 39 in 2011, two and a half times the 5.6 million just four years before, according to the data company I.M.S. Health. While this rise is generally attributed to the maturing of adolescents who have A.D.H.D. into young adults—combined with a greater recognition of adult A.D.H.D. in general—many experts caution that savvy college graduates, freed of parental oversight, can legally and easily obtain stimulant prescriptions from obliging doctors.

"Any step along the way, someone could have helped him—they were just handing out drugs," said Richard's father. Emphasizing that he had no intention of bringing legal action against any of the doctors involved, Mr. Fee said: "People have to know that kids are out there getting these drugs and getting addicted to them. And doctors are helping them do it."

•

". . . when he was in elementary school he fidgeted, daydreamed and got A's. he has been an A-B student until mid college when he became scattered and he wandered while reading He never had to study. Presently without medication, his mind thinks most of the time, he procrastinated, he multitasks not finishing in a timely manner."

Dr. Waldo M. Ellison
Richard Fee initial evaluation
Feb. 5, 2010

•

Richard began acting strangely soon after moving back home in late 2009, his parents said. He stayed up for days at a time, went from gregarious to grumpy and back, and scrawled compulsively in notebooks. His father, while trying to add Richard to his health insurance policy, learned that he was taking Vyvanse for A.D.H.D.

Richard explained to him that he had been having trouble concentrating while studying for medical school entrance exams the previous year and that he had seen a doctor and received a diagnosis. His father reacted with surprise. Richard had never shown any A.D.H.D. symptoms his entire life, from nursery school through high school, when he was awarded a full academic scholarship to Greensboro College in North Carolina. Mr. Fee also expressed concerns about the safety of his son's taking daily amphetamines for a condition he might not have.

"The doctor wouldn't give me anything that's bad for me," Mr. Fee recalled his son saying that day. "I'm not buying it on the street corner."

Richard's first experience with A.D.H.D. pills, like so many others', had come in college. Friends said he was a typical undergraduate user—when he needed to finish a paper or cram for exams, one Adderall capsule would jolt him with focus and purpose for six to eight hours, repeat as necessary.

So many fellow students had prescriptions or stashes to share, friends of Richard recalled in interviews, that guessing where he got his was futile. He was popular enough on campus—he was sophomore class president and played first base on the baseball team—that they doubted he even had to pay the typical $5 or $10 per pill.

"He would just procrastinate, wait till the last minute and then take a pill to study for tests," said Ryan Sykes, a friend. "It got to the point where he'd say he couldn't get anything done if he didn't have the Adderall."

Various studies have estimated that 8 percent to 35 percent of college students take stimulant pills to enhance school performance. Few students realize that giving or accepting even one Adderall pill from a friend with a prescription is a federal crime. Adderall and its stimulant siblings are classified by the Drug Enforcement Administration as Schedule II drugs, in the same category as cocaine, because of their highly addictive properties.

"It's incredibly nonchalant," Chris Hewitt, a friend of Richard, said of students' attitudes to the drug. "It's: 'Anyone have any Adderall? I want to study tonight,'" said Mr. Hewitt, now an elementary school teacher in Greensboro.

After graduating with honors in 2008 with a degree in biology, Richard planned to apply to medical schools and stayed in Greensboro to study for the entrance exams. He remembered how Adderall had helped him concentrate so well as an undergraduate, friends said, and he made an appointment at the nearby Triad Psychiatric and Counseling Center.

According to records obtained by Richard's parents after his death, a nurse practitioner at Triad detailed his unremarkable medical and psychiatric history before recording his complaints about "organization, memory, attention to detail." She characterized his speech as "clear," his thought process "goal directed" and his concentration "attentive."

Richard filled out an 18-question survey on which he rated various symptoms on a 0-to-3 scale. His total score of 29 led the nurse practitioner to make a diagnosis of "A.D.H.D., inattentive-type"—a type of A.D.H.D. without hyperactivity. She recommended Vyvanse, 30 milligrams a day, for three weeks.

Phone and fax requests to Triad officials for comment were not returned.

Some doctors worry that A.D.H.D. questionnaires, designed to assist and standardize the gathering of a patient's symptoms, are being used as a shortcut to diagnosis. C. Keith Conners, a longtime child psychologist who developed a popular scale similar to the one used with Richard, said in an interview that scales like his "have reinforced this tendency for quick and dirty practice."

Dr. Conners, an emeritus professor of psychiatry and behavioral sciences at Duke University Medical Center, emphasized that a detailed life history must be taken and other sources of information—such as a parent, teacher, or friend—must be pursued to learn the nuances of a patient's difficulties and to rule out other maladies before making a proper diagnosis of A.D.H.D. Other doctors interviewed said they would not prescribe medications on a patient's first visit, specifically to deter the faking of symptoms.

According to his parents, Richard had no psychiatric history, or even suspicion of problems, through college. None of his dozen high school and college acquaintances interviewed for this article said he had ever shown or mentioned behaviors related to A.D.H.D.—certainly not the "losing things" and "difficulty awaiting turn" he reported on the Triad questionnaire—suggesting that he probably faked or at least exaggerated his symptoms to get his diagnosis.

That is neither uncommon nor difficult, said David Berry, a professor and researcher at the University of Kentucky. He is a co-author of a 2010 study that compared two groups of college students—those with diagnoses of A.D.H.D. and others who were asked to fake symptoms— to see whether standard symptom questionnaires could tell them apart. They were indistinguishable.

"With college students," Dr. Berry said in an interview, "it's clear that it doesn't take much information for someone who wants to feign A.D.H.D. to do so."

Richard Fee filled his prescription for Vyvanse within hours at a local Rite Aid. He returned to see the nurse three weeks later and reported excellent concentration: "reading books—read 10!" her notes indicate. She increased his dose to 50 milligrams a day. Three weeks later, after Richard left a message for her asking for the dose to go up to 60, which is on the high end of normal adult doses, she wrote on his chart, "Okay rewrite."

Richard filled that prescription later that afternoon. It was his third month's worth of medication in 43 days.

"The patient is a 23-year-old Caucasian male who presents for refill of vyvanse—recently started on this while in NC b/c of lack of motivation/loss of drive. Has moved here and wants refill"

Dr. Robert M. Woodard
Notes on Richard Fee
Nov. 11, 2009

Richard scored too low on the MCAT in 2009 to qualify for a top medical school. Although he had started taking Vyvanse for its jolts of focus and purpose, their side effects began to take hold. His sleep patterns increasingly scrambled and his mood darkening, he moved back in with his parents in Virginia Beach and sought a local physician to renew his prescriptions.

A friend recommended a family physician, Dr. Robert M. Woodard. Dr. Woodard heard Richard describe how well Vyvanse was working for his A.D.H.D., made a diagnosis of "other malaise and fatigue" and renewed his prescription for one month. He suggested that Richard thereafter see a trained psychiatrist at Dominion Psychiatric Associates—only a five-minute walk from the Fees' house.

With eight psychiatrists and almost 20 therapists on staff, Dominion Psychiatric is one of the better-known practices in Virginia Beach, residents said. One of its better-known doctors is Dr. Waldo M. Ellison, a practicing psychiatrist since 1974.

In interviews, some patients and parents of patients of Dr. Ellison's described him as very quick to identify A.D.H.D. and prescribe medication for it. Sandy Paxson of nearby Norfolk said she took her 15-year-old son to see Dr. Ellison for anxiety in 2008; within a few minutes, Mrs. Paxson recalled, Dr. Ellison said her son had A.D.H.D. and prescribed him Adderall.

"My son said: 'I love the way this makes me feel. It helps me focus for school, but it's not getting rid of my anxiety, and that's what I need,'" Mrs. Paxson recalled. "So we went back to Dr. Ellison and told him that it wasn't working properly, what else could he give us, and he basically told me that I was wrong. He basically told me that I was incorrect."

Dr. Ellison met with Richard in his office for the first time on Feb. 5, 2010. He took a medical history, heard Richard's complaints regarding concentration, noted how he was drumming his fingers and made a diagnosis of A.D.H.D. with "moderate symptoms or difficulty functioning." Dominion Psychiatric records of that visit do not mention the use of any A.D.H.D. symptom questionnaire to identify particular areas of difficulty or strategies for treatment.

As the 47-minute session ended, Dr. Ellison prescribed a common starting dose of Adderall: 30 milligrams daily for 21 days. Eight days later, while Richard still had 13 pills remaining, his prescription was renewed for 30 more days at 50 milligrams.

Through the remainder of 2010, in appointments with Dr. Ellison that usually lasted under five minutes, Richard returned for refills of Adderall. Records indicate that he received only what was consistently coded as "pharmacologic management"—the official term for quick appraisals of medication effects—and none of the more conventional talk-based therapy that experts generally consider an important component of A.D.H.D. treatment.

His Adderall prescriptions were always for the fast-acting variety, rather than the extended-release formula that is less prone to abuse.

"PATIENT DOING WELL WITH THE MEDICATION, IS CALM, FOCUSED AND ON TASK, AND WILL RETURN TO OFFICE IN 3 MONTHS"

Dr. Waldo M. Ellison
Notes on Richard Fee
Dec. 11, 2010

Regardless of what he might have told his doctor, Richard Fee was anything but well or calm during his first year back home, his father said.

Blowing through a month's worth of Adderall in a few weeks, Richard stayed up all night reading and scribbling in notebooks, occasionally climbing out of his bedroom window and on to the roof to converse with the moon and stars. When the pills ran out, he would sleep for 48 hours straight and not leave his room for 72. He got so hot during the day that he walked around the house with ice packs around his neck—and in frigid weather, he would cool off by jumping into the 52-degree backyard pool.

As Richard lost a series of jobs and tensions in the house ran higher—particularly when talk turned to his Adderall—Rick and Kathy Fee continued to research the side effects of A.D.H.D. medication. They learned that stimulants are exceptionally successful at mollifying the impulsivity and distractibility that characterize classic A.D.H.D., but that they can cause insomnia, increased blood pressure and elevated body temperature. Food and Drug Administration warnings on packaging also note "high potential for abuse," as well as psychiatric side effects such as aggression, hallucinations and paranoia.

A 2006 study in the journal *Drug and Alcohol Dependence* claimed that about 10 percent of adolescents and young adults who misused A.D.H.D. stimulants became addicted to them. Even proper, doctor-supervised use of the medications can trigger psychotic behavior or suicidal thoughts in about 1 in 400 patients, according to a 2006 study in *The American Journal of Psychiatry*. So while a vast majority of stimulant users will not experience psychosis—and a doctor may never encounter it in decades of careful practice—the sheer volume of prescriptions leads to thousands of cases every year, experts acknowledged.

When Mrs. Fee noticed Richard putting tape over his computer's camera, he told her that people were spying on him. (He put tape on his fingers, too, to avoid leaving fingerprints.) He cut himself out of family pictures, talked to the television and became increasingly violent when agitated.

In late December, Mr. Fee drove to Dominion Psychiatric and asked to see Dr. Ellison, who explained that federal privacy laws forbade any discussion of an adult patient, even with the patient's father. Mr. Fee said he had tried unsuccessfully to detail Richard's bizarre behavior, assuming that Richard had not shared such details with his doctor.

"I can't talk to you," Mr. Fee recalled Dr. Ellison telling him. "I did this one time with another family, sat down and talked with them, and I ended up getting sued. I can't talk with you unless your son comes with you."

Mr. Fee said he had turned to leave but distinctly recalls warning Dr. Ellison, "You keep giving Adderall to my son, you're going to kill him."

Dr. Ellison declined repeated requests for comment on Richard Fee's case. His office records, like those of other doctors involved, were obtained by Mr. Fee under Virginia and federal law, which allow the legal representative of a deceased patient to obtain medical records as if he were the patient himself.

As 2011 began, the Fees persuaded Richard to see a psychologist, Scott W. Sautter, whose records note Richard's delusions, paranoia and "severe and pervasive mental disorder." Dr. Sautter recommended that Adderall either be stopped or be paired with a sleep aid "if not medically contraindicated."

Mr. Fee did not trust his son to share this report with Dr. Ellison, so he drove back to Dominion Psychiatric and, he recalled, was told by a receptionist that he could leave the information with her. Mr. Fee said he had demanded to put it in Dr. Ellison's hands himself and threatened to break down his door in order to do so.

Mr. Fee said that Dr. Ellison had then come out, read the report and, appreciating the gravity of the situation, spoken with him about Richard for 45 minutes. They scheduled an appointment for the entire family.

•

"meeting with parents—concern with 'metaphoric' speaking that appears to be outside the realm of appropriated one to one conversation. Richard says he does it on purpose—to me some of it sounds like pre-psychotic thinking."

Dr. Waldo M. Ellison
Notes on Richard Fee
Feb. 23, 2011

•

Dr. Ellison stopped Richard Fee's prescription—he wrote "no Adderall for now" on his chart and the next day refused Richard's phone request for more. Instead he prescribed Abilify and Seroquel, antipsychotics for schizophrenia that do not provide the bursts of focus and purpose that stimulants do. Richard became enraged, his parents recalled. He tried to back up over his father in the Dominion Psychiatric parking lot and threatened to burn the house down. At home, he took a baseball bat from the garage, smashed flower pots and screamed, "You're taking my medicine!"

Richard disappeared for a few weeks. He returned to the house when he learned of his grandmother's death, the Fees said.

The morning after the funeral, Richard walked down Potters Road to what became a nine-minute visit with Dr. Ellison. He left with two prescriptions: one for Abilify, and another for 50 milligrams a day of Adderall.

According to Mr. Fee, Richard later told him that he had lied to Dr. Ellison—he told the doctor he was feeling great, life was back on track and he had found a job in Greensboro that he would lose without Adderall. Dr. Ellison's notes do not say why he agreed to start Adderall again.

Richard's delusions and mood swings only got worse, his parents said. They would lock their bedroom door when they went to sleep because of his unpredictable rages. "We were scared of our own son," Mr. Fee said. Richard would blow through his monthly prescriptions in 10 to 15 days and then go through hideous withdrawals. A friend said that he would occasionally get Richard some extra pills during the worst of it, but that "it wasn't enough because he would take four or five at a time."

One night during an argument, after Richard became particularly threatening and pushed him over a chair, Mr. Fee called the police. They arrested Richard for domestic violence. The episode persuaded Richard to see another local psychiatrist, Dr. Charles Parker.

Mrs. Fee said she attended Richard's initial consultation on June 3 with Dr. Parker's clinician, Renee Strelitz, and emphasized his abuse of Adderall. Richard "kept giving me dirty looks," Mrs. Fee recalled. She said she had later left a detailed message on Ms. Strelitz's voice mail, urging her and Dr. Parker not to prescribe stimulants under any circumstances when Richard came in the next day.

Dr. Parker met with Richard alone. The doctor noted depression, anxiety and suicidal ideas. He wrote "no meds" with a box around it—an indication, he explained later, that he was aware of the parents' concerns regarding A.D.H.D. stimulants.

Dr. Parker wrote three 30-day prescriptions: Clonidine (a sleep aid), Venlafaxine (an antidepressant) and Adderall, 60 milligrams a day.

In an interview last November, Dr. Parker said he did not recall the details of Richard's case but reviewed his notes and tried to recreate his mind-set during that appointment. He said he must have trusted Richard's assertions that medication was not an issue, and must have figured that his parents were just philosophically anti-medication. Dr. Parker recalled that he had been reassured by Richard's intelligent discussions of the ins and outs of stimulants and his desire to pursue medicine himself.

"He was smart and he was quick and he had A's and B's and wanted to go to medical school—and he had all the deportment of a guy that had the potential to do that," Dr. Parker said. "He didn't seem like he was a drug person at all, but rather a person that was misunderstood, really desirous of becoming a physician. He was very slick and smooth. He convinced me there was a benefit."

Mrs. Fee was outraged. Over the next several days, she recalled, she repeatedly spoke with Ms. Strelitz over the phone to detail Richard's continued abuse of the medication (she found nine pills gone after 48 hours) and hand-delivered Dr. Sautter's appraisal of his recent psychosis. Dr. Parker confirmed that he had received this information.

Richard next saw Dr. Parker on June 27. Mrs. Fee drove him to the clinic and waited in the parking lot. Soon afterward, Richard returned and asked to head to the pharmacy to fill a prescription. Dr. Parker had raised his Adderall to 80 milligrams a day.

Dr. Parker recalled that the appointment had been a 15-minute "med check" that left little time for careful assessment of any Adderall addiction. Once again, Dr. Parker said, he must have believed Richard's assertions that he needed additional medicine more than the family's pleas that it be stopped.

"He was pitching me very well—I was asking him very specific questions, and he was very good at telling me the answers in a very specific way," Dr. Parker recalled. He added later, "I do feel partially responsible for what happened to this kid."

•

"Paranoid and psychotic . . . thinking that the computer is spying on him. He has also been receiving messages from stars at night and he is unable to be talked to in a reasonable fashion . . . The patient denies any mental health problems . . . fairly high risk for suicide."

Dr. John Riedler
Admission note for Richard Fee
Virginia Beach Psychiatric Center
July 8, 2011

•

The 911 operator answered the call and heard a young man screaming on the other end. His parents would not give him his pills. With the man's language scattered and increasingly threatening, the police were sent to the home of Rick and Kathy Fee.

The Fees told officers that Richard was addicted to Adderall, and that after he had received his most recent prescription, they allowed him to fill it through his mother's insurance plan on the condition that they hold it and dispense it appropriately. Richard was now demanding his next day's pills early.

Richard denied his addiction and threats. So the police, noting that Richard was an adult, instructed the Fees to give him the bottle. They said they would comply only if he left the house for good. Officers escorted Richard off the property.

A few hours later Richard called his parents, threatening to stab himself in the head with a knife. The police found him and took him to the Virginia Beach Psychiatric Center.

Described as "paranoid and psychotic" by the admitting physician, Dr. John Riedler, Richard spent one week in the hospital denying that he had any psychiatric or addiction issues. He was placed on two medications: Seroquel and the antidepressant Wellbutrin, no stimulants. In his discharge report, Dr. Riedler noted that Richard had stabilized but remained severely depressed and dependent on both amphetamines and marijuana, which he would smoke in part to counter the buzz of Adderall and the depression from withdrawal.

(Marijuana is known to increase the risk for schizophrenia, psychosis and memory problems, but Richard had smoked pot in high school and college with no such effects, several friends recalled. If that was the case, "in all likelihood the stimulants were the primary issue here," said Dr. Wesley Boyd, a psychiatrist at Children's Hospital Boston and Cambridge Health Alliance who specializes in adolescent substance abuse.)

Unwelcome at home after his discharge from the psychiatric hospital, Richard stayed in cheap motels for a few weeks. His Adderall prescription from Dr. Parker expired on July 26, leaving him eligible for a renewal. He phoned the office of Dr. Ellison, who had not seen him in four months.

•

"moved out of the house—doesn't feel paranoid or delusional. Hasn't been on meds for a while—working with a friend wiring houses for 3 months—doesn't feel he needs the abilify or seroquel for sleep."

Dr. Waldo M. Ellison
Notes on Richard Fee
July 25, 2011

•

The 2:15 p.m. appointment went better than Richard could have hoped. He told Dr. Ellison that the pre-psychotic and metaphoric thinking back in March had receded, and that all that remained was his A.D.H.D. He said nothing of his visits to Dr. Parker, his recent prescriptions or his week in the psychiatric hospital.

At 2:21 p.m., according to Dr. Ellison's records, he prescribed Richard 30 days' worth of Adderall at 50 milligrams a day. He also gave him prescriptions postdated for Aug. 23 and Sept. 21, presumably to allow him to get pills into late October without the need for followup appointments. (Virginia state law forbids the dispensation of 90 days of a controlled substance at one time, but does allow doctors to write two 30-day prescriptions in advance.)

Virginia is one of 43 states with a formal Prescription Drug Monitoring Program, an online database that lets doctors check a patient's one-year prescription history, partly to see if he or she is getting medication elsewhere. Although pharmacies are required to enter all prescriptions for controlled substances into the system, Virginia law does not require doctors to consult it.

Dr. Ellison's notes suggest that he did not check the program before issuing the three prescriptions to Richard, who filled the first within hours.

The next morning, during a scheduled appointment at Dr. Parker's clinic, Ms. Strelitz wrote in her notes: "Richard is progressing. He reported staying off of the Adderall and on no meds currently. Focusing on staying healthy, eating well and exercising."

About a week later, Richard called his father with more good news: a job he had found overseeing storm cleanup crews was going well. He was feeling much better.

But Mr. Fee noticed that the more calm and measured speech that Richard had regained during his hospital stay was gone. He jumped from one subject to the next, sounding anxious and rushed. When the call ended, Mr. Fee recalled, he went straight to his wife.

"Call your insurance company," he said, "and find out if they've filled any prescriptions for Adderall."

•

"spoke to father—richard was in VBPC [Virginia Beach Psychiatric Center] and OD on adderall—NO STIMULANTS—HE WAS ALSO SEEING DR. PARKER"

Dr. Waldo M. Ellison
Interoffice e-mail
Aug. 5, 2011

•

An insurance representative confirmed that Richard had filled a prescription for Adderall on July 25. Mr. Fee confronted Dr. Ellison in the Dominion Psychiatric parking lot.

Mr. Fee told him that Richard had been in the psychiatric hospital, had been suicidal and had been taking Adderall through June and July. Dr. Ellison confirmed that he had written not only another prescription but two others for later in August and September.

"He told me it was normal procedure and not 90 days at one time," Mr. Fee recalled. "I flipped out on him: 'You gave my son 90 days of Adderall? You're going to kill him!'"

Mr. Fee said he and Dr. Ellison had discussed voiding the two outstanding scripts. Mr. Fee said he had been told that it was possible, but that should Richard need emergency medical attention, it could keep him from getting what would otherwise be proper care or medication. Mr. Fee confirmed that with a pharmacist and decided to drive

to Richard's apartment and try to persuade him to rip up the prescriptions.

"I know that you've got these other prescriptions to get pills," Mr. Fee recalled telling Richard. "You're doing so good. You've got a job. You're working. Things with us are better. If you get them filled, I'm worried about what will happen."

"You're right," Mr. Fee said Richard had replied. "I tore them up and threw them away."

Mr. Fee spent two more hours with Richard making relative small talk—increasingly gnawed, he recalled later, by the sense that this was no ordinary conversation. As he looked at Richard he saw two images flickering on top of each other—the boy he had raised to love school and baseball, and the desperate addict he feared that boy had become.

Before he left, Mr. Fee made as loving a demand as he could muster.

"Please. Give them to me," Mr. Fee said.

Richard looked his father dead in the eye.

"I destroyed them," he said. "I don't have them. Don't worry."

•

"Richard said that he has stopped Adderall and wants to work on continuing to progress."

Renee Strelitz
Session notes
Sept. 13, 2011

•

Richard generally filled his prescriptions at a CVS on Laskin Road, less than three miles from his parents' home. But on Aug. 23, he went to a different CVS about 11 miles away, closer to Norfolk and farther from the locations that his father might have called to alert them to the situation. For his Sept. 21 prescription he traveled even farther, into Norfolk, to get his pills.

On Oct. 3, Richard visited Dr. Ellison for an appointment lasting 17 minutes. The doctor prescribed two weeks of Strattera, a medication for A.D.H.D. that contains no amphetamines and, therefore, is neither a controlled substance nor particularly prone to abuse. His records make no mention of the Adderall prescription Richard filled on Sept. 21; they do note, however, "Father says that he is crazy and abusive of the Adderall—has made directives with regard to giving Richard anymore stimulants—bringing up charges—I explained this to Richard."

Prescription records indicate that Richard did not fill the Strattera prescription before returning to Dr. Ellison's office two weeks later to ask for more stimulants.

"Patient took only a few days of Strattera 40 mg—it calmed him but not focusing," the doctor's notes read. "I had told him not to look for much initially—He would like a list of MD who could rx adderall."

Dr. Ellison never saw Richard again. Given his patterns of abuse, friends said, Richard probably took his last Adderall pill in early October. Because he abruptly stopped without the slow and delicate reduction of medication that is recommended to minimize major psychological risks, especially for instant-release stimulants, he crashed harder than ever.

Richard's lifelong friend Ryan Sykes was one of the few people in contact with him during his final weeks. He said that despite Richard's addiction to Adderall and the ease with which it could be obtained on college campuses nearby, he had never pursued it outside the doctors' prescriptions.

"He had it in his mind that because it came from a doctor, it was O.K.," Mr. Sykes recalled.

On Nov. 7, after arriving home from a weekend away, Mrs. Fee heard a message on the family answering machine from Richard, asking his parents to call him. She phoned back at 10 that night and left a message herself.

Not hearing back by the next afternoon, Mrs. Fee checked Richard's cellphone records—he was on her plan—and saw no calls or texts. At 9 p.m. the Fees drove to Richard's apartment in Norfolk to check on him. The lights were on; his car was in the driveway. He did not answer. Beginning to panic, Mr. Fee found the kitchen window ajar and climbed in through it.

He searched the apartment and found nothing amiss.

"He isn't here," Mr. Fee said he had told his wife.

"Oh, thank God," she replied. "Maybe he's walking on the beach or something."

They got ready to leave before Mr. Fee stopped.

"Wait a minute," he said. "I didn't check the closet."

•

"Spoke with Richard's mother, Kathy Fee, today. She reported that Richard took his life last November. Family is devasted and having a difficult time. Offerred assistance for family."

Renee Strelitz
Last page of Richard Fee file
June 21, 2012

•

Friends and former baseball teammates flocked to Richard Fee's memorial service in Virginia Beach. Most remembered only the funny and gregarious guy they knew in high school and college; many knew absolutely nothing of his last two years. He left no note explaining his suicide.

At a gathering at the Fees' house afterward, Mr. Fee told them about Richard's addiction to Adderall. Many recalled how they, too, had blithely abused the drug in college—to cram, just as Richard had—and could not help but wonder if they had played the same game of Russian roulette.

"I guarantee you a good number of them had used it for studying—that shock was definitely there in that room," said a Greensboro baseball teammate, Danny Michael, adding that he was among the few who had not. "It's so prevalent and widely used. People had no idea it could be abused to the point of no return."

Almost every one of more than 40 A.D.H.D. experts interviewed for this article said that worst-case scenarios like Richard Fee's can occur with any medication—and that people who do have A.D.H.D., or parents of children with the disorder, should not be dissuaded from considering the proven benefits of stimulant medication when supervised by a responsible physician.

Other experts, however, cautioned that Richard Fee's experience is instructive less in its ending than its evolution—that it underscores aspects of A.D.H.D. treatment that are mishandled every day with countless patients, many of them children.

"You don't have everything that happened with this kid, but his experience is not that unusual," said DeAnsin Parker, a clinical neuropsychologist in New York who specializes in young adults. "Diagnoses are made just this quickly, and medication is filled just this quickly. And the lack of therapy is really sad. Doctors are saying, 'Just take the meds to see if they help,' and if they help, 'You must have A.D.H.D.'"

Dr. Parker added: "Stimulants will help anyone focus better. And a lot of young people like or value that feeling, especially those who are driven and have ambitions. We have to realize that these are potential addicts—drug addicts don't look like they used to."

The Fees decided to go. The event was sponsored by the local chapter of Children and Adults with Attention Deficit Disorder (Chadd), the nation's primary advocacy group for A.D.H.D. patients. They wanted to attend the question-and-answer session afterward with local doctors and community college officials.

The evening opened with the local Chadd coordinator thanking the drug company Shire—the manufacturer of several A.D.H.D. drugs, including Vyvanse and extended-release Adderall—for partly underwriting the event. An hourlong film directed and narrated by two men with A.D.H.D. closed by examining some "myths" about stimulant medications, with several doctors praising their efficacy and safety. One said they were "safer than aspirin," while another added, "It's O.K.—there's nothing that's going to happen."

Sitting in the fourth row, Mr. Fee raised his hand to pose a question to the panel, which was moderated by Jeffrey Katz, a local clinical psychologist and a national board member of Chadd. "What are some of the drawbacks or some of the dangers of a misdiagnosis in somebody," Mr. Fee asked, "and then the subsequent medication that goes along with that?"

Dr. Katz looked straight at the Fees as he answered, "Not much."

Adding that "the medication itself is pretty innocuous," Dr. Katz continued that someone without A.D.H.D. might feel more awake with stimulants but would not consider it "something that they need."

"If you misdiagnose it and you give somebody medication, it's not going to do anything for them," Dr. Katz concluded. "Why would they continue to take it?"

Mr. Fee slowly sat down, trembling. Mrs. Fee placed her hand on his knee as the panel continued.

ALAN SCHWARZ is a Pulitzer Prize-nominated reporter for *The New York Times*.

Joshua Gowin

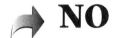

How "Smart Drugs" Enhance Us

If I only had a (better) brain.

The French Revolution was largely conceived in Parisian coffee houses such as Café Procope, where the radical journalist Jean-Paul Marat sipped java during his energetic diatribes and Robespierre's habitual consumption only increased his rebellious fervor. Voltaire reportedly guzzled over ten cups each day. Although they didn't know about caffeine at the time (it wasn't discovered until 1819, 30 years after the French Revolution), they certainly didn't overlook the stimulating effects of consuming a cup of perk. Some coffee-enthusiasts might suggest that imbibing the early-morning helper contributed to the monarchy's demise and the rise of the new Republic.

Our understanding of pharmacology has come a long way since the Reign of Terror. Recently, 'smart drugs' have been touted as a remedy to an array of problems, from bad moods to failing economies. What have we gained with the advent of modern cognitive enhancers?

A cup of coffee is a far cry from the sophisticated stimulants used by many on a daily basis. For example, Adderall and Ritalin, prescribed for the treatment of Attention-Deficit Hyperactivity Disorder (ADHD), work by helping individuals focus their attention without being easily distracted. For a child diagnosed with ADHD, these drugs can greatly improve both behavior and school performance. Adderall, composed of mixed amphetamine salts, and Ritalin, an amphetamine derivative, are also two of the drugs most widely used by healthy adults as purported brain boosters. Surveys at some universities have shown that up to 35% of students have obtained these drugs for use as a study aid, though most of them do not have ADHD (ADHD affects only 3–4% of people). For students without prescriptions, they usually have little trouble acquiring Ritalin or Adderall from friends or schoolmates. Students with prescriptions sometimes even sell their unneeded doses.

Given the dramatic rise in use for studying, ethicists have debated whether cognitive-enhancing drugs are unfair. Those who take them may have an advantage on tests versus students who attempt to study using their wits alone. If taking drugs could provide a cognitive edge, you might expect that these students would outperform their classmates. Some wonder if parents might begin forcing their children to take smart-drugs in order to maintain competitive grades.

In order to address this issue, The College Life Study began periodically surveying university students a few years ago to better understand how health-related behaviors, including all varieties of drug use, affect school performance and career development. At a recent conference, Amelia Arria, the lead researcher, presented data about the use of Ritalin and Adderall as study drugs. The students who used these drugs more often also tended to skip more classes and smoke more pot. In terms of performance, they tended to have lower GPAs, in the 2.0–3.0 range, not higher ones. It seems, rather than as a tool to get ahead, students used stimulants while cramming to catch up for lost study time. Students earning As were mostly doing so by steady work throughout the semester, without the assistance of modern medicine.

Of course, this finding merits some caveats. Maybe the students using cognitive-enhancers did better than they would have otherwise. Just because most students (without ADHD) who use pharmacological aids don't perform better, some users may see a dramatic improvement. Nonetheless, so far it appears that Ritalin and Adderall offer the greatest assistance to the people they're prescribed to, those diagnosed with ADHD. As for the rest of students, Adderall may not be an unequivocal performance enhancer. The results of this study suggest that if a gap exists, the students who don't take study drugs are edging out those who do.

Arria reminds that evidence has been inconclusive so far about whether the enhancement for studying is real or perceived in healthy adults. In another study, students were given pills labeled either 'Ritalin' or 'placebo' and asked to take a mock SAT examination. The students given pills labeled 'Ritalin' reported feeling greater focus and mental clarity but their scores weren't any better—perhaps because the labels were misleading: both groups actually received a placebo.

A third common cognitive-enhancer, modafinil, first entered the market to help people with narcolepsy stay awake. A great deal of research has since looked at the potential benefits of modafinil for a variety of purposes. In healthy adults who are sleep-deprived, modafinil can improve mood, provide 10–12 hours of wakeful, focused productivity and improve cognition to a similar extent as caffeine, but without the jitteriness—and the effects last longer. After working overnight in the emergency room, doctors who took a single dose of modafinil kept their eyes open more easily than doctors who didn't take modafinil during morning lectures. However, they were just as weary on the drive home, and they had more difficulty falling asleep once they finally made it to bed. For patients with traumatic brain injury, major depressive disorder or schizophrenia, modafinil had a substantial effect on reducing fatigue, excessive sleepiness and depression, but it did not provide any benefit greater than placebo. For well-rested, healthy adults, the benefits remain controversial. While some studies have demonstrated that well-rested individuals can show modest improvement on memory tasks with modafinil, there may be a ceiling effect. High-functioning, healthy adults with adequate sleep may not receive any noticeable benefit because they are already performing optimally.

What is the difference between cognitive-enhancers like modafinil or Adderall and predecessors like caffeine? The chemical compounds differ, and they have unique mechanisms of action. Pharmaceutical packaging gives them elegance and refinement. Most people believe they'll work, so they offer at minimum a placebo effect. Even if, at heart, they're simply newer, prettier double-shots of espresso, there may still be some advantages to taking these drugs, such as longer-lasting effects and no jitteriness.

Do these drugs make you smarter? More likely, they allow you to productively use your pre-existing intelligence, even if you didn't get a great night of rest beforehand. After ingesting one of these pills, an average person won't suddenly discover a cure for cancer or write a symphony that would make Beethoven envious. If someone is seeking a miraculous transformation, they're better off booking a room at a Holiday Inn Express or going about it the old-fashioned way-by signing a deal with the devil.

Joshua Gowin is a psychologist and former intern at *Psychology Today.*

EXPLORING THE ISSUE

Is the Use of "Smart" Pills for Cognitive Enhancement Dangerous?

Critical Thinking and Reflection

1. Why do so many young people fake symptoms in order to acquire "smart drugs"?
2. Describe the side effects of stimulant drugs such as Ritalin and Allderall. What are the effects that appeal to users?
3. What are the legitimate uses for stimulant drugs such as Ritalin and Allderall?

Is There Common Ground?

On some elite college campuses, up to 25 percent of students admit to nonmedical use of stimulant drugs. "Smart" drugs are also widely used off campus by business executives and others who wish to gain a competitive edge and to better meet deadlines. The drugs are becoming common and many people believe they have much to offer individuals and society and should be made more available. The benefits of enhancement drugs include increased alertness and focus and improvement in some types of memory. Among those who do not have ADHD, research has shown that stimulants consistently and significantly enhance learning of material recalled days later, an obvious advantage when studying for an exam. The drugs may even positively affect certain types of judgment. Improvements in memory and cognitive control have been reported in multiple studies, mainly using the drug Ritalin.

While the drugs may offer the benefit of cognitive enhancement, there is question as to whether their use is both cheating and drug abuse. Will there be pressure among students to take drugs just to keep up with their peers? One of the biggest concerns, however, is that cognitive enhancement may be wrong not because it is so physically risky or because it creates an unleveled playing field but because it redefines the nature of human achievement itself. The obvious parallel to performance-enhancing drug use among professional and amateur athletes is often made. While ethicists ponder this, the reality is that there are also health risks since the effects of chronic unregulated doses of stimulant drugs can be toxic. The drugs can also cause psychosis, actual cognitive deficits, and addiction.

Create Central

www.mhhe.com/createcentral

Additional Resources

Franke, A. G., Lieb, K., & Hildt, E. (2012). What users think about the differences between caffeine and illicit/prescription stimulants for cognitive enhancement. *PLoS One, 7,* 1–7.

Smith, M. E. & Farah, M. J. (2011). Are prescription stimulants "smart pills"? The epidemiology and cognitive neuroscience of prescription stimulant use by normal healthy individuals. *Psychological Bulletin, 137*(5), 717–741.

Varga, M. D. (2012). Adderall abuse on college campuses: A comprehensive literature review. *Journal of Evidence-Based Social Work, 9*(3), 293–313.

Vrecki, S. A. (2013). Just how cognitive is "cognitive enhancement"? On the significance of emotions in university students' experiences with study drugs. *AJOB Neuroscience, 4,* 4–12.

Webb, J. R., Valased, M. R., & North, C. S. (2013). Prevalence of stimulant use in a sample of US medical students. *Annals of Clinical Psychiatry, 25,* 27–32.

Internet References . . .

Food and Drug Administration

www.fda.gov

National Institute on Drug Abuse (NIDA)

www.nida.nih.gov

National Institutes of Mental Health (NIMH). Attention Deficit Hyperactivity Disorder (ADHD)

www.nimh.nih.gov/health/publications/index.shtml

Selected, Edited, and with issue Framing Material by:
Eileen Daniel, *SUNY College at Brockport*

ISSUE

Should Embryonic Stem Cell Research Be Permitted?

YES: Jeffrey Hart, from "NR on Stem Cells: The Magazine Is Wrong," *National Review* (April 19, 2004)

NO: Ramesh Ponnuru, from "NR on Stem Cells: The Magazine Is Right," *National Review* (April 19, 2004)

Learning Outcomes
After reading this issue, you should be able to:
• Discuss the basic characteristics of stem cells.
• Understand the potential benefits of stem cell therapy.
• Assess the difference between adult and embryonic stem cells.

ISSUE SUMMARY

YES: Professor Jeffrey Hart contends there are many benefits to stem cell research and that a ban on funded cloning research is unjustified.

NO: Writer Ramesh Ponnuru argues that a single-celled human embryo is a living organism, which directs its own development and should not be used for experimentation.

Research using human stem cells could one day lead to cures for diabetes, could restore mobility to paralyzed individuals, and may offer treatment for diseases such as Alzheimer's and Parkinson's. It may be possible for humans to regenerate body parts, or create new cells to treat disease. Stem cells, which have the potential to develop into many different cell types, serve as a type of repair system for the body. They can theoretically divide without limit to replenish other cells as long as the person or animal still lives. When a stem cell divides, each new cell has the potential to either remain a stem cell or become another type of cell with a more specialized function, such as a brain or blood cell.

There are two important characteristics of stem cells, which differentiate them from other types of cells. First, they are unspecialized cells that renew themselves for long periods through cell division. Second, under certain conditions, they can be become cells with special functions such as heart cells or the insulin-producing cells of the pancreas. Researchers mainly work with two kinds of stem cells from animals and humans: embryonic stem cells and adult stem cells, which have different functions and characteristics. Scientists learned different ways to get or derive stem cells from early rodent embryos over 20 years ago.

Detailed study of the biology of mouse stem cells led to the discovery, in 1998, of how to isolate stem cells from human embryos and grow the cells in the lab. The embryos used in these studies were created for infertility purposes through in vitro fertilization procedures and when no longer needed for that purpose, they were donated for research with the informed consent of the donor.

Researchers have hypothesized that embryonic stem cells may, at some point in the future, become the basis for treating diseases such as Parkinson's disease, diabetes, and heart disease. Scientists need to study stem cells to learn about their important properties and what makes them different from specialized cell types. As researchers discover more about stem cells, it may become possible to use the cells not just in cell-based therapies but also for screening new drugs and preventing birth defects.

Researching stem cells will allow scientists to understand how they transform into the array of specialized cells that make us human. Some of the most serious medical conditions, such as cancer and birth defects, are due to events that occur somewhere in this process. A better understanding of normal cell development will allow scientists to understand and possibly correct the errors that cause these conditions. Another potential application of stem cells is making cells and tissues for medical therapies. A type of stem cell, pluripotents, offers the possibility of a renewable source of replacement cells and tissues to treat a myriad of diseases, conditions, and disabilities including Parkinson's and Alzheimer's diseases, spinal cord injury, stroke, burns, heart disease, diabetes, and arthritis.

The Bush Administration did not support embryonic stem cell research, which they believed is experimentation on potential human life. As a result, researchers must rely on funding from business, private foundations, and other sources. While the potential for stem cells is great, there is not universal support for this research. In the YES and NO selections, Jeffrey Hart, a senior editor at *National Review*, contends that there are many benefits to stem cell research and that a federal ban on funded experimentation is unjustified. Ramesh Ponnuru argues that stem cell research is amoral since it involves the use of human embryos.

YES ⤶

Jeffrey Hart

NR on Stem Cells: The Magazine Is Wrong

National Review has consistently taken a position on stem-cell research that requires some discussion here. Three editorials early this year were based on the assertion that a single fertilized cell is a "human being." This premise—and the conclusions drawn from it—require challenge on conservative grounds, as they have never been approved by American law or accepted as common convention.

The first 2004 editorial appeared in the January 26 issue, and made a series of assertions about recent legislation in New Jersey. It included the notion that it is now "possible" to create a human embryo there—through cloning—that, at age eight months, could be sold for research. But this dystopian fantasy could become fact in no American jurisdiction.

In the March 8 NR we read another editorial; this one achieved greater seriousness. Still, it called for a "new law" that "would say that human beings, however small and young, may not be treated instrumentally and may not be deliberately destroyed."

In all of the editorials, we are asked to accept the insistent dogma that a single fertilized cell is a "human being, however small and young," and is not to be "deliberately destroyed."

This demand grates—because such "human beings" are deliberately destroyed all the time, and such "mass homicide" arouses no public outcry. In fact, there are about 100,000 fertilized cells now frozen in maternity clinics. These are the inevitable, and so deliberate, by-products of in vitro fertilization, accepted by women who cannot conceive children naturally. No wonder there has been no outcry: Where reality shows medical waste that would otherwise lie useless, NR's characterization of these frozen embryos as "small and young" makes one think of the Gerber baby.

The entire NR case against stem-cell research rests, like a great inverted pyramid, on the single assertion that these cells are "human beings"—a claim that is not self-evidently true. Even when the naked eye is aided by a microscope, these cells—"zygotes," to use the proper terminology—do not look like human beings. That resemblance does not emerge even as the zygote grows into the hundred-cell organism, about the size of a pinhead, called a "blastocyst." This is the level of development at which stem cells are produced: The researcher is not interested in larger embryos, much less full-blown, for-sale fetuses.

I myself have never met anyone who bites into an apple, gazes upon the seeds there, and sees a grove of apple trees. I think we must conclude, if we are to use language precisely, that the single fertilized cell is a *developing* or *potential* human being—many of which are destroyed during in vitro fertilization, and even in the course of natural fertilization. But just as a seed—a *potential* apple tree—is no orchard, a *potential* child is not yet a human being.

There is more to this matter than biology: In question is NR's very theory of—and approach to—politics. Classic and valuable arguments in this magazine have often taken the form of Idea (or paradigm) versus Actuality. Here are a few such debates that have shaped the magazine, a point of interest especially to new readers.

Very early in NR's history, the demand for indisputably conservative candidates gave way to William F. Buckley Jr.'s decisive formulation that NR should prefer "the most conservative electable candidate." WFB thus corrected his refusal to vote for Eisenhower, who was at least more conservative than Stevenson. Senior editor James Burnham, a realist, also voted for Ike; in his decision, Actuality won out.

In the 1956 crisis in Hungary, Burnham's profoundly held Idea about the necessity for Liberation in Europe contrasted with Eisenhower's refusal, based on Actuality, to intervene in a landlocked nation where Soviet ground and air superiority was decisive. But later on, Burnham, choosing Actuality over the Idea, saw much sooner than most conservatives that Nixon's containment and "Vietnamization" could not work in South Vietnam, which was a sieve. The "peace" that was "at hand" in 1972 was the peace of the grave.

A final example: In the late 1960s, senior editor Brent Bozell's theoretical demand for perfect Catholic morality—argued in a very fine exchange with another senior editor, Frank Meyer—was rejected by NR.

Thus the tension between Idea and Actuality has a long tradition at NR, revived by this question of stem cells. Ultimately, American constitutional decision-making rests upon the "deliberate consent" of a self-governing people. Such decision-making by consensus usually accords no participant everything he desires, and thus is non-utopian. Just try an absolute, ideological ban on in vitro fertilization, for example, and observe the public response.

In fact, an editorial (NR, August 6, 2001) has held that even in vitro fertilization is hard to justify morally. Understandably, NR has soft-pedaled this opinion: The magazine's view that a single cell is a "human being" has never been expressed in or embraced by American law. It represents an absolutization of the "human being" claim for a single cell. It stands in contradiction to the "deliberate sense" theory NR has heretofore espoused. And, at this very moment, it is being contradicted in the Actual world of research practice.

Recently, for instance, a Harvard researcher produced 17 stem-cell "lines" from the aforementioned left-over frozen cells. The researcher's goal is not homicide, of course, but the possible cure of dreadful diseases. It seems to me that the prospect of eliminating horrible, disabling ailments justifies, morally, using cells that are otherwise doomed. Morality requires the weighing of results, and the claim to a "right to life" applies in both directions. Those lifting that phrase from the Declaration of Independence do not often add "liberty and the pursuit of happiness," there given equal standing as "rights"—rights that might be more widely enjoyed in the wake of stem-cell advances.

As I said earlier, the evolution of NR as a magazine that matters has involved continuing arguments between Idea and Actuality. Here, the Idea that a single fertilized cell is a human being, and that destroying one is a homicide, is not sustainable. That is the basis—the only basis—for NR's position thus far on stem-cell research. Therefore NR's position on the whole issue is unsustainable.

Buckley has defined conservatism as the "politics of reality." That is the strength of conservatism, a Burkean strength, and an anti-utopian one. I have never heard a single cytologist affirming the proposition that a single cell is a "human being"; here, Actuality will prevail, as usual.

In recommending against federal funding for most stem-cell research, President Bush stated that 60 lines of stem cells that already exist are adequate for current research. The National Institutes of Health has said that this is incorrect. There are in fact 15 lines, and these are not adequate even for current research. The president was misinformed. But Actuality is gaining ground nonetheless: Harvard University has recently announced the formation of a $100 million Harvard Stem Cell Institute. And Harvard physicians are conducting community-education programs to counter misinformation (Reuters, March 3): "Scientists at Harvard University announced on Wednesday that they had created 17 batches of stem cells from human embryos in defiance of efforts by President Bush to limit such research. 'What we have done is to make use of previously frozen human fertilized eggs that otherwise were going to be discarded,' [Dr. Douglas] Melton told reporters in a tele-phone briefing."

Not unexpectedly, and after losing one of its top sci-entists in the field to Cambridge (England), the University of California, Berkeley, announced that it was pursuing stem-cell research. Other UCs also made such announce-ments, and California state funding has been promised. It is easy to see that major research universities across the nation—and in any nation that can afford them—will either follow or lose their top scientists in this field. Expe-rience shows that it is folly to reject medical investigation, a folly the universities and private-sector researchers will be sure to avoid.

Weak in theory, and irrelevant in practice, opposition to stem-cell research is now an irrelevance across the board; on this matter, even the president has made himself irrele-vant. All this was to be expected: The only surprise has been the speed with which American research is going forward. It is pleasant to have the private sector intervene, as at Har-vard, not to mention the initiatives of the states. In practi-cal terms, this argument is over. *National Review* should not make itself irrelevant by trying to continue it.

JEFFREY HART is a senior editor of the *National Review*.

Ramesh Ponnuru

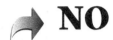 **NO**

NR on Stem Cells: The Magazine Is Right

National Review does not oppose stem-cell research. It approves of research on stem cells taken from adult somatic cells, or from umbilical cords. It opposes stem-cell research only when obtaining those cells destroys embryonic human beings, whether these beings are created through cloning, in vitro fertilization, or the old-fashioned way. Jeff Hart challenges NR's stance for three reasons: He disputes the idea that single-celled human embryos are human beings, he questions the prudence of advancing that idea, and he thinks the humanitarian goal of the research justifies the means.

Professor Hart starts his argument by noting that American law has never treated the single-celled embryo as a human being. This is true. But it never treated it as anything else, either. What would American law have had to say about the embryo in 1826, or, for that matter, in 1952?

The single-celled human embryo is neither dead nor inanimate. It is a living organism, not a functional part of another organism, and it directs its own development, according to its genetic template, through the embryonic, fetal, infant, and subsequent stages of development. (The terms "blastocyst," "adolescent," and "newborn" denote stages of development in a being of the same type, not different types of beings.) It is a *Homo sapiens,* not a member of some other species—which is why it is valuable to scientists in the first place. Strictly speaking, it is not even an "it": It has a sex.

"Even when the naked eye is aided by a microscope," writes Professor Hart, early embryos "do not look like human beings." Actually, they look *exactly* like human beings—the way human beings look at that particular stage of development. We all looked like that, at that age. Professor Hart believes that science can open up whole worlds of knowledge and possibility to us. He should be willing to entertain the possibility that among the insights we have gained is the revelation that human beings at their beginnings look like nothing we have ever seen before.

Professor Hart notes that many embryos die naturally. And so? Infant mortality rates have been very high in some societies; old people die all the time. That does not mean it is permissible to kill infants or old people.

I should also comment about the New Jersey law that makes it legally possible to create a human embryo through cloning, develop it through the fetal stage, and sell it for research purposes at eight months. Professor Hart writes that "this dystopian fantasy could become fact in no American jurisdiction." Sadly, this is untrue: In most American jurisdictions, no law on the books would prevent this scenario from taking place.

In the past, scientists have been quite interested in doing research on aborted fetuses. Right now, the early embryo is a hotter research subject. But neither Professor Hart nor I can rule out the possibility that research on cloned fetuses will be thought, in a few years, to hold great promise. If scientists want to conduct such research, the only legal obstacles will be the statutes of those states that have banned human cloning—the very laws that NR favors. New Jersey has brought this dystopia one step closer.

It would be possible for Professor Hart to concede that the history of a body begins with its conception—that we were all once one-celled organisms, in the sense that "we" were never a sperm cell and an egg cell—while still claiming that it would have been morally defensible to destroy us at that time. Our intrinsic moral worth came later, he might argue: when we developed sentience, abstract reasoning, relationships with others, or some other distinguishing attribute. According to this viewpoint, human beings as such have no intrinsic right to life; many human beings enjoy that right only by virtue of qualities they happen to possess.

The implications of this theory, however, extend beyond the womb. Infants typically lack the immediately exercisable capacity for abstract mental reasoning, too—which is how Peter Singer and others have justified infanticide. It is impossible to identify a non-arbitrary point at which there is "enough" sentience or meaningful interaction to confer a right to life. It is also impossible to explain why some people do not have basic rights more or less than other people depending on how much of the accidental quality they possess. In other words, the foundation of human equality is destroyed as soon as we suggest that private actors may treat some members of the human species as though they were mere things. The claim in the Declaration of Independence that "all men are created equal" becomes a self-evident lie.

Life comes before liberty and the pursuit of happiness in that declaration, and at no point is it suggested that liberty includes a right to kill, or that happiness may be pursued through homicide. Morality often "requires the weighing of results," as Professor Hart writes. But we would not kill one five-year-old child for the certain prospect of curing cancer, let alone the mere possibility—because the act would be intrinsically immoral. Or would we? Professor Hart writes that it is "folly to reject medical investigation." So much for restrictions on human experimentation.

Apple seeds are not a grove of trees. An infant is not an adult, either, just a potential adult, but that doesn't mean you can kill it. Professor Hart objects to the use of the words "young" and "small" to characterize the entities whose destruction we are debating. Since the argument for terminating them turns precisely on their having 100 cells or fewer (they're small), and on their not yet having advanced to later stages of human development (they're young), it's hard to see his point.

Let me turn now to the question of the politics of Actuality. NR is, in principle, against the intentional destruction of human embryos. But we have been quite mindful of political circumstances. As Professor Hart notes, we have not said much about regulating the practices of fertility clinics. (He faults us for both running wild with ideas and prudently declining to do so; also, freezing something is not the same as destroying it.) Prudence has kept us from urging the president to fight for a ban on all research that destroys human embryos. We have principally asked for two things: a ban on governmental funding of such research, and a ban on human cloning—even suggesting a simple moratorium on cloning as a compromise. We are not calling, to pursue one of Professor Hart's analogies, for an invasion of Hungary here. But neither are we suggesting that we are indifferent to the Soviet domination of Eastern Europe.

Our position on cloning is not that of some political fringe: It is the position of President Bush. It is the position of the House of Representatives, which has twice voted to ban human cloning. It is a position that, depending on the wording of the poll question, somewhere between one-third and two-thirds of the public shares. It is the position of the governments of Canada and Germany. NR has fought lonelier battles.

We are sometimes told that, in a pluralistic society in which many people have different views about such matters as the moral status of the human embryo, we cannot impose public policies that assume the correctness of some views over others. I cannot agree. Some people will not accept the justice of a ban on cloning for research; few policies command the full assent of all people of good will. But disagreement about the requirements of justice is no excuse for failing to do it.

RAMESH PONNURU is a senior editor at the *National Review*.

EXPLORING THE ISSUE

Should Embryonic Stem Cell Research Be Permitted?

Critical Thinking and Reflection

1. What are the differences between adult and embryonic stem cells?
2. Why are many individuals opposed to stem cell research?
3. Why did the government under the Bush Administration deny funding for stem cell research?

Is There Common Ground?

Many scientists believe that human embryonic stem cell research could one day lead to a cure for a variety of diseases that plague humans. While a cure for diabetes, cancer, Parkinson's, and other diseases would greatly benefit humanity, there are many who believe that it is amoral to use human embryos for this purpose. These individuals believe that every human being begins as a single-cell zygote, and develops into an embryo, fetus, and then is born. To destroy the embryonic stem cell is to destroy a potential life, which many cannot justify. The Bush Administration supported these beliefs and enacted a moratorium on U.S. federal funding for embryonic stem cell research. When Barack Obama became president, he issued an executive order that lifted restrictions on U.S. federal funding for research on human embryonic stem cells (ESCs). The advocates of stem cell research celebrated the issuance of the order. However, the order is sparsely worded and leaves the details to be worked out by the National Institutes of Health.

In "Distinctly Human: The When, Where & How of Life's Beginnings," John Collins Harvey (*Commonweal*, February 8, 2002) asserts that the human embryo is a living human being from the moment of conception. As such, it should never be used as an object or considered as a means to an end. It should not be killed so that parts of it can be used for the benefit of another person. That sentiment is echoed by William Sanders in "Embryology: Inconvenient Facts," *First Things* (December 2004), who believes that adult human stems cells have been proven to have great value in the invention of new and better medical treatments, but the value of ESCs is theoretical and cannot justify killing an embryo. In "Many Say Adult Stem Cell Reports Overplayed," *Journal of the American Medical Association* (2001), the value of adult stem cells is debated.

Create Central

www.mhhe.com/create central

Additional Resources

Hug, K. & Hermerén, G. (2011). Do we still need human embryonic stem cells for stem cell-based therapies? Epistemic and ethical aspects. *Stem Cell Reviews & Reports, 7*(4), 761–774.

Kolios, G. & Moodley, Y. (2012). Introduction to stem cells and regenerative medicine. *Respiration, 85*(1), 3–10.

Mitrečić, D. & Šepac, A. (2013). Current perspective of stem cells in the treatment of heart failure. *Cardiologia Croatica, 8*(1/2), 40–43.

Mukhopadhyay, C. S., Tokas, J., & Mathur, P. D. (2011). Prospects and ethical concerns of embryonic stem cells research—a review. *Veterinary World, 4*(6), 281–286.

Robertson, J. A. (2010). Embryo stem cell research: Ten years of controversy. *Journal of Law, Medicine & Ethics, 38*(2), 191–203.

Internet References . . .

International Society for Stem Cell Research

www.isscr.org/

National Bioethics Advisory Commission: Publications

www.bioethics.gov/pubs.html

U.S. National Institutes of Health (NIH)

www.nih.gov

Unit 3

Mind–Body Relationships

Humans have long sought to extend life, eliminate disease, and prevent sickness. In modern times, people depend on technology to develop creative and innovative ways to improve health, extend life, and treat disease. However, as true cures for diseases such as AIDS, cancer, and heart disease continue to elude scientists and doctors, many people question whether or not modern medicine has reached a plateau in improving health. As a result, over the last decade, an emphasis has been placed on prevention as a way to maintain wellness. Prevention includes maintaining a healthy mind, body, and spirit. In addition, the theme of healing prayer is very common in the history of spirituality.

Selected, Edited, and with Issue Framing Material by:
Eileen Daniel, *SUNY College at Brockport*

ISSUE

Should Addiction to Drugs Be Labeled a Brain Disease?

YES: **Alan I. Leshner,** from "Addiction Is a Brain Disease," *Issues in Science and Technology* (Spring 2001)

NO: **Alva Noë,** from "Addiction Is Not a Disease of the Brain," *National Public Radio* (September 9, 2011)

Learning Outcomes
After reading this issue, you should be able to: • Discuss the causes of drug addiction.   • Discuss the argument that addiction is a disease and not a behavioral issue.   • Understand the various types of treatment for drug and alcohol addiction.

ISSUE SUMMARY

YES: Alan I. Leshner, director of the National Institute on Drug Abuse at the National Institutes of Health, believes that addiction to drugs and alcohol is not a behavioral condition but a treatable disease.

NO: Professor Alva Noë counters that addiction is a phenomenon that can only be understood in terms of the life choices, needs, and understanding of the whole person.

There are many different theories as to why some individuals become addicted to alcohol or other drugs. Historically, drug and alcohol dependency has been viewed as either a disease or a moral failing. In more recent years, other theories of addiction have been developed, including behavioral, genetic, socio-cultural, and psychological theories.

The view that drug addiction and alcoholism are moral failings maintains that abusing drugs is voluntary behavior that the user chooses to do. Users choose to over-indulge in such a way that they create suffering for themselves and others. American history is marked by repeated and failed government efforts to control this abuse by eliminating drug and alcohol use with legal sanctions, such as the enactment of Prohibition in the late 1920s and the punishment of alcoholics and drug users via jail sentences and fines. However, there seem to be several contradictions to this behavioral model of addiction. Addiction may be a complex condition that is caused by multiple factors, including environment, biology, and others. It is not totally clear that addiction is voluntary behavior. And from a historical perspective, punishing alcoholics and drug addicts has been ineffective.

In the United States today, the primary theory for understanding the causes of addiction is the disease model rather than the moral model. Borrowing from the modern mental health movement, addiction as a disease has been promoted by mental health advocates who tried to change the public's perception of severe mental illness. Diseases like bipolar disorder and schizophrenia were defined as the result of brain abnormalities rather than environmental factors or poor parenting. Likewise, addiction was not a moral weakness but a brain disorder that could be treated. In 1995 the National Institute of Drug Addiction (NIDA) supported the idea that drug addiction was a type of brain disorder. Following NIDA's support, the concept of addiction as a brain disease has become more widely accepted.

This model has been advocated by the medical and alcohol treatment communities as well as self-help groups such as Alcoholics Anonymous and Narcotics Anonymous. The disease model implies that addiction is not the result of voluntary behavior or lack of self-control; it is caused by biological factors, which are treatable. While there are somewhat different interpretations of this theory, it generally refers to addiction as an organic brain syndrome with biological and genetic origins rather than voluntary and behavioral origins.

Alan Leshner believes that taking drugs causes changes in neurons in the central nervous system that compel the individual to use drugs. These neurological changes, which are not reversible, force addicts to continue to take drugs. Professor Alva Noë disagrees. He believes that most addicts are not innocent victims of chronic disease but individuals who are responsible for their illness and recovery.

YES ⤶

Alan I. Leshner

Addiction Is a Brain Disease

The United States is stuck in its drug abuse metaphors and in polarized arguments about them. Everyone has an opinion. One side insists that we must control supply, the other that we must reduce demand. People see addiction as either a disease or as a failure of will. None of this bumpersticker analysis moves us forward. The truth is that we will make progress in dealing with drug issues only when our national discourse and our strategies are as complex and comprehensive as the problem itself.

A core concept that has been evolving with scientific advances over the past decade is that drug addiction is a brain disease that develops over time as a result of the initially voluntary behavior of using drugs. The consequence is virtually uncontrollable compulsive drug craving, seeking, and use that interferes with, if not destroys, an individual's functioning in the family and in society. This medical condition demands formal treatment.

We now know in great detail the brain mechanisms through which drugs acutely modify mood, memory, perception, and emotional states. Using drugs repeatedly over time changes brain structure and function in fundamental and long-lasting ways that can persist long after the individual stops using them. Addiction comes about through an array of neuroadaptive changes and the laying down and strengthening of new memory connections in various circuits in the brain. We do not yet know all the relevant mechanisms, but the evidence suggests that those long-lasting brain changes are responsible for the distortions of cognitive and emotional functioning that characterize addicts, particularly including the compulsion to use drugs that is the essence of addiction. It is as if drugs have highjacked the brain's natural motivational control circuits, resulting in drug use becoming the sole, or at least the top, motivational priority for the individual. Thus, the majority of the biomedical community now considers addiction, in its essence, to be a brain disease: a condition caused by persistent changes in brain structure and function.

This brain-based view of addiction has generated substantial controversy, particularly among people who seem able to think only in polarized ways. Many people erroneously still believe that biological and behavioral explanations are alternative or competing ways to understand phenomena, when in fact they are complementary and integratable. Modern science has taught that it is much too simplistic to set biology in opposition to behavior or to pit willpower against brain chemistry. Addiction involves inseparable biological and behavioral components. It is the quintessential biobehavioral disorder.

Many people also erroneously still believe that drug addiction is simply a failure of will or of strength of character. Research contradicts that position. However, the recognition that addiction is a brain disease does not mean that the addict is simply a hapless victim. Addiction begins with the voluntary behavior of using drugs, and addicts must participate in and take some significant responsibility for their recovery. Thus, having this brain disease does not absolve the addict of responsibility for his or her behavior, but it does explain why an addict cannot simply stop using drugs by sheer force of will alone. It also dictates a much more sophisticated approach to dealing with the array of problems surrounding drug abuse and addiction in our society.

The Essence of Addiction

The entire concept of addiction has suffered greatly from imprecision and misconception. In fact, if it were possible, it would be best to start all over with some new, more neutral term. The confusion comes about in part because of a now archaic distinction between whether specific drugs are "physically" or "psychologically" addicting. The distinction historically revolved around whether or not dramatic physical withdrawal symptoms occur when an individual stops taking a drug; what we in the field now call "physical dependence."

However, 20 years of scientific research has taught that focusing on this physical versus psychological distinction is off the mark and a distraction from the real issues. From both clinical and policy perspectives, it actually does not matter very much what physical withdrawal symptoms occur. Physical dependence is not that important, because even the dramatic withdrawal symptoms of heroin and alcohol addiction can now be easily managed with appropriate medications. Even more important, many of the most dangerous and addicting drugs, including methamphetamine and crack cocaine, do not produce very severe physical dependence symptoms upon withdrawal.

What really matters most is whether or not a drug causes what we now know to be the essence of addiction:

Leshner, Alan I. From *California Society of Addiction Medicine Legislative Day Information Book,* February 1, 2006, pp. 92–98. Published by the National Institute on Drug Abuse.

uncontrollable, compulsive drug craving, seeking, and use, even in the face of negative health and social consequences. This is the crux of how the Institute of Medicine, the American Psychiatric Association, and the American Medical Association define addiction and how we all should use the term. It is really only this compulsive quality of addiction that matters in the long run to the addict and to his or her family and that should matter to society as a whole. Compulsive craving that overwhelms all other motivations is the root cause of the massive health and social problems associated with drug addiction. In updating our national discourse on drug abuse, we should keep in mind this simple definition: Addiction is a brain disease expressed in the form of compulsive behavior. Both developing and recovering from it depend on biology, behavior, and social context.

It is also important to correct the common misimpression that drug use, abuse, and addiction are points on a single continuum along which one slides back and forth over time, moving from user to addict, then back to occasional user, then back to addict. Clinical observation and more formal research studies support the view that, once addicted, the individual has moved into a different state of being. It is as if a threshold has been crossed. Very few people appear able to successfully return to occasional use after having been truly addicted. Unfortunately, we do not yet have a clear biological or behavioral marker of that transition from voluntary drug use to addiction. However, a body of scientific evidence is rapidly developing that points to an array of cellular and molecular changes in specific brain circuits. Moreover, many of these brain changes are common to all chemical addictions, and some also are typical of other compulsive behaviors such as pathological overeating.

Addiction should be understood as a chronic recurring illness. Although some addicts do gain full control over their drug use after a single treatment episode, many have relapses. Repeated treatments become necessary to increase the intervals between and diminish the intensity of relapses, until the individual achieves abstinence.

The complexity of this brain disease is not atypical, because virtually no brain diseases are simply biological in nature and expression. All, including stroke, Alzheimer's disease, schizophrenia, and clinical depression, include some behavioral and social aspects. What may make addiction seem unique among brain diseases, however, is that it does begin with a clearly voluntary behavior—the initial decision to use drugs. Moreover, not everyone who ever uses drugs goes on to become addicted. Individuals differ substantially in how easily and quickly they become addicted and in their preferences for particular substances. Consistent with the biobehavioral nature of addiction, these individual differences result from a combination of environmental and biological, particularly genetic, factors. In fact, estimates are that between 50 and 70 percent of the variability in susceptibility to becoming addicted can be accounted for by genetic factors.

Over time the addict loses substantial control over his or her initially voluntary behavior, and it becomes compulsive. For many people these behaviors are truly uncontrollable, just like the behavioral expression of any other brain disease. Schizophrenics cannot control their hallucinations and delusions. Parkinson's patients cannot control their trembling. Clinically depressed patients cannot voluntarily control their moods. Thus, once one is addicted, the characteristics of the illness—and the treatment approaches—are not that different from most other brain diseases. No matter how one develops an illness, once one has it, one is in the diseased state and needs treatment.

Moreover, voluntary behavior patterns are, of course, involved in the etiology and progression of many other illnesses, albeit not all brain diseases. Examples abound, including hypertension, arteriosclerosis and other cardiovascular diseases, diabetes, and forms of cancer in which the onset is heavily influenced by the individual's eating, exercise, smoking, and other behaviors.

Addictive behaviors do have special characteristics related to the social contexts in which they originate. All of the environmental cues surrounding initial drug use and development of the addiction actually become "conditioned" to that drug use and are thus critical to the development and expression of addiction. Environmental cues are paired in time with an individual's initial drug use experiences and, through classical conditioning, take on conditioned stimulus properties. When those cues are present at a later time, they elicit anticipation of a drug experience and thus generate tremendous drug craving. Cue-induced craving is one of the most frequent causes of drug use relapses, even after long periods of abstinence, independently of whether drugs are available.

The salience of environmental or contextual cues helps explain why reentry to one's community can be so difficult for addicts leaving the controlled environments of treatment or correctional settings and why aftercare is so essential to successful recovery. The person who became addicted in the home environment is constantly exposed to the cues conditioned to his or her initial drug use, such as the neighborhood where he or she hung out, drug-using buddies, or the lamppost where he or she bought drugs. Simple exposure to those cues automatically triggers craving and can lead rapidly to relapses. This is one reason why someone who apparently overcame drug cravings while in prison or residential treatment could quickly revert to drug use upon returning home. In fact, one of the major goals of drug addiction treatment is to teach addicts how to deal with the cravings caused by inevitable exposure to these conditioned cues.

Implications

Understanding addiction as a brain disease has broad and significant implications for the public perception of addicts and their families, for addiction treatment practice, and for some aspects of public policy. On the other hand, this biomedical view of addiction does not speak directly to and is unlikely to bear significantly on many other issues, including specific strategies for controlling the supply of drugs and whether initial drug use should be legal or not. Moreover, the brain disease model of addiction does not address the question of whether specific drugs of abuse can also be potential medicines. Examples abound of drugs that can be both highly addicting and extremely effective medicines. The best-known example is the appropriate use of morphine as a treatment for pain. Nevertheless, a number of practical lessons can be drawn from the scientific understanding of addiction.

It is no wonder addicts cannot simply quit on their own. They have an illness that requires biomedical treatment. People often assume that because addiction begins with a voluntary behavior and is expressed in the form of excess behavior, people should just be able to quit by force of will alone. However, it is essential to understand when dealing with addicts that we are dealing with individuals whose brains have been altered by drug use. They need drug addiction treatment. We know that, contrary to common belief, very few addicts actually do just stop on their own. Observing that there are very few heroin addicts in their 50s or 60s, people frequently ask what happened to those who were heroin addicts 30 years ago, assuming that they must have quit on their own. However, longitudinal studies find that only a very small fraction actually quit on their own. The rest have either been successfully treated, are currently in maintenance treatment, or (for about half) are dead. Consider the example of smoking cigarettes: Various studies have found that between 3 and 7 percent of people who try to quit on their own each year actually succeed. Science has at last convinced the public that depression is not just a lot of sadness; that depressed individuals are in a different brain state and thus require treatment to get their symptoms under control. The same is true for schizophrenic patients. It is time to recognize that this is also the case for addicts.

The role of personal responsibility is undiminished but clarified. Does having a brain disease mean that people who are addicted no longer have any responsibility for their behavior or that they are simply victims of their own genetics and brain chemistry? Of course not. Addiction begins with the voluntary behavior of drug use, and although genetic characteristics may predispose individuals to be more or less susceptible to becoming addicted, genes do not doom one to become an addict. This is one major reason why efforts to prevent drug use are so vital to any comprehensive strategy to deal with the nation's drug problems. Initial drug use is a voluntary, and therefore preventable, behavior.

Moreover, as with any illness, behavior becomes a critical part of recovery. At a minimum, one must comply with the treatment regimen, which is harder than

it sounds. Treatment compliance is the biggest cause of relapses for all chronic illnesses, including asthma, diabetes, hypertension, and addiction. Moreover, treatment compliance rates are no worse for addiction than for these other illnesses, ranging from 30 to 50 percent. Thus, for drug addiction as well as for other chronic diseases, the individual's motivation and behavior are clearly important parts of success in treatment and recovery.

Implications for treatment approaches and treatment expectations. Maintaining this comprehensive biobehavioral understanding of addiction also speaks to what needs to be provided in drug treatment programs. Again, we must be careful not to pit biology against behavior. The National Institute on Drug Abuse's recently published Principles of Effective Drug Addiction Treatment provides a detailed discussion of how we must treat all aspects of the individual, not just the biological component or the behavioral component. As with other brain diseases such as schizophrenia and depression, the data show that the best drug addiction treatment approaches attend to the entire individual, combining the use of medications, behavioral therapies, and attention to necessary social services and rehabilitation. These might include such services as family therapy to enable the patient to return to successful family life, mental health services, education and vocational training, and housing services.

That does not mean, of course, that all individuals need all components of treatment and all rehabilitation services. Another principle of effective addiction treatment is that the array of services included in an individual's treatment plan must be matched to his or her particular set of needs. Moreover, since those needs will surely change over the course of recovery, the array of services provided will need to be continually reassessed and adjusted.

What to do with addicted criminal offenders. One obvious conclusion is that we need to stop simplistically viewing criminal justice and health approaches as incompatible opposites. The practical reality is that crime and drug addiction often occur in tandem: Between 50 and 70 percent of arrestees are addicted to illegal drugs. Few citizens would be willing to relinquish criminal justice system control over individuals, whether they are addicted or not, who have committed crimes against others. Moreover, extensive real-life experience shows that if we simply incarcerate addicted offenders without treating them, their return to both drug use and criminality is virtually guaranteed.

A growing body of scientific evidence points to a much more rational and effective blended public health/public safety approach to dealing with the addicted offender. Simply summarized, the data show that if addicted offenders are provided with well-structured drug treatment while under criminal justice control, their recidivism rates can be reduced by 50 to 60 percent for subsequent drug use and by more than 40 percent for further criminal behavior. Moreover, entry into drug treatment need not be completely voluntary in order for it to work. In fact, studies suggest that increased pressure to stay in treatment—whether from the legal system or from family members or employers—actually increases the amount of time patients remain in treatment and improves their treatment outcomes.

Findings such as these are the underpinning of a very important trend in drug control strategies now being implemented in the United States and many foreign countries. For example, some 40 percent of prisons and jails in this country now claim to provide some form of drug treatment to their addicted inmates, although we do not know the quality of the treatment provided. Diversion to drug treatment programs as an alternative to incarceration is gaining popularity across the United States. The widely applauded growth in drug treatment courts over the past five years—to more than 400—is another successful example of the blending of public health and public safety approaches. These drug courts use a combination of criminal justice sanctions and drug use monitoring and treatment tools to manage addicted offenders.

Updating the Discussion

Understanding drug abuse and addiction in all their complexity demands that we rise above simplistic polarized thinking about drug issues. Addiction is both a public health and a public safety issue, not one or the other. We must deal with both the supply and the demand issues with equal vigor. Drug abuse and addiction are about both biology and behavior. One can have a disease and not be a hapless victim of it.

We also need to abandon our attraction to simplistic metaphors that only distract us from developing appropriate strategies. I, for one, will be in some ways sorry to see the War on Drugs metaphor go away, but go away it must. At some level, the notion of waging war is as appropriate for the illness of addiction as it is for our War on Cancer, which simply means bringing all forces to bear on the problem in a focused and energized way. But, sadly, this concept has been badly distorted and misused over time, and the War on Drugs never became what it should have been: the War on Drug Abuse and Addiction. Moreover, worrying about whether we are winning or losing this war has deteriorated to using simplistic and inappropriate measures such as counting drug addicts. In the end, it has only fueled discord. The War on Drugs metaphor has done nothing to advance the real conceptual challenges that need to be worked through.

I hope, though, that we will all resist the temptation to replace it with another catchy phrase that inevitably will devolve into a search for quick or easy-seeming solutions to our drug problems. We do not rely on simple metaphors or strategies to deal with our other major national problems such as education, health care, or national security.

We are, after all, trying to solve truly monumental, multidimensional problems on a national or even international scale. To devalue them to the level of slogans does our public an injustice and dooms us to failure.

Understanding the health aspects of addiction is in no way incompatible with the need to control the supply of drugs. In fact, a public health approach to stemming an epidemic or spread of a disease always focuses comprehensively on the agent, the vector, and the host. In the case of drugs of abuse, the agent is the drug, the host is the abuser or addict, and the vector for transmitting the illness is clearly the drug suppliers and dealers that keep the agent flowing so readily. Prevention and treatment are the strategies to help protect the host. But just as we must deal with the flies and mosquitoes that spread infectious diseases, we must directly address all the vectors in the drug-supply system.

In order to be truly effective, the blended public health/public safety approaches advocated here must be implemented at all levels of society—local, state, and national. All drug problems are ultimately local in character and impact, since they differ so much across geographic settings and cultural contexts, and the most effective solutions are implemented at the local level. Each community must work through its own locally appropriate antidrug implementation strategies, and those strategies must be just as comprehensive and science-based as those instituted at the state or national level.

The message from the now very broad and deep array of scientific evidence is absolutely clear. If we as a society ever hope to make any real progress in dealing with our drug problems, we are going to have to rise above moral outrage that addicts have "done it to themselves" and develop strategies that are as sophisticated and as complex as the problem itself. Whether addicts are "victims" or not, once addicted they must be seen as "brain disease patients."

Moreover, although our national traditions do argue for compassion for those who are sick, no matter how they contracted their illnesses, I recognize that many addicts have disrupted not only their own lives but those of their families and their broader communities, and thus do not easily generate compassion. However, no matter how one may feel about addicts and their behavioral histories, an extensive body of scientific evidence shows that approaching addiction as a treatable illness is extremely cost-effective, both financially and in terms of broader societal impacts such as family violence, crime, and other forms of social upheaval. Thus, it is clearly in everyone's interest to get past the hurt and indignation and slow the drain of drugs on society by enhancing drug use prevention efforts and providing treatment to all who need it.

ALAN I. LESHNER is the director of the National Institute on Drug Abuse.

Alva Noë

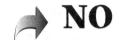 **NO**

Addiction Is Not a Disease of the Brain

Addiction has been moralized, medicalized, politicized, and criminalized.

And, of course, many of us are addicts, have been addicts or have been close to addicts. Addiction runs very hot as a theme.

Part of what makes addiction so compelling is that it forms a kind of conceptual/political crossroads for thinking about human nature. After all, to make sense of addiction we need to make sense of what it is to be an agent who acts, with values, in the face of consequences, under pressure, with compulsion, out of need and desire. One needs a whole philosophy to understand addiction.

Today I want to respond to readers who were outraged by my willingness even to question whether addiction is a disease of the brain.

Let us first ask: what makes something—a substance or an activity—addictive? Is there a property shared by all the things to which we can get addicted?

Unlikely. Addictive substances such as alcohol, heroin and nicotine are chemically distinct. Moreover, activities such as gambling, eating, sex—activities that are widely believed to be addictive—have no ingredients.

And yet it is remarkable—as Gene Heyman notes in his excellent book on addiction—that there are only 20 or so distinct activities and substances that produce addiction. There must be something in virtue of which these things, and these things alone, give rise to the distinctive pattern of use and abuse in the face of the medical, personal and legal perils that we know can stem from addiction.

What do gambling, sex, heroin and cocaine—and the other things that can addict us—have in common?

One strategy is to look not to the substances and activities themselves, but to the effects that they produce in addicts. And here neuroscience has delivered important insights.

If you feed an electrical wire through a rat's skull and onto a short dopamine release circuit that connects the VTA (ventral tegmental area) and the nucleus accumbens, and if you attach that wire to a lever-press, the rat will self-stimulate—press the lever to produce the increase in dopamine—and it will do so basically forever, forgoing food, sex, water and exercise. Addiction, it would seem, is produced by direct action on the brain!

And indeed, there is now a substantial body of evidence supporting the claim that all drugs or activities of abuse (as we can call them) have precisely this kind of effect on this dopamine neurochemical circuit.

When the American Society of Addiction Medicine recently declared addiction to be a brain disease their conclusion was based on findings like this. Addiction is an effect brought about in a neurochemical circuit in the brain. If true, this is important, for it means that if you want to treat addiction, you need to find ways to act on this neural substrate.

All the rest—the actual gambling or drug taking, the highs and lows, the stealing, lying and covering up, the indifference to work and incompetence in the workplace, the self-loathing and anxiety about getting high, or getting discovered, or about trying to stop, and the loss of friends and family, the life stories and personal and social pressures—all these are merely symptoms of the underlying neurological disease.

But not so fast. Consider:

All addictive drugs and activities elevate the dopamine release system. Such activation, we may say, is a necessary condition of addiction. But it is very doubtful that it is sufficient. Neuroscientists refer to the system in question as the "reward-reinforcement pathway" precisely because all rewarding activities, including nonaddictive ones like reading the comics on Sunday morning or fixing the leaky pipe in the basement, modulate its activity. Elevated activity in the reward-reinforcement pathway is a normal concomitant of healthy, nonaddictive, engaged life.

Neuroscientists like to say that addictive drugs and activities, but not the nonaddictive ones, "highjack" the reward-reinforcement pathway, they don't merely activate it. This is the real upshot of the rat example. The rat preferred lever-pressing to everything; it dis-valued everything in comparison with lever-pressing. And not because of the intrinsic value of lever-pressing, but because of the link artificially established between the lever-pressing and the dopamine release.

If this is right, then we haven't discovered, in the reward reinforcement system, a neurochemical signature of addiction. We haven't discovered the place where addiction happens in the brain. After all, the so-called highjacking of the reward system is not itself a neurochemical process; it is a process whereby neurochemical events get entrained within in a larger pattern of action and decision making.

Is addiction a disease of the brain? That's a bit like saying that eating is a phenomenon of the stomach. The stomach is an important part of the story. But don't forget the mouth, the intestines, the blood, and don't forget the hunger, and also the whole socially-sustained practice of producing, shopping for and cooking food.

And so with addiction. The neural events in VTA clearly belong to the underlying mechanisms of addiction. They are necessary, but not sufficient; they are only part of the story.

Remember: normally there is a dynamic quality to our actions and preferences, just as there is with those of rats. We enjoy exercising, but we soon get tired or bored. But rest, too, soon loses its appeal. We eat, and then we are sated. And then we are ready for the treadmill again. And so on. Things have gradually changing and complementary values. In addiction, this dynamic goes rigid. The addict's goal assumes a fixed value, and the value of everything shrinks to zero, and with terrible costs.

Our strategy was to look for systematic effects that all and only the addictive drugs and activities have on addicts. And we've found what we were looking for. The effects are behavioral and experiential. The things that addict us all produce a very distinctive breakdown in the organization of our preferences, actions and choices.

Is addiction a disease of the brain? This strikes me as a dubious falsification of what is, really, a phenomenon that can only be understood in terms of the life choices, needs and understanding of the whole person.

ALVA NOË is a professor of philosophy at the University of California, Berkeley. The main focus of his work is the theory of perception and consciousness. He earned a PhD from Harvard University.

EXPLORING THE ISSUE

Should Addiction to Drugs Be Labeled a Brain Disease?

Critical Thinking and Reflection

1. What are the root causes of drug and alcohol addiction?
2. What are the benefits to labeling addiction a brain disease?
3. Why could it be harmful to label addiction a brain disease?
4. Describe the types of treatment for alcohol and drug addiction.

Is There Common Ground?

One of the most valuable aspects of labeling addiction a disease is that it removes alcohol and drugs from the moral realm. It is proposed that addiction sufferers should be treated and helped, rather than scorned and punished. Though the moral model of addiction has by no means disappeared in the United States, today more resources are directed toward rehabilitation than punishment. Increasingly, it is being recognized and understood that fines, victim-blaming, and imprisonment do little to curb alcohol and drug addiction in society.

An article, "New Insights into the Genetics of Addiction" (*Nature Reviews Genetics*, April 2009) indicates that genetics contributes significantly to susceptibility to this disorder, but identification of vulnerable genes has lagged. In "It's Time for Addiction Science to Supersede Stigma" (*Science News*, November 8, 2009), the author discusses advances made in the scientific community in studying *addictions*, and says that people should regard drug addicts the same they regard other people with *brain diseases*. To do this, it should be recognized that *addictions* are a form of *brain disease*, and rather than blaming people for becoming addicted, energy should be spent on finding solutions.

Critics argue, however, that this belief either underemphasizes or ignores the impact of self-control, learned behaviors, and many other factors which lead to alcohol and drug abuse. Furthermore, most treatment programs in the United States are based on the concept of addiction as a brain disease, and most are considered to be generally ineffective when judged by their high relapse rates. Many researchers claim that advances in neuroscience are changing the way mental health issues such as addiction

are understood and addressed as brain diseases. While calling addiction a brain disease and medical condition legitimizes it, many scientists do not completely support this model.

It appears that the causes of addiction are complex and that brain, mind, and behavioral specialists are rethinking the whole notion of addiction. With input from neuroscience, biology, pharmacology, psychology, and genetics, they're questioning assumptions and identifying some common characteristics among addicts, which will, it is hoped, improve treatment outcomes and even prevent people from using drugs in the first place.

Create Central

www.mhhe.com/createcentral

Additional Resources

Alavi, S., Ferdosi, M., Jannatifard, F., Eslami, M., Alaghemandan, H., & Setare, M. (2012). Behavioral addiction versus substance addiction: Correspondence of psychiatric and psychological views. *International Journal of Preventive Medicine, 3*(4), 290–294.

Karim, R. & Chaudhri, P. (2012). Behavioral addictions: An overview. *Journal of Psychoactive Drugs, 44*(1), 5–17.

Miller, W. (2011). *Treating addictions: A guide for professionals.* New York, NY: Guilford Press.

Vrecko, S. (2010). Birth of a brain disease: Science, the state and addiction neuropolitics. *History of the Human Sciences, 23*(4), 52–67.

Internet References . . .

American Psychological Association (APA)

Offers information on a variety of mental health topics with multiple links.

www.apa.org

National Institutes of Health: National Institute on Drug Abuse

Offers information on drug abuse directed at a variety of constituents: professionals, researchers, teachers, parents, students, and young adults.

www.drugabuse.gov/nidahome.html

Web of Addictions

The Web of Addictions site is dedicated to providing accurate information about alcohol and other drug addictions. The site was developed to provide data about drugs of abuse and to provide a resource for teachers, students, and others who needed factual information about abused drugs.

www.well.com/user/woa

Selected, Edited, and with Issue Framing Material by:
Eileen Daniel, *SUNY College at Brockport*

ISSUE

Do Religion and Prayer Benefit Health?

YES: **Thomas J. Cottle**, from "Our Thoughts and Our Prayers," *The Antioch Review* (Spring 2010)

NO: **Michael Shermer**, from "Prayer and Healing: The Verdict Is in and the Results Are Null," *Skeptic* (vol. 12, no. 3, 2006)

Learning Outcomes
After reading this issue, you should be able to: • Discuss the benefits of prayer for those suffering from an illness. • Discuss the argument that the relationship between prayer and health cannot adequately be measured. • Discuss the ways in which prayer could be used as part of a treatment program.

ISSUE SUMMARY

YES: Psychologist and educator Thomas J. Cottle believes that prayer can fill patients with a spirit of security when confronted with illness.

NO: Author Michael Shermer contends that intercessory prayer offered by strangers on the health and recovery of patients undergoing coronary bypass surgery is ineffective. He also addresses flaws in studies showing a relationship between prayer and health.

Practitioners of holistic medicine believe that people must take responsibility for their own health by practicing healthy behaviors and maintaining positive attitudes instead of relying on health providers. They also believe that physical disease has behavioral, psychological, and spiritual components. These spiritual components can be explained by the relationship between beliefs, mental attitude, and the immune system. Until recently, few studies existed to prove a relationship between religion and health.

Much of modern medicine has spent the past century ridding itself of mysticism and relying on science. Twenty years ago, no legitimate physician would have dared to study the effects of religion on disease. Recently, however, at the California Pacific Medical Center in San Francisco, California, Elisabeth Targ, clinical director of psychosocial oncology research, has recruited 20 faith healers to determine if prayer can affect the outcome of disease. Targ states that her preliminary results are encouraging. In addition to Targ's study, other research has shown that religion and spirituality can help determine

health and well-being. According to a 1995 investigation at Dartmouth College, one of the strongest predictors of success after open-heart surgery was the level of comfort patients derived from religion and spirituality. Other recent studies have linked health with church attendance, religious commitment, and spirituality. There are, however, other studies that have not been as successful; a recent one involving the effects of prayer on alcoholics found no relationship.

Can spirituality or prayer in relation to health and healing be explained scientifically? Prayer or a sense of spirituality may function in a similar manner as stress management or relaxation. Spirituality or prayer may cause the release of hormones that help lower blood pressure or produce other benefits. Although science may never be able to exactly determine the benefits of spirituality, it does appear to help some people.

In the YES and NO selections, Thomas J. Cottle states that prayer can have a significant influence over the body. Michael Shermer argues that religious prayer does not heal the sick and the studies showing the relationship between religion and healing are flawed.

YES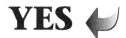

Thomas J. Cottle

Our Thoughts and Our Prayers

Little grates on me as much as the clichés hurled again and again on television. Families in mourning have to hear about this closure business, whatever it means. Or those ubiquitous questions, When you heard that your parents had died, what was going through your mind? When the flood destroyed your community, what was that like?

Another one that has always rankled me is the predictable statement following the announcement of a death: "Our thoughts and prayers go out to the families." One would think that intelligent people could come up with something more thoughtful, sensitive, caring. But then the words were addressed to me.

I felt obliged to tell a patient of mine that I would have to call him regarding our next appointment as I was about to undergo surgery and didn't know how long a recuperation period I was facing. Seemingly without thinking, he looked at me and said softly, "I'll pray for you, Doc." His words had no sooner filled the air than I felt the tears. Apparently, the prayers of this man were exactly what I wanted. A devout Catholic tells me, a Jew, he will pray for me, and at once I am filled with some peculiar spirit of security, or is it a release from something? A release, perhaps, from a lifetime void of the spiritual? Normally I will think, pray what you wish, my friend, but just don't mention the name of your Lord. But this time that thought never emerged, and it was not because he was my patient; I had no desire to censure a single word, a single holy name. I felt filled up, somehow, with the mere statement that he would pray for me. And I have no idea what praying actually means, much less whether there really is something called a power that emanates from this activity.

In the hospital, on the morning following surgery, I obeyed orders and walked the floor. Around and around the nurses' station, pitiful laps in corridors that remind one of anything but a walking track. But it is here that one meets the other lap walkers, the other post-surgery folks. And the talk goes right to the heart of the medical matter, names rarely exchanged. This one has cells dying in his prostate, each cellular death causing exquisite pain. I ask about his PSA readings and hear a number that astonishes me; it is in the high fifties. I have a macabre urge to tell him if it gets to sixty he might want to sell. And this one, a strong looking man pushing an IV stand in front of him, was doing so well, even with a blood thinner issue

from a previous cardiac condition threatening his surgery and recovery that the doctors sent him home. Three hours later he couldn't eliminate fluids and here he was back on the same floor, walking the track.

Then I met Sammy, a man in his early sixties who told me he had survived prostate cancer, colon cancer, and was living with diabetes. He had just been operated on yet again for another problem. Sammy is an educator, a father of six, a truly good man, and a man of God. "God is good," he said, seemingly a hundred times during our laps together. "He looks out for us; He has shaped the whole thing." Prostate cancer, colon cancer, diabetes, another operation, God is good. God was still good when later that first post-operative day Sammy suddenly couldn't eliminate fluids and had to be catheterized. Of course God was still good. The words are intended merely as a pronouncement of healing.

My assurance to Sammy that he was going to be fine paled next to his spiritually founded assurances. "God doesn't want me yet. Nor you. He wants you," Sammy said, "to keep educating people." And do you know, when he said those words, I believed him. I believed him not in the spirit of, well, you have to have faith in something and I don't see any rabbi with an enlarged prostate walking the corridor. I believed him as if a scientist had recited unalloyed scientific facts to me. Fact One: God doesn't want you. Fact Two: Water is two parts hydrogen, one part oxygen.

Sammy grew tired and I walked him to his room where slowly, laboriously, he climbed onto his bed. He knew I was there watching him. "I will come to you later," he whispered. "We'll pray together." Once again, I felt comforted. I wanted that praying together moment more than I wanted a sumptuous meal. I hoped he would remember his promise.

Americans, I have learned recently, pray a great deal. Seventy-seven percent of people pray outside of any religious service. Even people who don't believe in God pray. They may even pray all the time. Inexact, the numbers coming from a national poll, it is strange to think that so many people call themselves spiritual, not necessarily religious.

Two-thirds of the people in the poll said they pray because it makes them feel secure, comforted, hopeful. Whereas twenty-one percent reported that they pray they might possess material things, seventy-two percent pray for the well-being of others. Fewer people, actually, are attending religious services now that they are caught up in a strangling recession, but still they pray. "Our thoughts and prayers go out to the families."

The little I have read offers mixed reviews on the subject of whether praying for another actually makes a difference. Some research alleges that prayer is so powerful it affects even those who have no knowledge anyone is praying for them. Other research suggests that if you think it works then it works. And still other research cannot find a shred of evidence that prayer does anything other than gratify the person praying. I don't know what to think. No, that's not true; I do know one thing. I know my patient and Sammy prayed for me, believed in their prayers, and believed, moreover, that their prayers would help me, not just them. "I'll pray for you, Doc," and "I will come to your room and we will pray together," I choose to believe, were proffered as gifts, pure, simple gifts, one human to another. There wasn't a single shard of selfishness, I choose to believe, in either of these utterances.

Prayer, evidently, is about contemplation, philosophical, theological, personal. It is not about conversation. In some corners of the theological world, as, for example, in the mysticism of the Kabbalah, reality itself is meant to be altered, restructured by prayer. And if the universe, the very fabric of creation, is to be repaired by prayer, then why not the single self?

It is written by philosophers and psychologists that identity, whatever is meant by that term, is the *sine qua non* of human nature. Our subjective experiencing of the world, our so-called experiential knowledge, our ability to genuinely understand our own selves, much less have empathy for the selves of others, all are part of this identity business. Can we recognize our selves, psychologists ask, and is there some sub-set of experiences that makes us feel as though we are acting genuinely, or authentically?

Many people actually are able to describe that event or moment when they truly felt they had become the person they were meant to be. As Karl Jaspers wrote, these must be moments when they have a stake in what is happening. It is not too different from the great drama that inevitably finds characters with huge stakes in the outcome of the plot. Perhaps it is in periods of illness, or recovery, when we beg—or is it pray?—to transform situations, transform reality, when we are most likely to turn to prayer. Perhaps we feel we are losing something, something appears to be slipping away from us, and all that is left is to redefine reality or turn to some activity that convinces us that we still maintain ownership of the situation. Needless to say, our self, or more accurately our sense of self, always remains center stage.

In a sense, the self is little more than a theory, or a narrative, that we constantly construct out of our thoughts and feelings, if in fact we can even separate these two activities. Ceaselessly, we look outside ourselves, often using people as mirrors, as Jacques Lacan wrote, and inside ourselves to formulate this mutable theory that appears to come to us replete with all sorts of assessments and testable hypotheses. Seemingly, we cannot inhibit our urge to make sense of our worlds, and our selves. Rollo May postulated that the notion of repression refers to an inability or unwillingness to become aware of our self, containing as it does our authentic potentials. In a word, if the self represents a mediator between a person and the situation in which he is embedded, like an illness, then perhaps prayer is the method of communication for this mediation.

But prayer seems to require another soul. It evokes in us that sense of needing to speak to someone, or at least know that someone might hear our entreaties. We wonder, perhaps, whether we are even entitled to have our thoughts and feelings if someone is no longer present to hear them. It is often through prayer that we imagine that we can shape some small piece of our reality and thereby regain a sense of worth, competence, or agency. In some instances, and I believe I experienced this, the prayer reminds me that I am still alive; there is still hope upon which to draw life. Dear Someone: Please let my narrative continue. Please let me know that even in illness I may remain somewhat recognizable. Dare I ask to be perceived as distinctive? Is anyone there?

We change, and the landscape changes, and rarely do we experience these changes more vividly than when we enter hospitals. Both our illness and the hospital setting encompass us. Here we are, precisely as Jaspers described, rooted in the world of illness and the treatment, a world that feels simultaneously surreal and infinitely practical. We reflect on it, we pray on it; we cannot deny the utterly real constituents of it. We are defined, in part, by our illness, by our healers, by technology, and by our abilities to draw from what Martha Nussbaum has called our narrative imaginations. Our personal stories, one might say, have taken unpredictable, albeit not wholly unfamiliar turns. We know these stories from others, and we perhaps have always dreaded the moment when these narratives would be about us.

Then suddenly we are members of a new club, a new totality, a new historic unity dominated ironically, not by fellow members, but by ideas. If Jaspers remains a reasonable guide, we have entered the spiritual mode of encompassing; we have entered the realm of the transcendent wherein we exist as beings beyond all objectivity. As I say, it is not unfamiliar territory to us; through art, morality, religion, fantasy, we have been here before. What makes this moment unique is that it has been launched by illness and surgical invasion.

In turning my body over to the surgeon, an act occurring, moreover, during a protracted period of unconsciousness that I shall not remember, I am acknowledging what is labeled the boundary experience. I cannot affect this experience; I cannot influence it. I am left only to suffer, struggle, and pray. I can make it lucid only to myself. No matter the fright, no matter the dread, I feel required to keep my eyes wide open, Sometimes I may achieve transcendence through knowledge, sometimes, as the existentialists write, I can only hope to grasp it through my being, for it forever lies outside my sphere of influence. The meanings are something other than myself, more than mere expressions of myself, more than mere projections of myself. They push me toward meanings outside of myself, like the meaning of death.

But to give life meaning, I must transcend the limits of my physical life, which means my illness and its attendant treatment. I cannot allow myself to once again become the adolescent wondering whether he might live forever. I cannot let myself grapple with that question of whether I will still be, somehow, after life. Or can I? I must recognize, however, that in transcendence, arrived at in part through prayer, I may just have urged my self to reach the core of authentic resilience. I convince myself that I am back creating a trajectory for my life. I am back at work on the narrative that was interrupted by illness, and my fright. Choice and will have been part of my activity, and hence through prayer I feel a certain sense that the power of agency has returned. Or is it that I experience agency as never before?

Thrown into the realm of the spiritual, I pray. One way or another, as Robert Kegan has written, I must make meaning of my illness and treatment, or at least find some context where I imagine, or pray, that a meaning may emerge. When the shallow life doesn't work, Abraham Maslow taught, there occurs a call to fundamentals. But these fundamentals refer to the experience of being. Said simply, fundamentals make us aware of our very being, if we dare to cease our need to constantly evaluate or criticize, and instead remain vulnerable to the world around us, and within us. Prayer, somehow, aids in this effort.

So now I wonder, do I require these experiences, must I grow ill, must I face death, or the dread of it, merely to encounter the transcendent, and hence my real self? William James was right: these sorts of prayerful contemplations demand supreme mental effort. It isn't at all easy to insist that one's mind attend and hold fast to the boundary situation. It isn't easy to keep one's eyes wide open. How ironic that in some mysterious manner, I feel obliged to close my eyes in prayer in order to achieve a state of mind that will allow me to reopen them. It has become evident that my praying is also a way of offering consent to a particular reality. It is the best I can do, apparently, in wishing to become heroic. Through prayer I imagine that I have launched myself into what Carl Rogers called the stream of life. I have chosen not to surrender, but to become. Which in part means that I am not shaped even by seemingly implacable reality. Prayer, I have convinced myself, is not merely a coping mechanism; it is a mode of being that protects me. It ignites resilience.

The self, Robert Nozick wrote, is in part constituted by its process of change. It is not simply influenced by the world; it changes and ignites changes and then appears to run itself according to these changes. In a word, it dwells in its own capacity to change. Nozick believed that we aim our selves at developing themselves. We long to have our deepest parts connect with, or at least resonate to, what we imagine to be the highest things there are, thereby rendering us the highest things that we can be. This may very well be what we seek through prayer, realizing it is only the medium of prayer that will yield this prize. In fact, we may well be performing at the highest level, and hence feel in touch with our most authentic self precisely when we experience the resiliency of transcendence offered up by prayer. For it is in this act of prayer that we imagine we have reached the highest order of our narratives, and hence confronted the outline of the divine. How precious, therefore, the opportunity provided by adversity.

Sammy did remember. I stopped by his room, the light dim, the ambience antiseptic. He struggled to get out of bed disregarding my protestation. Near the door, he put his arm over my shoulder, held me close, and closed his eyes. I put my arm around his big back, feeling his skin through the opening in his hospital gown. I can't remember, precisely, what he asked of his Lord, but clearly he was urging a power he so trusts to look out for a man he had met, what, three hours before. He was petitioning God, entreating God in my behalf. As he spoke, I wondered how I would react when, ineluctably, he would speak the name of his God. And then I stopped wondering and let his words, how I dread this phrase, flow into me. "I ask this for Tom in the spirit of our Lord Jesus Christ."

We just stood there, the door to the corridor wide open, holding one another. I think I probably was praying, pitiful as it sounds, that his prayers, his acts of interceding, would make a difference. Probably I was praying that I needed his words to heal me as badly as I needed the skills and demonstration of care from the surgeon, residents, and nurses. Count me among the two-thirds of the people in the poll who said they pray because it makes them feel secure, comforted, hopeful. Perhaps I should worship the God Sammy.

But now, as I end, I fear that it can be said that my words here contain clichés as jaded and empty as "Our thoughts and prayers go out to the families." Still, I choose to believe, once again, that both Sammy and my patient clearly considered their prayers to be the most powerful acts they could perform in my behalf. Not because they were founded in religion, nor in ritualistic behavior that has been emulated for centuries, but because, in the same way that blood carries oxygen to the cells, prayers carry love to and from the soul. In fact, merely to open myself to my patient and Sammy was to give permission to entreat my own soul to be acknowledged, then nourished. And yes, I did notice that I commenced a sentence that prayer opens the soul with the words *in fact*.

Thomas J. Cottle is a sociologist and licensed clinical psychologist and professor of education at Boston University. He holds a PhD from the University of Chicago.

Michael Shermer

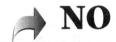 **NO**

Prayer and Healing: The Verdict Is in and the Results Are Null

In a long-awaited comprehensive scientific study on the effects of intercessory prayer on the health and recovery of 1,802 patients undergoing coronary bypass surgery in six different hospitals, prayers offered by strangers had no effect. In fact, contrary to common belief, patients who knew they were being prayed for had a higher rate of postoperative complications such as abnormal heart rhythms, possibly the result of anxiety caused by learning that they were being prayed for and thus their condition was more serious than anticipated.

The study, which cost $2.4 million (mast of which came from the John Templeton Foundation), was begun almost a decade ago and was directed by Harvard University Medical School cardiologist Dr. Herbert Benson and published in *The American Heart Journal*. It was by far the most rigorous and comprehensive study on the effects of intercessory prayer on the health and recovery of patients ever conducted. In addition to the numerous methodological flaws in the previous research corrected for in the Benson study. Dr. Richard Sloan, a professor of behavioral medicine at Columbia and author of the forthcoming book, *Blind Faith: The Unholy Alliance of Religion and Medicine*, explained: "The problem with studying religion scientifically is that you do violence to the phenomenon by reducing it to basic elements that can be quantified, and that makes for bad science and bad religion."

The 1,802 patients were divided into three groups, two of which were prayed for by members of three congregations: St. Paul's Monastery in St. Paul, MN; the Community of Teresian Carmelites in Worcester, MA; and Silent Unity, a Missouri prayer ministry near Kansas City, MO. The prayers were allowed to pray in their own manner, but they were instructed to include the following phrase in their prayers: "for a successful surgery with a quick, healthy recovery and no complications." Prayers began the night before the surgery and continued daily for two weeks after. Half the prayer-recipient patients were told that they were being prayed for while the other half were told that they might or might not receive prayers. The researchers monitored the patients for 30 days after the operations.

Results showed no statistically significant differences between the prayed-for and non-prayed-for groups. Although the following findings were not statistically significant, 59% of patients who knew that they were being prayed for suf-

fered complications, compared with 51% of those who were uncertain whether they were being prayed for or not; and 18% in the uninformed prayer group suffered major complications such as heart attack or stroke, compared with 13% in the group that received no prayers.

This study is particularly significant because Herbert Benson has long been sympathetic to the possibility that intercessory prayer can positively influence the health of patients. His team's rigorous methodologies overcame the numerous flaws that called into question previously published studies. The most commonly cited study in support of the connection between prayer and healing is Randolph C. Byrd's "Positive Therapeutic Effects of Intercessory Prayer in a Coronory Care Unit Population," *Southern Medical Journal* 81 (1998): 826–829. The two best studies on the methodological problems with prayer and healing are the following: Richard Sloan, E. Bagiella, and T. Powell, 1999. "Religion, Spirituality, and Medicine," *The Lancet*, Feb. 20, Vol. 353: 664–667; and: John T. Chibnall, Joseph M. Jeral, Michael Cerullo, 2001. "Experiments on Distant Intercessory Prayer," *Archives of Internal Medicine*, Nov. 26, Vol. 161: 2529–2536. . . .

The Most Significant Flaws in All Such Studies Include the Following:

1. *Fraud.* In 2001, the *Journal of Reproductive Medicine* published a study by three Columbia University researchers claiming that prayer for women undergoing in-vitro fertilization resulted in a pregnancy rate of 50%, double that of women who did not receive prayer. Media coverage was extensive. ABC News medical correspondent Dr. Timothy Johnson, for example, reported, "A new study on the power of prayer over pregnancy reports surprising results; but many physicians remain skeptical." One of those skeptics was University of California Clinical Professor of Gynecology and Obstetrics Bruce Flamm, who not only found numerous methodological errors in the experiment, but also discovered that one of the study's authors, Daniel Wirth (AKA "John Wayne Truelove"), is not an M.D., but an M.S. in parapsychology who has since been indicted on felony charges

for mail fraud and theft, for which he pleaded guilty. The other two authors have refused comment, and after three years of inquiries from Flamm the journal removed the study from its website and Columbia University has launched an investigation.

2. *Lack of Controls.* Many of these studies failed to control for such intervening variables as age, sex, education, ethnicity, socioeconomic status, marital standing, degree of religiosity, and the fact that most religions have sanctions against such behaviors as sexual promiscuity, alcohol and drug abuse, and smoking. When such variables are controlled for, the formerly significant results disappear. One study on recovery from hip surgery in elderly women failed to control for age; another study on church attendance and illness recovery did not consider that people in poorer health are less likely to attend church; a related study failed to control for levels of exercise.

3. *Outcome differences.* In one of the most highly publicized studies of cardiac patients prayed for by born-again Christians, 29 outcome variables were measured but on only six did the prayed-for group show improvement. In related studies, different outcome measures were significant. To be meaningful, the same measures need to be significant across studies, because if enough outcomes are measured some will show significant correlations by chance.

4. *Selective Reporting.* In several studies on the relationship between religiosity and mortality (religious people allegedly live longer), a number of religious variables were used, but only those with significant correlations were reported. Meanwhile, other studies using the same religiosity variables found different correlations and, of course, only reported those. The rest were filed away in the drawer of non-significant findings. When all variables are factored in together, religiosity and mortality show no relationship.

5. *Operational definitions.* When experimenting on the effects of prayer, what, precisely, is being studied? For example, what type of prayer is being employed? (Are Christian, Jewish, Muslim, Buddhist, Wiccan, and Shaman prayers equal?) Who or what is being prayed to? (Are God, Jesus, and a universal life force equivalent?) What is the length and frequency of the prayer? (Are two 10-minute prayers equal to one 20-minute prayer?) How many people are praying and does their status in the religion matter? (Is one priestly prayer identical to ten parishioner prayers?) Most prayer studies either lack such operational definitions, or there is no consistency across studies in such definitions.

6. *Theological implications.* The ultimate flaw in all such studies is theological. If God is omniscient and omnipotent why should he need to be reminded or inveigled that someone needs healing? Scientific prayer makes God a celestial lab rat, leading to bad science and worse religion.

MICHAEL SHERMER is a science writer and the editor-in-chief of *Skeptic*.

EXPLORING THE ISSUE

Do Religion and Prayer Benefit Health?

Critical Thinking and Reflection

1. Why is scientifically measuring the impact of prayer so challenging?
2. Describe possible mechanisms in which prayer and religion may benefit health.
3. What might be the downside of relying on prayer for healing?

Is There Common Ground?

Can we influence the course of our own illnesses? Can emotions, stress management, and prayer prevent or cure disease? In a telephone poll of 1,004 Americans conducted by *Time/CNN* in June 1996, 82 percent indicated that they believed in the healing power of personal prayer. Three-fourths felt that praying for someone else could help cure their illness. Interestingly, fewer than two-thirds of doctors say they believe in God. Benson, who developed the "relaxation response," thinks there is a strong link between religious commitment and good health. He contends that people do not have to have a professed belief in God to reap the psychological and physical rewards of the "faith factor."

Benson defined the faith factor as the combined force of the relaxation response and the placebo effect. In "God at the Bedside" (*New England Journal of Medicine*, March 18, 2004), physician Jerome Groopman is asked by a patient to pray for her after receiving a diagnosis of cancer. Dr. Groopman, although religious, considers prayer and religion a private matter. He debated over whether or not he should sidestep the patient's request or should he cross a boundary from the purely professional to the personal and join her in prayer. The article addresses his solution to dealing with this difficult issue.

Dr. Bernard Siegel, writing in his bestseller *Love, Medicine and Miracles* (Harper & Row, 1986), argues that there are no "incurable diseases, only incurable people" and that illness is a personality flaw. In "Welcome to the Mind/Body Revolution," *Psychology Today* (July/August 1993), author Marc Barash further discusses how the mind and immune system influence each other. The journal *Social Science and Medicine* published a literature review in July 2006 entitled "Do Religious/Spiritual Coping Strategies Affect Illness Adjustment in Patients with Cancer? A Systematic Review of the Literature." The study found mixed results. Some researchers determined that religion influenced the outcome of disease while other did not. The authors also found that many of the studies showed methodological flaws, echoed by Michael Shermer. Mixed results were also found in a study that reviewed the effects of prayer on coping after open heart surgery. The authors determined that despite the growing evidence for effects of religious factors on cardiac health, findings are not always consistent, especially among older and sicker populations. See "Long Term Adjustment After Surviving Open Heart Surgery: The Effect of Using Prayer for Coping Replicated in a Prospective Design," *Gerontologist*, December 2010.

In *You Don't Have to Die: Unraveling the AIDS Myth* (Burton Goldberg Group, 1994), a chapter entitled "Mind-Body Medicine" discusses the body's innate healing capabilities and the role of self-responsibility in the healing process. A long-term AIDS survivor who traveled the country interviewing other long-term survivors found that the one thing they all shared was the belief that AIDS was survivable. They all also accepted the reality of their diagnosis but refused to see their condition as a death sentence.

Create Central

www.mhhe.com/createcentral

Additional Resources

Ferguson, J. K., Willemsen, E. W., & Castañeto, M. V. (2010). Centering prayer as a healing response to everyday stress: A psychological and spiritual process. *Pastoral Psychology, 59*(3), 305–329.

Güthlin, C., Anton, A., Kruse, J., & Walach, H. (2012). Subjective concepts of chronically ill patients using distant healing. *Qualitative Health Research, 22*(3), 320–331.

Mouch, C. & Sonnega, A. (2012). Spirituality and recovery from cardiac surgery: A review. *Journal of Religion & Health, 51*(4), 1042–1060.

Poloma, M. M. (2012). Testing prayer: Science and healing. *Journal for the Scientific Study of Religion, 51*(4), 825–827.

Internet References . . .

Ethics in Medicine: Spirituality and Medicine

http://eduserv.hscer.Washington.edu/bioethics/topics/spirit.html

WebMD

Can prayer heal?

www.webmd.com/balance/features/can-prayer-heal

MedScape: The Online Resource for Better Patient Care

www.medscape.com

Unit 4

Sexuality and Gender Issues

*F*ew issues could be of greater controversy than those concerning gender and sexuality. Recent generations of Americans have rejected "traditional" sexual roles and values, which have resulted in more opportunities and great equality for women. On the other hand, societal changes have seen a significant increase in babies born out of wedlock, the spread of sexually transmitted diseases, and a rise in legal abortions. Many of these issues such as abortion, birth control, and right to life versus pro-choice remain controversial and may never be fully resolved. This section addresses many of the concerns associated with sexuality, gender, and health.

Selected, Edited, and with Issue Framing Material by:
Eileen Daniel, *SUNY College at Brockport*

ISSUE

Is It Necessary for Pregnant Women to Completely Abstain from All Alcoholic Beverages?

YES: Melinda Beck, from "Stricter Thinking on Alcohol During Pregnancy," *The Wall Street Journal* (January 24, 2012)

NO: Julia Moskin, from "The Weighty Responsibility of Drinking for Two," *The New York Times* (November 29, 2006)

Learning Outcomes

After reading this issue, you should be able to:

- Discuss the risks associated with alcohol consumption during pregnancy.
- Discuss the characteristics of fetal alcohol syndrome.
- Assess the argument that limited amounts of alcohol during pregnancy may not be harmful to the child.

ISSUE SUMMARY

YES: Journalist Melinda Beck provides evidence that even moderate quantities of alcohol can damage a developing fetus and cites new research indicating that even small amounts of alcoholic beverages consumed during pregnancy may be harmful.

NO: Journalist Julia Moskin argues that there are almost no studies on the effects of moderate drinking during pregnancy and that small amounts of alcohol are unlikely to have much effect.

In 1973, a paper was published in the British medical journal *The Lancet*. It described a pattern of birth defects that occurred among children born of alcoholic women and was called "fetal alcohol syndrome" or FAS ("Recognition of the Fetal Alcohol Syndrome in Early Infancy, *Lancet*, vol. 2, 1973). Since that time, thousands of studies have supported the relationship between heavy alcohol consumption during pregnancy and resulting birth defects. One controversial point related to FAS, however, is the amount of alcohol that must be consumed to cause danger to the developing baby. It seems that some threshold must exist though it's unclear what that is.

In their 1973 study, Jones and Smith correlated FAS only among children born to alcohol abusing women. While the researchers were successful in bringing the syndrome to international attention, it also created apprehension that any amount of alcohol consumption during pregnancy could cause danger to the child. Many doctors and researchers believe that even minute levels of alcohol intake during pregnancy can cause FAS, causing

a panic that may have exaggerated the dangers of *any* consumption.

Fortunately, FAS is relatively uncommon, though the United States has one of the highest rates in the developed world. This may be related to the pattern of alcohol consumption in this country. In many European countries, alcohol is often consumed daily, whereas in the United States, alcohol intake is more confined to weekends. This results in higher blood alcohol levels on those days. In addition, there are other variables that increase the risk of FAS, which cannot be linked solely to the amount of alcohol consumed. For example, women who binge drink are much more likely to bear children with the pattern of birth defects linked to FAS than women who consume the same total amount of alcohol over a period of time. In addition to binge drinking, a pregnant woman's health is another significant factor. Women who bear children with FAS often have liver disease, nutritional deficiencies including anemia, infections, and other conditions that exacerbate alcohol's effects on the fetus. Older mothers and those who have given birth to several children are also at greater risk to have children with FAS. While binge drinking, other health issues, and age are important risk factors, the two most significant conditions along with alcohol consumption are low income and cigarette smoking. Low income is related to poor diet, smoking, and other drug use, and exposure to pollutants such as lead. Smoking is also a factor in FAS because it contains toxins which reduce blood flow and level of oxygen available to the fetus.

While it appears that heavy alcohol consumption, particularly binge drinking, combined with smoking, poor diet, low income, and concomitant health problems increases the risk of FAS, is there an absolutely safe level of consumption during pregnancy? Two recent studies suggest that alcohol use during pregnancy may be more dangerous for the child than previously thought. In one study, researchers found symptoms of FAS in children whose mothers drank two drinks per day at certain stages of pregnancy. The children born of these women were found to be unusually small and/or had learning or behavioral problems. The researchers also found other defects associated with FAS at a higher rate than expected. ("Epidemiology of FASD in a Province in Italy: Prevalence and Characteristics of Children in a Random Sample of Schools," *Alcoholism: Clinical and Experimental Research*, September 2006). A second study confirmed that FAS is not the only concern associated with alcohol consumption during pregnancy. It's also a risk factor for alcohol abuse among the children born of these women ("In Utero Alcohol Exposure and Prediction of Alcohol Disorders in Early Adulthood: A Birth Cohort Study," *Archives of General Psychiatry*, September 2006).

It's apparent that heavy use of alcohol during pregnancy increases the risk of FAS. What is unclear is the risk associated with any amount of alcohol. A 25-year study of babies born to mothers who were social drinkers found that even low intakes of alcohol had measurable effects on their babies. The study concluded that no minimum level of drinking was absolutely safe. See "When Two Drinks Are Too Many," *Psychology Today* (May/June 2004).

The YES and NO selections address whether it is safe for pregnant women to drink during pregnancy. Melinda Beck argues that even a small amount of alcohol can damage a developing fetus and cites new research, which indicates that moderate consumption of alcoholic beverages during pregnancy may be harmful and that it's safer to avoid drinking.

Journalist Julia Moskin counters that there are almost no studies on the effects of moderate drinking during pregnancy and that small amounts of alcohol consumed during pregnancy are unlikely to have much harmful effect.

YES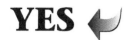

Melinda Beck

Stricter Thinking on Alcohol During Pregnancy

In the sixth to 12th week of pregnancy, a fetus's bones, brain and central nervous system are forming. Buds blossom into arms and legs, and internal organs start to function. A face with eyelids, lips and other features appears.

This is also the time when a mother's alcohol consumption poses the greatest risk of doing lifelong physical damage to her baby, according to a new study of nearly 1,000 women who drank at least once in their pregnancies.

On average, the women drank a small fraction of a drink a day. But some downed as many as 12 drinks a day—well above the amount considered safe for the women's own health—and binged frequently.

For each drink consumed each day over the daily average in the second half of the first trimester, the women's babies were 12% more likely to have a small head circumference, 16% more likely to have low birth weight and over 20% more likely to have a very thin upper lip or lack a vertical indentation between their noses and lips. While seemingly minor, those characteristics are typical of fetal alcohol syndrome, or FAS, and frequently presage cognitive and behavior problems later in life.

Overall, the more the women drank, the more likely their babies were to have such problems, according to the study published last week in the journal *Alcoholism: Clinical and Experimental Research.* Some who averaged less than one drink a day still had babies with some FAS characteristics.

"We found that there is no safe amount of alcohol to drink during pregnancy," says lead author Haruna Sawada Feldman, a postdoctoral student at the University of California, San Diego.

A few studies have found a drink or two a week seemed to have little effect on babies. But most of those relied on mothers' recall after giving birth, while the UC San Diego researchers interviewed subjects throughout their pregnancies.

Fetal alcohol syndrome—an array of physical and mental abnormalities including learning disabilities, language delays, poor concentration and low IQ—was first recognized in the early 1970s. Experts have never pinpointed how much alcohol it takes to cause damage, so the U.S. Surgeon General, the Centers for Disease Control

and Prevention and the March of Dimes all urge women not to drink at all if they are or might become pregnant.

Some women drink anyway—in part because friends, family members and even some obstetricians say an occasional drink isn't likely to cause harm.

"We know that alcohol crosses the placenta; we know that it's linked to mental and physical problems; so why risk it?" says Tom Donaldson, president of the National Organization for Fetal Alcohol Syndrome, or NOFAS, a nonprofit advocacy group.

In government surveys, about 12% of pregnant women in the U.S. report drinking some alcohol in the past 30 days and about 2% report drinking five or more drinks at a time. The CDC estimates that of approximately four million U.S. infants born each year, between 1,000 and 6,000 fit the criteria for FAS. Experts think as many as 40,000 a year have some neurological or behavior issues caused by prenatal alcohol exposure, a broader, less well-defined range of conditions known as fetal alcohol spectrum disorder, or FASD.

Why alcohol seemingly affects some unborn babies but not others remains a mystery.

"There's a huge amount that we still don't know about this disorder," says Kenneth Lyons Jones, one of the physicians who first recognized the danger of alcohol in pregnancy when he and a colleague noticed that eight children in a Seattle clinic all had similar facial features and developmental problems and discovered that all had been born to alcoholic mothers.

Dr. Jones, now a professor of pediatrics at UC San Diego and a co-author of the study, speculates that genetic differences may at least partly explain why some babies are more affected than others. He and other researchers are also investigating whether a mother's health and nutrition may play a role, studying pregnant women in Ukraine where the incidence of FAS is high.

In the U.S., experts say most children who fit the criteria for FAS or FASD never get a formal diagnosis. Many of the cognitive and behavioral problems are common in the general population and some are subtle enough to go unrecognized. Mothers who drank during pregnancy are often reluctant to admit it and physicians are often loath to voice suspicions, experts say. What's more, there are no blood tests or other biomarkers to show alcohol exposure in the womb.

But the damage can last a lifetime.

Researchers at Emory University in Atlanta have been following a group of alcohol-affected children born between 1980 and 1986 into young adulthood. ("In those days, mothers told us everything," says Claire Coles, a professor of psychiatry at Emory and the project leader.)

Not all those whose mothers drank have suffered physical or cognitive damage. One recently graduated from Princeton University, says Dr. Coles. But many have visual and spatial difficulties and trouble encoding memories. Functional MRI studies have found that corresponding areas of their brains are abnormal. Many also have trouble with math concepts, starting around age 5. "You can get them to say that 2 plus 2 equals 4, but they don't know what that means," says Dr. Coles.

She and others have designed learning programs that address the specific needs FAS children have—but she stresses that it's important to identify them early, when their brains are most adaptable. Other experts agree. The American Academy of Pediatrics plans to issue new guidelines this year urging pediatricians to look for signs of FAS and FASD in their young patients and urge parents to seek help.

Admitting that their drinking may have caused their children's problems can be difficult for mothers, however.

"It takes a lot of courage to own this and tell people, 'Yes, I drank while I was pregnant,'" says Kathy Mitchell, who had three children by the time she was 20 years old in the 1970s and drank wine with each pregnancy. Two of them are healthy, but one daughter, now 37, has severe FAS. Two other children died in infancy, which Ms. Mitchell also attributes to her drinking.

Now a recovering alcoholic and spokeswoman for NOFAS, Ms. Mitchell works with families who have adopted FAS children, knowingly or unknowingly, as well as birth mothers who are "stunned and remorseful and full of guilt," she says.

"No one intentionally sets out to harm her children," says Ms. Mitchell. "Most birth families who receive the diagnosis don't tell anyone. But it's not going to get prevented if we call it something else."

MELINDA BECK is a health columnist at *The Wall Street Journal* and a graduate of Yale University.

Julia Moskin

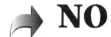 **NO**

The Weighty Responsibility of Drinking for Two

It happens at coffee bars. It happens at cheese counters. But most of all, it happens at bars and restaurants. Pregnant women are slow-moving targets for strangers who judge what we eat—and, especially, drink.

"Nothing makes people more uncomfortable than a pregnant woman sitting at the bar," said Brianna Walker, a bartender in Los Angeles. "The other customers can't take their eyes off her."

Drinking during pregnancy quickly became taboo in the United States after 1981, when the Surgeon General began warning women about the dangers of alcohol. The warnings came after researchers at the *University of Washington* identified Fetal Alcohol Syndrome, a group of physical and mental birth defects caused by alcohol consumption, in 1973. In its recommendations, the government does not distinguish between heavy drinking and the occasional beer: all alcohol poses an unacceptable risk, it says.

So those of us who drink, even occasionally, during pregnancy face unanswerable questions, like why would anyone risk the health of a child for a passing pleasure like a beer?

"It comes down to this: I just don't buy it," said Holly Masur, a mother of two in Deerfield, Ill., who often had half a glass of wine with dinner during her pregnancies, based on advice from both her mother and her obstetrician. "How can a few sips of wine be dangerous when women used to drink martinis and smoke all through their pregnancies?"

Many American obstetricians, skeptical about the need for total abstinence, quietly tell their patients that an occasional beer or glass of wine—no hard liquor—is fine.

"If a patient tells me that she's drinking two or three glasses of wine a week, I am personally comfortable with that after the first trimester," said Dr. Austin Chen, an obstetrician in TriBeCa. "But technically I am sticking my neck out by saying so."

Americans' complicated relationship with food and drink—in which everything desirable is also potentially dangerous—only becomes magnified in pregnancy.

When I was pregnant with my first child in 2001 there was so much conflicting information that doubt became a reflexive response. Why was tea allowed but not coffee? How could all "soft cheeses" be forbidden if cream cheese was recommended? What were the real risks of having a glass of wine on my birthday?

Pregnant women are told that danger lurks everywhere: listeria in soft cheese, mercury in canned tuna, *salmonella* in fresh-squeezed orange juice. Our responsibility for minimizing risk through perfect behavior feels vast.

Eventually, instead of automatically following every rule, I began looking for proof.

Proof, it turns out, is hard to come by when it comes to "moderate" or "occasional" drinking during pregnancy. Standard definitions, clinical trials and long-range studies simply do not exist.

"Clinically speaking, there is no such thing as moderate drinking in pregnancy," said Dr. Ernest L. Abel, a professor at Wayne State University Medical School in Detroit, who has led many studies on pregnancy and alcohol. "The studies address only heavy drinking"—defined by the *National Institutes of Health* as five drinks or more per day—"or no drinking."

Most pregnant women in America say in surveys that they do not drink at all—although they may not be reporting with total accuracy. But others make a conscious choice not to rule out drinking altogether.

For me, the desire to drink turned out to be all tied up with the ritual of the table—sitting down in a restaurant, reading the menu, taking that first bite of bread and butter. That was the only time, I found, that sparkling water or nonalcoholic beer didn't quite do it. And so, after examining my conscience and the research available, I concluded that one drink with dinner was an acceptable risk.

My husband, frankly, is uncomfortable with it. But he recognizes that there is no way for him to put himself in my position, or to know what he would do under the same circumstances.

While occasional drinking is not a decision I take lightly, it is also a decision in which I am not (quite) alone. Lisa Felter McKenney, a teacher in Chicago whose first child is due in January, said she feels comfortable at her current level of three drinks a week, having been grudgingly cleared by her obstetrician. "Being able to look forward to a beer with my husband at the end of the day really helps me deal with the horrible parts of being pregnant," she said. "It makes me feel like myself: not the alcohol, but the ritual. Usually I just take a few sips and that's enough."

Ana Sortun, a chef in Cambridge, Mass., who gave birth last year, said that she (and the nurse practitioner who delivered her baby) both drank wine during their pregnancies. "I didn't do it every day, but I did it often," she said. "Ultimately I trusted my own instincts, and my doctor's, more than anything else. Plus, I really believe all that stuff about the European tradition."

Many women who choose to drink have pointed to the habits of European women who legendarily drink wine, eat raw-milk cheese and quaff Guinness to improve breast milk production, as justification for their own choices in pregnancy.

Of course, those countries have their own taboos. "Just try to buy unpasteurized cheese in England, or to eat salad in France when you're pregnant," wrote a friend living in York, England. (Many French obstetricians warn patients that raw vegetables are risky.) However, she said, a drink a day is taken for granted. In those cultures, wine and beer are considered akin to food, part of daily life; in ours, they are treated more like drugs.

But more European countries are adopting the American stance of abstinence. Last month, France passed legislation mandating American-style warning labels on alcohol bottles, beginning in October 2007.

If pregnant Frenchwomen are giving up wine completely (although whether that will happen is debatable—the effects of warning labels are far from proven), where does that leave the rest of us?

"I never thought it would happen," said Jancis Robinson, a prominent wine critic in Britain, one of the few countries with government guidelines that still allow pregnant women any alcohol—one to two drinks per week. Ms. Robinson, who spent three days tasting wine for her Masters of Wine qualification in 1990 while pregnant with her second child, said that she studied the research then available and while she was inclined to be cautious, she didn't see proof that total abstinence was the only safe course.

One thing is certain: drinking is a confusing and controversial choice for pregnant women, and among the hardest areas in which to interpret the research.

Numerous long-term studies, including the original one at the University of Washington at Seattle, have established beyond doubt that heavy drinkers are taking tremendous risks with their children's health.

But for women who want to apply that research to the question of whether they must refuse a single glass of Champagne on New Year's Eve or a serving of rum-soaked Christmas pudding, there is almost no information at all.

My own decision came down to a stubborn conviction that feels like common sense: a single drink—sipped slowly, with food to slow the absorption—is unlikely to have much effect.

Some clinicians agree with that instinct. Others claim that the threat at any level is real.

"Blood alcohol level is the key," said Dr. Abel, whose view, after 30 years of research, is that brain damage and other alcohol-related problems most likely result from the spikes in blood alcohol concentration that come from binge drinking—another difficult definition, since according to Dr. Abel a binge can be as few as two drinks, drunk in rapid succession, or as many as 14, depending on a woman's physiology.

Because of ethical considerations, virtually no clinical trials can be performed on pregnant women.

"Part of the research problem is that we have mostly animal studies to work with," Dr. Abel said. "And who knows what is two drinks, for a mouse?"

Little attention has been paid to pregnant women at the low end of the consumption spectrum because there isn't a clear threat to public health there, according to Janet Golden, a history professor at Rutgers who has written about Americans' changing attitudes toward drinking in pregnancy.

The research—and the public health concern—is focused on getting pregnant women who don't regulate their intake to stop completely.

And the public seems to seriously doubt whether pregnant women can be trusted to make responsible decisions on their own.

"Strangers, and courts, will intervene with a pregnant woman when they would never dream of touching anyone else," Ms. Golden said.

Ms. Walker, the bartender, agreed. "I've had customers ask me to tell them what the pregnant woman is drinking," she said. "But I don't tell them. Like with all customers, unless someone is drunk and difficult it's no one else's business—or mine."

Julia Moskin is a reporter for *The New York Times*.

EXPLORING THE ISSUE

Is It Necessary for Pregnant Women to Completely Abstain from All Alcoholic Beverages?

Critical Thinking and Reflection

1. What are the short- and long-term effects of fetal alcohol syndrome?
2. Will consuming small amounts of alcohol necessarily cause damage to a developing fetus? Explain.
3. Why is it so difficult to determine a safe level of alcohol consumption during pregnancy?

Is There Common Ground?

Since its medical recognition in 1973, FAS has progressed from a little-known condition to a major public health issue. The condition has been characterized by exaggerated and unproved claims, particularly the cause and impact of the condition. For further reading on FAS see "Fetal Alcohol Syndrome: A Cautionary Note," *Current Pharmaceutical Design* (vol. 12, 2006). The author discusses the fact that there is likely a safe threshold for alcohol consumption during pregnancy and that FAS typically occurs among women who consume the highest amount of alcohol and/or binge drink. Binge drinking among women of childbearing age is common in the United States, which has one of the world's highest rates of FAS. In a recent study, researchers determined that one in six women in the United States continues to drink during pregnancy and one in seven consumes more than seven drinks per week; 3 percent drink more than 14 drinks per week. Thirteen percent of U.S. women aged 18–44 binge drink. The estimated number of childbearing-age women engaged in binge drinking rose from 6.2 million in 2001 to 7.1 million in 2003, an increase of .9 million. A study involving over 4,000 randomly selected women showed that 30.3 percent of all women reported drinking alcohol at some time during pregnancy, of whom 8.3 percent reported binge drinking (4+ drinks on one occasion) ("Alcohol Consumption by Women Before and During Pregnancy," *Maternal and Child Health Journal*, March 2009).

Fortunately, most women who use alcohol reduce their intake dramatically once they realize they are pregnant. A recent article, however, indicated that among 12,611 mothers from Maryland who gave birth to live infants between 2001 and 2008, nearly 8 percent of the study subjects admitted to drinking alcoholic beverages during the last 3 months of their pregnancy (*Obstetrics & Gynecology*, February 2011). But doctors still don't know that risk or harm, if any, results from light to moderate alcohol intake during pregnancy, which is why they caution pregnant women to abstain. For ethical reasons, there have been few, if any, studies conducted on pregnant women to determine if small to moderate intakes of alcohol are harmful. And to confuse the issue, some effects of alcohol consumption during pregnancy may not be apparent until a child starts school or even later in life. Child developmental and behavioral characteristics were examined from the 9-month data point of the Early Childhood Longitudinal Studies—Birth Cohort, a prospective nationally representative study. Several findings showed clear patterns between the amount of prenatal alcohol consumed and sensory regulation, mental, and motor development outcomes. Undesirable social engagement and child interaction were found to be statistically significant at the prenatal alcohol level of one to three drinks per week. Children exposed to four or more drinks per week showed statistically significant and clinically passive behavior on three sensory regulation variables ("Maternal Alcohol Consumption During Pregnancy and Infant Social, Mental, and Motor Development," *Journal of Early Intervention*, March, 2010). Clearly, excessive alcohol consumption during pregnancy has negative effects on fetal growth and development. Less consistent relationships have been shown for the correlation between light and moderate maternal alcohol consumption during pregnancy with health outcomes in the offspring. Researchers in the study "Associations of Light and Moderate Maternal Alcohol Consumption with Fetal Growth Characteristics in Different Periods of Pregnancy: The Generation R Study" examined the associations of light to moderate maternal alcohol consumption with various fetal growth characteristics measured in different periods of pregnancy and found various levels of impairment among the children of women who consumed alcohol during their pregnancies (*International Journal of Epidemiology*, June 2010).

Although individual differences in reaction to alcohol prevent determining a "safe level" of drinking for all pregnant women, encouraging total abstinence from alcohol during pregnancy is prudent though not necessarily based on research. The changes in fetal activity associated with one or two drinks clearly indicate that the fetus reacts to low levels of alcohol. But these changes don't necessarily mean the fetus is damaged. Until relationships are considerably stronger than the evidence now indicates, the research does not support the consensus that low levels of alcohol intake pose a danger to the developing baby. Even though scientists can't prove small amounts of alcohol are harmful, they can't prove they aren't. On the other hand, setting a realistic threshold may be more effective than encouraging women to completing forgo alcohol. Setting a definite limit, two or less drinks per day, for example, may be more realistic to those women who continue to drink during pregnancy. Prevention efforts have not been particularly effective among women who drink at levels that pose the greatest risk to their fetus ("Motivational Interventions in Prenatal Clinics," *Alcohol Research & Health*, vol. 25, 2001). They may be able to reduce rather than eliminate all alcohol, which could result in a reduced risk for FAS.

Create Central

www.mhhe.com/createcentral

Additional Resources

Buxton, B. (2005). *Damaged angels: An adoptive mother discovers the tragic toll of alcohol in pregnancy*. New York, NY: Carroll & Graf.

Chen, J. (2012). Maternal alcohol use during pregnancy, birth weight and early behavioral outcomes. *Alcohol & Alcoholism, 47*(6), 649–656.

Powers, J., Mcdermott, L., Loxton, D., & Chojenta, C. (2013). A prospective study of prevalence and predictors of concurrent alcohol and tobacco use during pregnancy. *Maternal & Child Health Journal, 17*(1), 76–84.

Sullum, J. (2012). Drink up, moms! *Reason, 44*(5), 13–14.

Internet References . . .

National Clearinghouse for Alcohol and Drug Information

www.health.org

March of Dimes Foundation

www.marchofdimes.com

National Organization on Fetal Alcohol Syndrome: NOFAS

www.nofas.org/

Selected, Edited, and with Issue Framing Material by:
Eileen Daniel, *SUNY College at Brockport*

ISSUE

Should Pro-Life Health Providers Be Allowed to Deny Prescriptions on the Basis of Conscience?

YES: John A. Menges, from "Public Hearing on HB4346 Before the House State Government Administration Committee," Illinois House State Government Administration Committee (February 15, 2006)

NO: R. Alta Charo, from "The Celestial Fire of Conscience—Refusing to Deliver Medical Care," *The New England Journal of Medicine* (June 16, 2005)

Learning Outcomes

After reading this issue, you should be able to:

- Discuss why some pharmacists refuse to dispense certain medications.
- Understand the mechanisms of the morning after pill.
- Assess the legality of a pharmacist refusing to filling prescriptions.

ISSUE SUMMARY

YES: Pharmacist John A. Menges believes that it is his right to refuse to dispense any medication that is designed to end a human life.

NO: Attorney R. Alta Charo argues that health care professionals who protect themselves from the moral consequences of their actions may do so at their patients' risk.

A trend has been making news recently. The Pharmacists' Refusal Clause also known as the Conscience Clause allows pharmacists to refuse to fill certain prescriptions because of their own moral objections to the medication. These medications are mostly birth control pills and the "morning after pill," which can be used as emergency contraception. Though nearly all states offer some type of legal protection for health care providers who refuse to provide certain women's health care services, only three states—Arkansas, Mississippi, and South Dakota—specifically protect pharmacists who refuse to dispense birth control and emergency contraceptive pills. While only a limited number of states have passed refusal clause legislation specific to pharmacists, more and more states are considering adding it.

In the past several years there have been reports of pharmacists who refused to fill prescriptions for birth control and emergency contraceptive pills. In some of these instances, the pharmacists who refused service were fired, but in others, no legal action was taken. As a result, some women have left their drug stores without getting their pills and not sure where to go to have their prescriptions filled.

While doctors may refuse to perform abortions or other procedures that they morally object to, should pharmacists have the same right? They are members of the health care team and should be treated as medical professionals. Society does not demand that professionals abandon their morals as a condition of their employment. On the other hand, there are a number of reasons against a pharmacist's right to object. First and foremost is the right of a patient to receive timely medical treatment. Pharmacists may refuse to fill prescriptions for emergency contraception because they believe that drug ends a life. Although the patient may disapprove of abortion, she may not share the pharmacist's beliefs about birth control. If she becomes pregnant, she may then consider abortion, an issue she could have avoided if allowed to fill prescriptions for the morning after pill. Other concerns include the time-sensitive nature of the morning after pill, which must be taken within 72 hours of intercourse to effectively prevent pregnancy. Women who are refused the medication by one pharmacist may not be able to get the drug from another. This is especially true if she lives in an area with only one pharmacy. Also, low-income women may not have the time or resources to locate a pharmacy that would fill the prescription.

Other potential abuses could also arise. For instance, some pharmacists may object to filling drugs to treat AIDS if they believe HIV-positive individuals are engaged in behaviors they consider immoral such as IV drug use or homosexual relations. A pharmacist who does not believe in extramarital sex might refuse to fill a prescription for Viagra for an unmarried man. Could a pharmacist's objec-tions here be considered invasive? Further, because a phar-macist does not have access to a patient's medical records or history, refusing to fill a prescription could be medically harmful.

While arguments could be made for both sides, it appears that there needs to be a compromise between the needs of a patient and the moral beliefs of a pharmacist. In the YES and NO selections, physician John Menges argues that health providers' consciences must be respected. R. Alta Charo counters that a provider's conscience can be in conflict with legitimate medical needs of a patient.

YES ↵

John A. Menges

Public Hearing on HB4346 Before the House State Government Administration Committee

[I am] one of the 4 fired Walgreens pharmacists. I was fired for not signing a policy saying that I would indeed fill a prescription if presented with it. I did not see a prescription! Walgreens does not respect a pharmacist's right to choose. I was one of Walgreens' best pharmacists prior to this issue. I had no problem with telling someone when a pharmacist would be available to fill a prescription. I can not fill the prescriptions myself but I try to the best of my ability to not take a side because I want to be able to tell people that this drug can end a life if a woman does have questions. By taking the position I take I find women asking questions. I believe many women wouldn't use this drug if they knew how it can work. If a woman is going to make a real choice as the other side says then the woman needs to have access to both "pro-choice" pharmacist and pro-life pharmacist like myself, so her choice is an informed choice. I pray that by trying to take a neutral position on this issue that some women will listen and some children will live.

The one thing I could not be neutral on is the issue of dispensing. When my three supervisors fired me, I told them "It feels very good knowing that my Faith and Religion is more important to me than a paycheck."

The following is a testimony I gave on a House bill earlier this year [2006].

Testimony

I would like to thank Rep. Granberg for introducing this bill and all members of this committee for giving me the opportunity to speak to you today.

My name is JOHN A. MENGES and I am a licensed pharmacist in the state of Illinois. I am one of the four pharmacists who lost my job with Walgreens for failing to sign an Emergency Contraceptive Policy that violated my religious beliefs. To make things clear to all members of this committee during the 8 months I worked following the Governor's mandate I was not presented with a prescription to fill. During the 3 years I worked at Walgreens I can only recall being presented with prescriptions for this medication 3 times and during that time I estimate that I filled over 71,000 prescriptions.

I am here today because I can not dispense any drug designed to end a human life. Before I enter any discussion of these drugs I would like to try to clarify some terminology. For me human life begins when fertilization occurs. Fertilization is the point at which the sperm penetrates the egg. Life for me is the issue. The redefining of the terms "pregnancy" and "conception" in 1965 by the American College of Obstetricians and Gynecologists only confuse this life issue more. Prior to 1965 "pregnancy" and "conception" began at fertilization when life begins. Now "pregnancy" and "conception" begins at implantation of the embryo in the uterus. This still doesn't negate the fact that embryologists world-wide agree unanimously that human life begins at fertilization. This does explain why the morning after pill is classified as a contraceptive by the FDA and not as an abortafacient and I hope this clarifies why many say this drug doesn't end a pregnancy. Understanding the terminology enables one to realize how confusing the words fertilization, pregnancy, and conception have become. With this very simple explanation of the terminology I want to remind you that the beginning of human life at the point of fertilization is the issue for me. I hold human life at this stage in development with the same respect I hold for any human life.

The drugs I was referring to as I tried to explain some definitions are classified as "emergency contraceptives" by the FDA. Presently "Plan B" also known as the "morning after pill" is the only drug approved to be used for emergency contraception but most oral contraceptives can be dosed to work as emergency contraception. Emergency contraceptive doses are doses that are higher than doses of regular birth control. To simplify my discussion of emergency contraceptives I will limit my discussion to "Plan B." Plan B consists of two Progestin tablets containing 0.75 mg of levonorgestrel. The first tablet is to be taken within 72 hours of intercourse and the second tablet 12 hours after the first dose. Without getting into too much detail here the problem I have is the significant post-fertilization mechanism of action by which these drugs work. The mechanisms of action stated in the manufacturers prescribing information include preventing ovulation, altering tubal transport of sperm and/or ova, or inhibiting implantation by altering the endometrium.

Menges, John A. Illinois House State Government Administration Committee, February 15, 2006.

The time during a woman's menstrual cycle plays an important role in what mechanism of action is at work. The menstrual cycle can last anywhere from 21 to 40 days. Ovulation usually occurs 14 to 15 days before the end of the cycle. If emergency contraception is given early in the cycle it is more likely to prevent ovulation. But during this time ovulation and pregnancy are less likely to occur anyway. As the time for ovulation nears the chance for emergency contraception to prevent ovulation will lessen to the effect that ovulation can occur in some instances after emergency contraception has been taken. Once ovulation has occurred and fertilization has taken place any mechanism that prevents this implantation is the ending of human life.

So what am I doing as a pharmacist if I can't dispense a drug approved by the FDA? Believe me I asked myself this question when the first emergency contraceptive was approved by the FDA in 1998. I was a pharmacy manager in a supermarket pharmacy at the time. My number one priority as pharmacy manager is the same as it is today and that is customer service to my patients. I have always made it known to my employees, supervisors, and patients that I work first for the patient. My employer was a direct beneficiary of this as I always made them look good. The day the first emergency contraceptive was approved I talked with the staff pharmacist who worked with me about his thoughts. Neither of us could dispense emergency contraceptives as it went against everything we believed in. The question I and many pharmacists had to answer was which patient do we serve? Do we serve the women requesting emergency contraceptive or the human life she could be carrying? I could not make a decision to participate in ending any human life so my decision was to refer women and answer any questions they might have if and when the situation arose.

So here I am almost 8 years after the first emergency contraceptives were approved and I can only recall 5 times that I have been faced with prescriptions. Three of those prescriptions I saw while employed with Walgreens. Not that a person can derive any statistical conclusions from 5 prescriptions but I didn't have incident with any of those encounters. In fact I have been thanked for my willingness to talk about emergency contraceptives as many pharmacists avoid the issue. This leads me to the moral issue I read about in different editorials. My choice to step aside and not fill these prescriptions in no way is a reflection of me trying to push my morals on others. It is my upholding my moral beliefs for myself. Our government allows women to make this choice and my actions have never prevented any women from exercising her choice. I have a choice too and my choice is not to dispense any medication that will end a human life. Those are morals that I have to live up to. The people who think I try to push my morals on others need to ask themselves why I dispense medication to patients who have just had an abortion for pain and bleeding. I give these patients the same respect I give every patient. The answers are simple as I went into pharmacy to help people not hurt people. I don't ask questions as to why people need my help because morals don't play a role in my helping people. I went into pharmacy to care for people and help them improve their lives. I love the profession of pharmacy because of all the good I am able to do as a pharmacist. Pharmacy goes beyond the counseling, recommendations and referrals I give. It is much more than my filling prescriptions fast and accurately. It is the respect I give every patient. I listen to my patients and help them when I can. I will never intentionally do any harm to any patient.

On November 28th of last year I lost my job because of my conscience objective to filling a medication that ends human life. My employer fired me for not signing policy asking me to violate my conscience. During the 8 months following the Governor's mandate I was not presented with a prescription to fill. Even though I believe I am currently covered under The Health Care Right of Conscience Act, I would like to ask every member of the house to vote YES on HB 4346. I am one of a small minority of pharmacists in this state who can't fill these medications. By voting YES on HB 4346 you will protect other pharmacists from having to endure what I, my wife, and my 2 children have had to endure these past months. It is difficult to explain my feelings. It hurts.

Without saying anymore I would like to answer any questions members might have. Thank You.

JOHN A. MENGES is a licensed pharmacist.

R. Alta Charo

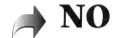

The Celestial Fire of Conscience—Refusing to Deliver Medical Care

Apparently heeding George Washington's call to "labor to keep alive in your breast that little spark of celestial fire called conscience," physicians, nurses, and pharmacists are increasingly claiming a right to the autonomy not only to refuse to provide services they find objectionable, but even to refuse to refer patients to another provider and, more recently, to inform them of the existence of legal options for care.

Largely as artifacts of the abortion wars, at least 45 states have "conscience clauses" on their books—laws that balance a physician's conscientious objection to performing an abortion with the profession's obligation to afford all patients nondiscriminatory access to services. In most cases, the provision of a referral satisfies one's professional obligations. But in recent years, with the abortion debate increasingly at the center of wider discussions about euthanasia, assisted suicide, reproductive technology, and embryonic stem-cell research, nurses and pharmacists have begun demanding not only the same right of refusal, but also—because even a referral, in their view, makes one complicit in the objectionable act—a much broader freedom to avoid facilitating a patient's choices.

A bill recently introduced in the Wisconsin legislature, for example, would permit health care professionals to abstain from "participating" in any number of activities, with "participating" defined broadly enough to include counseling patients about their choices. The privilege of abstaining from counseling or referring would extend to such situations as emergency contraception for rape victims, in vitro fertilization for infertile couples, patients' requests that painful and futile treatments be withheld or withdrawn, and therapies developed with the use of fetal tissue or embryonic stem cells. This last provision could mean, for example, that pediatricians—without professional penalty or threat of malpractice claims—could refuse to tell parents about the availability of varicella vaccine for their children, because it was developed with the use of tissue from aborted fetuses.

This expanded notion of complicity comports well with other public policy precedents, such as bans on federal funding for embryo research or abortion services, in which taxpayers claim a right to avoid supporting objectionable practices. In the debate on conscience clauses, some professionals are now arguing that the right to practice their religion requires that they not be made complicit in any practice to which they object on religious grounds.

Although it may be that, as Mahatma Gandhi said, "in matters of conscience, the law of majority has no place," acts of conscience are usually accompanied by a willingness to pay some price. Martin Luther King, Jr., argued, "An individual who breaks a law that conscience tells him is unjust, and who willingly accepts the penalty of imprisonment in order to arouse the conscience of the community over its injustice, is in reality expressing the highest respect for law."

What differentiates the latest round of battles about conscience clauses from those fought by Gandhi and King is the claim of entitlement to what newspaper columnist Ellen Goodman has called "conscience without consequence."

And of course, the professionals involved seek to protect only themselves from the consequences of their actions—not their patients. In Wisconsin, a pharmacist refused to fill an emergency-contraception prescription for a rape victim; as a result, she became pregnant and subsequently had to seek an abortion. In another Wisconsin case, a pharmacist who views hormonal contraception as a form of abortion refused not only to fill a prescription for birth-control pills but also to return the prescription or transfer it to another pharmacy. The patient, unable to take her pills on time, spent the next month dependent on less effective contraception. Under Wisconsin's proposed law, such behavior by a pharmacist would be entirely legal and acceptable. And this trend is not limited to pharmacists and physicians; in Illinois, an emergency medical technician refused to take a woman to an abortion clinic, claiming that her own Christian beliefs prevented her from transporting the patient for an elective abortion.

At the heart of this growing trend are several intersecting forces. One is the emerging norm of patient autonomy, which has contributed to the erosion of the professional stature of medicine. Insofar as they are reduced to mere purveyors of medical technology, doctors no longer have extraordinary privileges, and so their notions of extraordinary duty—house calls, midnight duties, and charity care—deteriorate as well. In addition, an emphasis on mutual responsibilities has been gradually supplanted by an emphasis on individual rights. With autonomy and rights as the preeminent social values comes a devaluing of relationships and a diminution of the difference between our personal lives and our professional duties.

Finally, there is the awesome scale and scope of the abortion wars. In the absence of legislative options for outright prohibition, abortion opponents search for proxy wars, using debates on research involving human embryos, the donation of organs from anencephalic neonates, and the right of persons in a persistent vegetative state to die as opportunities to rehearse arguments on the value of biologic but nonsentient human existence. Conscience clauses represent but another battle in these so-called culture wars.

Most profoundly, however, the surge in legislative activity surrounding conscience clauses represents the latest struggle with regard to religion in America. Should the public square be a place for the unfettered expression of religious beliefs, even when such expression creates an oppressive atmosphere for minority groups? Or should it be a place for religious expression only if and when that does not in any way impinge on minority beliefs and practices? This debate has been played out with respect to blue laws, school prayer, Christmas crèche scenes, and workplace dress codes.

Until recently, it was accepted that the public square in this country would be dominated by Christianity. This long-standing religious presence has made atheists, agnostics, and members of minority religions view themselves as oppressed, but recent efforts to purge the public square of religion have left conservative Christians also feeling subjugated and suppressed. In this culture war, both sides claim the mantle of victimhood—which is why health care professionals can claim the right of conscience as necessary to the nondiscriminatory practice of their religion, even as frustrated patients view conscience clauses as legalizing discrimination against them when they practice their own religion.

For health care professionals, the question becomes: What does it mean to be a professional in the United States? Does professionalism include the rather old-fashioned notion of putting others before oneself? Should professionals avoid exploiting their positions to pursue an agenda separate from that of their profession? And perhaps most crucial, to what extent do professionals have a collective duty to ensure that their profession provides nondiscriminatory access to all professional services?

Some health care providers would counter that they distinguish between medical care and nonmedical care that uses medical services. In this way, they justify their willingness to bind the wounds of the criminal before sending him back to the street or to set the bones of a battering husband that were broken when he struck his wife. Birth control, abortion, and in vitro fertilization, they say, are lifestyle choices, not treatments for diseases.

And it is here that licensing systems complicate the equation: such a claim would be easier to make if the states did not give these professionals the exclusive right to offer such services. By granting a monopoly, they turn the profession into a kind of public utility, obligated to provide service to all who seek it. Claiming an unfettered right to personal autonomy while holding monopolistic control over a public good constitutes an abuse of the public trust—all the worse if it is not in fact a personal act of conscience but, rather, an attempt at cultural conquest.

Accepting a collective obligation does not mean that all members of the profession are forced to violate their own consciences. It does, however, necessitate ensuring that a genuine system for counseling and referring patients is in place, so that every patient can act according to his or her own conscience just as readily as the professional can. This goal is not simple to achieve, but it does represent the best effort to accommodate everyone and is the approach taken by virtually all the major medical, nursing, and pharmacy societies. It is also the approach taken by the governor of Illinois, who is imposing an obligation on pharmacies, rather than on individual pharmacists, to ensure access to services for all patients.

Conscience is a tricky business. Some interpret its personal beacon as the guide to universal truth. But the assumption that one's own conscience is the conscience of the world is fraught with dangers. As C.S. Lewis wrote, "Of all tyrannies, a tyranny sincerely exercised for the good of its victims may be the most oppressive. It would be better to live under robber barons than under omnipotent moral busybodies. The robber baron's cruelty may sometimes sleep, his cupidity may at some point be satiated; but those who torment us for our own good will torment us without end for they do so with the approval of their own conscience."

R. Alta Charo teaches law and bioethics at the University of Wisconsin Law and Medical Schools.

IE ISSUE

Life Health Providers Be
Deny Prescriptions on the
s of Conscience?

on

ng after pills lead to a "slippery slope"?
right to refuse to provide medical care or dispense medications they do

macists have the right to refuse to fill all prescriptions?

Is There Common Ground?

In the years since *Roe v. Wade*, state and federal legislatures have seen a growth in conscience clauses. Many pro-choice advocates perceive these clauses as another way to limit a woman's right to choose. Within weeks of the *Roe* decision in the early 1970s, Congress adopted legislation that permitted individual health care providers receiving federal funding or working for organizations receiving such funding to refuse to perform or assist in performing abortions or sterilizations if these procedures violated their moral or religious beliefs. The provision also prohibited discrimination against these providers because of the refusal to perform abortions or sterilizations. Currently, 45 states allow health care providers to refuse to be involved in abortions. Also, 12 states allow health care providers to refuse to provide sterilization, while 13 states allow providers to refuse to provide contraceptive services or information related to contraception.

Pharmacists who refuse to fill prescriptions for birth control pills or emergency contraception largely believe that these medications are actually a method of abortion. In a paper published in the *Archives of Family Medicine* (2000), physicians Walter Larimore and Joseph B. Stanford stated that birth control pills have the potential of interrupting development of the fertilized egg after fertilization. Emergency contraception or the morning after pill also has been seen as a means of abortion. It prevents pregnancy by either preventing fertilization or preventing implantation of a fertilized egg in the uterus. The morning after pill is often confused with RU-486, which is clearly a method of abortion. Unlike RU-486, emergency contraception cannot disrupt an established pregnancy and cannot cause an abortion. Clearly, better education about the methods of action of these drugs would be valuable.

Solutions have been proposed to enable patients to receive the drugs prescribed by their physicians. As a rule, it would make sense for pharmacists who will not dispense a drug to have an obligation to meet their customers'

needs by referring them to other pharmacies. Pharmacists who object to filling prescriptions for birth control pills or emergency contraception might ensure that there is a pharmacist on duty who will fill the prescription or refer their customers elsewhere.

In some countries, customers can purchase the drug without a prescription. In the United States, a prescription can only be filled by a licensed pharmacist. As a result, pharmacists are the last link in the chain of delivery. The author believes it is not acceptable to allow refusals in urban areas where pharmacies are plentiful, but forbid them in rural settings, where pharmacies are scarce. Rather, there should be strong public policy requiring that all pharmacists dispense emergency contraception to customers who request it, regardless of pharmacists' moral or religious objections. In "Claims of Conscience: Setting the Ground Rules When Rights Collide," *Humanist* (September/October 2009), the author discusses right of conscience claims, which allow pharmacists to refuse to fill morning-after pill prescriptions. The author notes that these claims can be taken too far. It takes a result-oriented approach to the ethical argument so that if another pharmacist is available to fill the legal prescription, it would allow a conscience refusal but not otherwise. See also "Pharmacist Conscience Clauses and Access to Oral Contraceptives" (*Journal of Medical Ethics*, July 2008). This paper examines the pharmacists' role and their professional and moral obligations to patients in the light of recent refusals by pharmacists to dispense oral contraceptives.

This issue raises important questions about public health and individual rights. Should pharmacists have a right to reject prescriptions for birth control pills, emergency contraception, Viagra, or any other drug that may be morally objectionable to them?

Create Central

www.mhhe.com/createcentral

Additional Resources

Davidson, L. A., Pettis, C. T., Joiner, A. J., Cook, D. M., & Klugman, C. M. (2010). Religion and conscientious objection: A survey of pharmacists' willingness to dispense medications. *Social Science & Medicine, 71*(1), 161–165.

Kelleher, J. (2010). Emergency contraception and conscientious objection. *Journal of Applied Philosophy, 27*(3), 290–304.

Lewis, J. D. & Sullivan, D. M. (2012). Abortifacient potential of emergency contraceptives. *Ethics & Medicine: An International Journal of Bioethics, 28*(3), 113–120.

Marshall, C. (2013). The spread of conscience clause legislation. *Human Rights, 39*(2), 15–16.

Internet References . . .

American Pharmacists Association

www.aphanet.org/

National Right to Life

www.nrlc.org/

Pharmacists for Life International

www.pfli.org/

Selected, Edited, and with Issue Framing Material by:
Eileen Daniel, *SUNY College at Brockport*

ISSUE

Should the Cervical Cancer Vaccine for Girls Be Compulsory?

YES: Cynthia Dailard, from "Achieving Universal Vaccination Against Cervical Cancer in the United States: The Need and the Means," *Guttmacher Policy Review* (Fall 2006)

NO: Gail Javitt, Deena Berkowitz, and Lawrence O. Gostin, from "Assessing Mandatory HPV Vaccination: Who Should Call the Shots?" *Journal of Law, Medicine & Ethics* (Summer 2008)

Learning Outcomes
After reading this issue, you should be able to: • Discuss why many parents oppose having their daughters vaccinated against cervical cancer.   • Assess the risk associated with contracting the HPV virus.   • Identify the side effects associated with the vaccine.

ISSUE SUMMARY

YES: The late Cynthia Dailard, a senior public policy associate at the Guttmacher Institute, argues that universal vaccination is needed because virtually all cases of cervical cancer are linked to the human papillomavirus. Most infected people are unaware of their infection, which is linked to nearly 10,000 cases of cervical cancer.

NO: Professors Gail Javitt, Deena Berkowitz, and Lawrence Gostin believe that mandating the cervical cancer vaccine raises significant legal, ethical, and social concerns. They are also concerned about the long-term safety and effectiveness of the vaccine.

A number of infectious diseases are almost completely preventable through childhood immunization. These include diphtheria, meningitis, pertussis (whooping cough), tetanus, polio, measles, mumps, and rubella (German measles). Largely as a result of widespread vaccination, these once-common diseases have become relatively rare. Before the introduction of the polio vaccine in 1955, polio epidemics occurred each year. In 1952, a record 20,000 cases were diagnosed, as compared to the last outbreak in 1979, when only 10 cases were identified.

While vaccination is a life saver, it may also be controversial. In June 2006, the Food and Drug Administration approved a new immunization called Gardisil, used to prevent diseases caused by the sexually transmitted human papillomavirus (HPV). The virus causes genital warts and cervical cancer. The Centers for Disease Control and Prevention has determined that up to 50 percent of all sexually active men and women in the United States will be infected with HPV at some time in their

life. The infection is especially common among women aged 20–24. About 20 states are considering making the vaccination a requirement, while Texas has already done so. Many parents and lawmakers are opposed to the mandatory vaccination for a variety of reasons: the vaccine doesn't target all types of HPV, it doesn't prevent diseases caused by these other types, and while HPV affects both sexes, It's usually recommended. Other reasons for the opposition include the relatively high cost of the vaccine, the fact that many people don't understand that HPV causes cervical cancer, and questions about its long-term safety.

The Centers for Disease Control and Prevention supports getting as many girls vaccinated as early and as fast as possible. They believe this vaccination will reduce the incidence and prevalence of cervical cancer among older women and lessen the spread of this highly infectious disease. The American Cancer Society also supports early and widespread vaccination of young girls.

In the United States it is believed that a valid way to lower the expense of the HPV vaccine and to educate the public on the advantages of vaccination is to make it compulsory for girls entering school. Mumps, measles, rubella, and hepatitis B (which is also sexually transmitted) are currently required. While there is value in preventing cervical cancer, which is estimated to be the most common sexually transmitted infection in the United States, many parents have concerns over mandatory vaccination to prevent a sexually transmitted disease. Some parents believe that young girls should be encouraged to abstain from sexual relations rather than being forced to receive the vaccination.

In the YES and NO selections, the late Cynthia Dailard, a senior public policy associate at the Guttmacher Institute, argued that universal vaccination was needed because virtually all cases of cervical cancer are linked to the human papillomavirus. Most infected people are unaware of their infection, which is linked to nearly 10,000 cases of cervical cancer. Professors Gail Javitt, Deena Berkowitz, and Lawrence Gostin believe that mandating the cervical cancer vaccine raises significant legal, ethical, and social concerns. They are also concerned over the long-term safety and effectiveness of the relatively new vaccine.

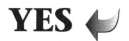

YES

Cynthia Dailard

Achieving Universal Vaccination Against Cervical Cancer in the United States: The Need and the Means

The advent of a vaccine against the types of human papillomavirus (HPV) linked to most cases of cervical cancer is widely considered one of the greatest health care advances for women in recent years. Experts believe that vaccination against HPV has the potential to dramatically reduce cervical cancer incidence and mortality particularly in resource-poor developing countries where cervical cancer is most common and deadly. In the United States, the vaccine's potential is likely to be felt most acutely within low-income communities and communities of color, which disproportionately bear the burden of cervical cancer.

Because HPV is easily transmitted through sexual contact, the vaccine's full promise may only be realized through near-universal vaccination of girls and young women prior to sexual activity—a notion reflected in recently proposed federal guidelines. And history, as supported by a large body of scientific evidence, suggests that the most effective way to achieve universal vaccination is by requiring children to be inoculated prior to attending school. Yet the link between HPV and sexual activity—and the notion that HPV is different than other infectious diseases targeted by vaccine school entry requirements—tests the prevailing justification for such efforts. Meanwhile, any serious effort to achieve universal vaccination among young people with this relatively expensive vaccine will expose holes in the public health safety net that, if left unaddressed, have the potential to exacerbate longstanding disparities in cervical cancer rates among American women.

The Case for Universal Vaccination

Virtually all cases of cervical cancer are linked to HPV, an extremely common sexually transmitted infection (STI) that is typically asymptomatic and harmless; most people never know they are infected, and most cases resolve on their own. It is estimated that approximately three in four Americans contract HPV at some point in their lives, with most cases acquired relatively soon after individuals have sex for the first time. Of the approximately 30 known types of HPV that are sexually transmitted, more than 13 are associated with cervical cancer. Yet despite the prevalence of HPV, cervical cancer is relatively rare in the United States; it generally occurs only in the small proportion of cases where a persistent HPV infection goes undetected over many years. This is largely due to the widespread availability of Pap tests, which can detect precancerous changes of the cervix that can be treated before cancer sets in, as well as cervical cancer in its earliest stage, when it is easily treatable.

Still, the American Cancer Society estimates that in 2006, almost 10,000 cases of invasive cervical cancer will occur to American women, resulting in 3,700 deaths. Significantly, more than half of all U.S. women diagnosed with cervical cancer have not had a Pap test in the last three years. These women are disproportionately low income and women of color who lack access to affordable and culturally competent health services. As a result, the incidence of cervical cancer is approximately 1.5 times higher among African American and Latina women than among white women; women of color are considerably more likely than whites to die of the disease as well. Two new HPV vaccines—Gardasil, manufactured by Merck & Company, and Cervarix, manufactured by GlaxoSmithKline—promise to transform this landscape. Both are virtually 100% effective in preventing the two types of HPV responsible for 70% of all cases of cervical cancer; Gardasil also protects against two other HPV types associated with 90% of all cases of genital warts. Gardasil was approved by the federal Food and Drug Administration (FDA) in June; GlaxoSmithKline is expected to apply for FDA approval of Cervarix by year's end.

Following FDA approval, Gardasil was endorsed by the Centers for Disease Control and Prevention's Advisory Committee on Immunization Practices (ACIP), which is responsible for maintaining the nation's schedule of recommended vaccines. ACIP recommended that the vaccine be routinely administered to all girls ages 11–12, and as early as age nine at a doctor's discretion. Also, it recommended vaccination of all adolescents and young women ages 13–26 as part of a national "catch-up" campaign for those who have not already been vaccinated.

The ACIP recommendations, which are closely followed by health care professionals, reflect the notion that to eradicate cervical cancer, it will be necessary to achieve near-universal vaccination of girls and young women prior to sexual activity, when the vaccine is most effective. Experts believe that such an approach has the potential to significantly reduce cervical cancer deaths in this country and around the world. Also, high vaccination rates will significantly reduce the approximately 3.5 million abnormal Pap results experienced by American women each year, many of which are caused by transient or persistent HPV infections. These abnormal Pap results require millions of women to seek follow-up care, ranging from additional Pap tests to more invasive procedures such as colposcopies and biopsies. This additional care exacts a substantial emotional and even physical toll on women, and costs an estimated $6 billion in annual health care expenditures. Finally, widespread vaccination fosters "herd immunity," which is achieved when a sufficiently high proportion of individuals within a population are vaccinated that those who go unvaccinated—because the vaccine is contraindicated for them or because they are medically underserved, for example—are essentially protected.

The Role of School Entry Requirements

Achieving high vaccination levels among adolescents, however, can be a difficult proposition. Unlike infants and toddlers, who have frequent contact with health care providers in the context of well-child visits, adolescents often go for long stretches without contact with a health care professional. In addition, the HPV vaccine is likely to pose particular challenges, given that it must be administered three times over a six-month period to achieve maximum effectiveness.

A large body of evidence suggests that the most effective means to ensure rapid and widespread use of childhood or adolescent vaccines is through state laws or policies that require children to be vaccinated prior to enrollment in day care or school. These school-based immunization requirements, which exist in some form in all 50 states, are widely credited for the success of immunization programs in the United States. They have also played a key role in helping to close racial, ethnic and socioeconomic gaps in immunization rates, and have proven to be far more effective than guidelines recommending the vaccine for certain age-groups or high-risk populations. Although each state decides for itself whether a particular vaccine will be required for children to enroll in school, they typically rely on ACIP recommendations in making their decision.

In recent months, some commentators have noted that as a sexually transmitted infection, HPV is "different" from other infectious diseases such as measles, mumps or whooping cough, which are easily transmitted in a school setting or threaten school attendance when an outbreak occurs. Some socially conservative advocacy groups accordingly argue that the HPV vaccine does not meet the historical criteria necessary for it to be required for children attending school; many of them also contend that abstinence outside of marriage is the real answer to HPV. They welcome the advent of the vaccine, they say, but will oppose strenuously any effort to require it for school enrollment.

This position reflects only a limited understanding of school-based vaccination requirements. These requirements do not exist solely to prevent the transmission of disease in school or during childhood. Instead, they further society's strong interest in ensuring that people are protected from disease throughout their lives and are a highly efficient means of eradicating disease in the larger community. For example, states routinely require school-age children to be vaccinated against rubella (commonly known as German measles), a typically mild illness in children, to protect pregnant women in the community from the devastating effects the disease can have on a developing fetus. Similarly, states currently require vaccination against certain diseases, such as tetanus, that are not "contagious" at all, but have very serious consequences for those affected. And almost all states require vaccination against Hepatitis B, a blood borne disease which can be sexually transmitted.

Moreover, according to the National Conference of State Legislatures (NCSL), all 50 states allow parents to refuse to vaccinate their children on medical grounds, such as when a vaccine is contraindicated for a particular child due to allergy, compromised immunity or significant illness. All states except Mississippi and West Virginia allow parents to refuse to vaccinate their children on religious grounds. Additionally, 20 states go so far as to allow parents to refuse to vaccinate their children because of a personal, moral or other belief. Unlike a medical exemption, which requires a parent to provide documentation from a physician, the process for obtaining nonmedical exemptions can vary widely by state.

NCSL notes that, in recent years, almost a dozen states considered expanding their exemption policy. Even absent any significant policy change, the rate of parents seeking exemptions for nonmedical reasons is on the rise. This concerns public health experts. Research shows that in states where exemptions are easier to obtain, a higher proportion of parents refuse to vaccinate their children; research further shows that these states, in turn, are more likely to experience outbreaks of vaccine-preventable diseases, such as measles and whooping cough. Some vaccine program administrators fear that because of the social sensitivities surrounding the HPV vaccine, any effort to require the vaccine for school entry may prompt legislators to amend their laws to create nonmedical exemptions where they do not currently exist or to make existing exemptions easier to obtain. This has the potential not only to thwart the effort to stem the tide of cervical cancer, but to foster the spread of other vaccine-preventable diseases as well.

Financing Challenges Laid Bare

Another barrier to achieving universal vaccination of girls and young women will be the high price of the vaccine. Gardasil is expensive by vaccine standards, costing approximately $360 for the three-part series of injections. Despite this high cost, ACIP's endorsement means that Gardasil will be covered by most private insurers; in fact, a number of large insurers have already announced they will cover the vaccine for girls and young women within the ACIP-recommended age range. Still, the Institute of Medicine estimates that approximately 11% of all American children have private insurance that does not cover immunization, and even those with insurance coverage may have to pay deductibles and copayments that create a barrier to care.

Those who do not have private insurance or who cannot afford the out-of-pocket costs associated with Gardasil will need to rely on a patchwork system of programs that exist to support the delivery of subsidized vaccines to low-income and uninsured individuals. In June, ACIP voted to include Gardasil in the federal Vaccines for Children program (VFC), which provides free vaccines largely to children and teenagers through age 18 who are uninsured or receive Medicaid. The program's reach is significant: In 2003, 43% of all childhood vaccine doses were distributed by the VFC program.

The HPV vaccine, however, is not just recommended for children and teenagers; it is also recommended for young adult women up through age 26. Vaccines are considered an "optional" benefit for adults under Medicaid, meaning that it is up to each individual state to decide whether or not to cover a given vaccine. Also, states can use their own funds and federal grants to support the delivery of subsidized vaccines to low-income or uninsured adults. Many states, however, have opted instead to channel these funds toward childhood-vaccination efforts, particularly as vaccine prices have grown in recent years. As a result, adult vaccination rates remain low and disparities exist across racial, ethnic and socioeconomic groups—mirroring the disparities that exist for cervical cancer.

In response to all this, Merck in May announced it would create a new "patient assistance program," designed to provide all its vaccines free to adults who are uninsured, unable to afford the vaccines and have an annual household income below 200% of the federal poverty level ($19,600 for individuals and $26,400 for couples). To receive free vaccines, patients will need to complete and fax forms from participating doctors' offices for processing by Merck during the patients' visits. Many young uninsured women, however, do not seek their care in private doctors' offices, but instead rely on publicly funded family planning clinics for their care, suggesting the impact of this program may be limited (see box).

Thinking Ahead

Solutions to the various challenges presented by the HPV vaccine are likely to have relevance far beyond cervical cancer. In the coming years, scientific breakthroughs in the areas of immunology, molecular biology and genetics will eventually permit vaccination against a broader range of acute illnesses as well as chronic diseases. Currently, vaccines for other STIs such as chlamydia, herpes and HIV are in various stages of development. Also under study are

---

THE POTENTIAL ROLE OF FAMILY PLANNING CLINICS IN AN HPV VACCINE "CATCH-UP" CAMPAIGN

Family planning clinics, including those funded under Title X of the Public Health Service Act, have an important role to play in a national "catch-up" campaign to vaccinate young women against HPV. This is particularly true for women ages 19–26, who are too old to receive free vaccines through the federal Vaccines for Children program but still fall within the ACIP-recommended age range for the HPV vaccine.

Almost 4,600 Title X–funded family planning clinics provide subsidized family planning and related preventive health care to just over five million women nationwide. In theory, Title X clinics are well poised to offer the HPV vaccine, because they already are a major provider of STI services and cervical cancer screening, providing approximately six million STI (including HIV) tests and 2.7 million Pap tests in 2004 alone. Because Title X clients are disproportionately low income and women of color, they are at particular risk of developing cervical cancer later in life. Moreover, most Title X clients fall within the ACIP age recommendations of 26 and under for the HPV vaccine (59% are age 24 or younger, and 18% are ages 25–29); many of these women are uninsured and may not have an alternative source of health care.

Title X funds may be used to pay for vaccines linked to improved reproductive health outcomes, and some Title X clinics offer the Hepatitis B vaccine (which can be sexually transmitted). Although many family planning providers are expressing interest in incorporating the HPV vaccine into their package of services, its high cost—even at a discounted government purchase price—is likely to stand in the way. Clinics that receive Title X funds are required by law to charge women based on their ability to pay, with women under 100% of the federal poverty level (representing 68% of Title X clients) receiving services completely free of charge and those with incomes between 100–250% of poverty charged on a sliding scale. While Merck has expressed an interest in extending its patient assistance program to publicly funded family planning clinics, it makes no promises. In fact, a statement on the company's Web site says that "Due to the complexities associated with vaccine funding and distribution in the public sector, as well as the resource constraints that typically exist in public health settings, Merck is currently evaluating whether and how a vaccine assistance program could be implemented in the public sector."

vaccines for Alzheimer's disease, diabetes and a range of cancers. Vaccines for use among adolescents will also be increasingly common. A key question is, in the future, will individuals across the economic spectrum have access to these breakthrough medical advances or will disadvantaged individuals be left behind?

When viewed in this broader context, the debate over whether the HPV vaccine should be required for school enrollment may prove to be a healthy one. If the HPV vaccine is indeed "the first of its kind," as some have characterized it, it has the potential to prompt communities across the nation to reconsider and perhaps reconceive the philosophical justification for school entry requirements. Because the U.S. health care system is fragmented, people have no guarantee of health insurance coverage or access to affordable care. School entry requirements might therefore provide an important opportunity to deliver public health interventions that, like the HPV vaccine, offer protections to individuals who have the potential to become disconnected from health care services later in life. Similar to the HPV vaccine's promise of cervical cancer prevention, these benefits may not be felt for many years, but nonetheless may be compelling from a societal standpoint. And bearing in mind that school dropout rates begin to climb as early as age 13, middle school might be appropriately viewed as the last public health gate that an entire age-group of individuals pass through together—regardless of race, ethnicity or socioeconomic status.

Meanwhile, the cost and affordability issues raised by the HPV vaccine may help draw attention to the need to reform the vaccine-financing system in this country. In 2003, the Institute of Medicine proposed a series of reforms designed to improve the way vaccines are financed and distributed. They included a national insurance benefit mandate that would apply to all public and private health care plans and vouchers for uninsured children and adults to receive immunizations through the provider of their choice. Legislation introduced by Rep. Henry Waxman (D-CA) and Sen. Edward Kennedy (D-MA), called the Vaccine Access and Supply Act, adopts a different approach. The bill would expand the Vaccines for Children program, create a comparable Vaccines for Adults program, strengthen the vaccine grant program to the states and prohibit Medicaid cost-sharing requirements for ACIP-recommended vaccines for adults.

Whether the HPV vaccine will in fact hasten reforms of any kind remains to be seen. But one thing is clear: If the benefits of this groundbreaking vaccine cannot be enjoyed by girls and women who are disadvantaged by poverty or insurance status, then it will only serve to perpetuate the disparities in cervical cancer rates that have persisted in this country for far too long.

Cynthia Dailard was a senior public policy associate at the Guttmacher Institute and a NEPRHA Board member.

Gail Javitt, Deena Berkowitz,
and Lawrence O. Gostin

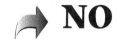 **NO**

Assessing Mandatory HPV Vaccination: Who Should Call the Shots?

I. Introduction

The human papillomavirus (HPV) is the most common sexually transmitted infection worldwide. In the United States, more than six million people are infected each year. Although most HPV infections are benign, two strains of HPV cause 70 percent of cervical cancer cases.[1] Two other strains of HPV are associated with 90 percent of genital warts cases.[2]

In June 2006, the Food and Drug Administration (FDA) approved the first vaccine against HPV. Sold as Gardasil, the quadrivalent vaccine is intended to prevent four strains of HPV associated with cervical cancer, precancerous genital lesions, and genital warts.[3] Following FDA approval, the national Advisory Committee on Immunization Practices (ACIP) recommended routine vaccination for girls ages 11–12 with three doses of quadrivalent HPV vaccine.[4] Thereafter, state legislatures around the country engaged in an intense effort to pass laws mandating vaccination of young girls against HPV. This activity was spurred in part by an intense lobbying campaign by Merck, the manufacturer of the vaccine.[5]

The United States has a robust state-based infrastructure for mandatory vaccination that has its roots in the 19th century. Mandating vaccination as a condition for school entry began in the early 1800s and is currently required by all 50 states for several common childhood infectious diseases.[6] Some suggest that mandatory HPV vaccination for minor females fits squarely within this tradition.

Nonetheless, state efforts to mandate HPV vaccination in minors have raised a variety of concerns on legal, ethical, and social grounds. Unlike other diseases for which state legislatures have mandated vaccination for children, HPV is neither transmissible through casual contact nor potentially fatal during childhood. It also would be the first vaccine to be mandated for use exclusively in one gender. As such, HPV vaccine presents a new context for considering vaccine mandates.

In this paper, we review the scientific evidence supporting Gardasil's approval and the legislative actions in the states that followed. We then argue that mandatory HPV vaccination at this time is both unwarranted and unwise. While the emergence of an HPV vaccine refects a potentially significant public health advance, the vac-

cine raises several concerns. First, the long-term safety and effectiveness of the vaccine are unclear, and serious adverse events reported shortly after the vaccine's approval raise questions about its short-term safety as well. In light of unanswered safety questions, the vaccine should be rolled out slowly, with risks carefully balanced against benefits in individual cases. Second, the legal and ethical justifications that have historically supported state-mandated vaccination do not support mandating HPV vaccine. Specifically, HPV does not threaten an imminent and significant risk to the health of others. Mandating HPV would therefore constitute an expansion of the state's authority to interfere with individual and parental autonomy. Engaging in such expansion in the absence of robust public discussion runs the risk of creating a public backlash that may undermine the goal of widespread HPV vaccine coverage and lead to public distrust of established childhood vaccine programs for other diseases. Third, the current sex-based HPV vaccination mandates present constitutional concerns because they require only girls to be vaccinated. Such concerns could lead to costly and protracted legal challenges. Finally, vaccination mandates will place economic burdens on federal and state governments and individual practitioners that may have a negative impact on the provision of other health services. In light of these potentially adverse public health, economic, and societal consequences, we believe that it is premature for states to add HPV to the list of state-mandated vaccines.

II. Background

Before discussing in detail the basis for our opposition to mandated HPV vaccination, it is necessary to review the public health impact of HPV and the data based on which the FDA approved the vaccine. Additionally, to understand the potentially widespread uptake of HPV vaccine mandates, we review the state legislative activities that have occurred since the vaccine's approval.

A. HPV Epidemiology

In the United States, an estimated 20 million people, or 15 percent of the population, are currently infected with HPV.[7] Modeling studies suggest that up to 80 percent of

Javitt, Gail, et al. From *Journal of Law, Medicine & Ethics*, vol. 36, issue 2, Summer 2008, pp. 384–395. Copyright © 2008 by American Society of Law, Medicine & Ethics. Reprinted by permission.

sexually active women will have become infected with the virus at some point in their lives by the time they reach age 50.[8] Prevalence of HPV is highest among sexually active females ages 14–19.[9]

Human papillomavirus comprises more than 100 different strains of virus, of which more than 30 infect the genital area.[10] The majority of HPV infections are transient, asymptomatic, and cause no clinical problems. However, persistent infection with high risk types of HPV is the most important risk factor for cervical cancer precursors and invasive cervical cancer. Two strains in particular, 16 and 18, have been classified as carcinogenic to humans by the World Health Organization's international agency for research on cancer.[11] These strains account for 70 percent of cervical cancer cases[12] and are responsible for a large proportion of anal, vulvar, vaginal, penile, and urethral cancers.[13]

More than 200,000 women die of cervical cancer each year.[14] The majority of these deaths take place in developing countries, which lack the screening programs and infrastructure for diagnosis, treatment, and prevention that exist in the United States. In the U.S., it is estimated that there were about 9,700 cases of invasive cervical cancer and about 3,700 deaths from cervical cancer in 2006, as compared with 500,000 cases and 288,000 deaths worldwide.[15]

Two other HPV types, 6 and 11, are associated with approximately 90 percent of anogenital warts. They are also associated with low grade cervical disease and recurrent respiratory papillomatosis (RRP), a disease consisting of recurrent warty growths in the larynx and respiratory tract. Juvenile onset RRP (JORRP), a rare disorder caused by exposure to HPV during the peripartum period, can cause significant airway obstruction or lead to squamous cell carcinoma with poor prognosis.[16]

Although HPV types 6, 11, 16, and 18 are associated with significant morbidity and mortality, they have a fairly low prevalence in the U.S. population. One study of sexually active women ages 18 to 25 found HPV 16 and 18 prevalence to be 7.8 percent.[17] Another study found overall prevalence of types 6, 11, 16, and 18 to be 1.3 percent, 0.1 percent, 1.5 percent, and 0.8 percent, respectively.[18]

B. Gardasil Safety and Effectiveness

Gardasil was approved based on four randomized, double blind, placebo-controlled studies in 21,000 women ages 16 to 26. Girls as young as nine were included in the safety and immunogenicity studies but not the efficacy studies. The results demonstrated that in women without prior HPV infection, Gardasil was nearly 100 percent effective in preventing precancerous cervical lesions, precancerous vaginal and vulvar lesions, and genital warts caused by vaccine-type HPV. Although the study period was not long enough for cervical cancer to develop, the prevention of these cervical precancerous lesions was considered a valid surrogate marker for cancer prevention. The studies also show that the vaccine is only effective when given prior to infection with high-risk strains.[19]

Gardasil is the second virus-like particle (VLP) vaccine to be approved by the FDA; the first was the Hepatitis B vaccine. VLPs consist of viral protein particles derived from the structural proteins of a virus. These particles are nearly identical to the virus from which they were derived but lack the virus's genetic material required for replication, so they are noninfectious and nononcogenic. VLPs offer advantages over more traditional peptide vaccines as the human body is more highly attuned to particulate antigens, which leads to a stronger immune response since VLP vaccines cannot revert to an infectious form, such as attenuated particles or incompletely killed particles.

No serious Gardasil-related adverse events were observed during clinical trials. The most common adverse events reported were injection site reactions, including pain, redness, and swelling.[20] The most common systemic adverse reactions experienced at the same rate by both vaccine and placebo recipients were headache, fever, and nausea. Five vaccine recipients reported adverse vaccine-related experiences: bronchospasm, gastroenteritis, headache with hypertension, joint movement impairment near injection site, and vaginal hemorrhage. Women with positive pregnancy tests were excluded from the studies, as were some women who became pregnant following receipt of either vaccine or placebo. The incidence of spontaneous pregnancy loss and congenital anomalies were similar in both groups.[21] Gardasil was assigned pregnancy risk category B by the FDA on the basis that animal reproduction studies failed to demonstrate a risk to the fetus.[22]

As of June 2007, the most recent date for which CDC has made data available, there were 1,763 reports of potential side effects following HPV vaccination made to the CDC's Vaccine Adverse Event Reporting System (VAERS). Ninety-four of these were defined as serious, including 13 unconfirmed reports of Guillain-Barre syndrome (GBS), a neurological illness resulting in muscle weakness and sometimes in paralysis. The CDC is investigating these cases. Seven deaths were also reported among females who received the vaccine, but the CDC stated that none of these deaths appeared to be caused by vaccination.[23]

Although the FDA approved the vaccine for females ages 9–26, based on the data collected in those age groups, the ACIP recommendation for vaccination is limited to females ages 11–12. This recommendation was based on several considerations, including age of sexual debut in the United States and the high probability of HPV acquisition within several years of sexual debut, cost-effectiveness evaluations, and the established young adolescent health care visit at ages 11–12 when other vaccines are also recommended.

C. State Legislative Activities

Since the approval of Gardasil, legislators in 41 states and the District of Columbia have introduced legislation addressing the HPV vaccine.[24] Legislative responses to

Gardasil have focused on the following recommendations: (1) mandating HPV vaccination of minor girls as a condition for school entrance; (2) mandating insurance coverage for HPV vaccination or providing state funding to defray or eliminate cost of vaccination; (3) educating the public about the HPV vaccine; and/or (4) establishing committees to make recommendations about the vaccine.

In 2007, 24 states and the District of Columbia introduced legislation specifically to mandate the HPV vaccine as a condition for school entry.[25] Of these, only Virginia and Washington, D.C. passed laws requiring HPV vaccination. The Virginia law requires females to receive three properly spaced doses of HPV vaccine, with the first dose to be administered before the child enters sixth grade. A parent or guardian may refuse vaccination for his child after reviewing "materials describing the link between the human papillomavirus and cervical cancer approved for such use by the Board of Health."[26] The law will take effect October 1, 2008.

Additionally, the D.C. City Council passed the HPV Vaccination and Reporting Act of 2007, which directs the mayor to establish an HPV vaccination program "consistent with the standards set forth by the Centers for Disease Control for all females under the age of 13 who are residents of the District of Columbia."[27] The program includes a "requirement that the parent or legal guardian of a female child enrolling in grade 6 for the first time submit certification that the child has received the HPV vaccine" and a provision that "allows a parent or guardian to opt out of the HPV vaccination requirement." It also directs the mayor to develop reporting requirements "for the collection and analyzation [sic] of HPV vaccination data within the District of Columbia Department of Health," including "annual reporting to the Department of Health as to the immunization status of each female child entering grade 6." The law requires Congressional approval in order to take effect.

In contrast, an Executive Order issued by the Texas governor was thwarted by that state's legislature. Executive Order 4, signed by Governor Rick Perry on February 4, 2007, would have directed the state's health department to adopt rules mandating the "age appropriate vaccination of all female children for HPV prior to admission to the sixth grade."[28] It would have allowed parents to "submit a request for a conscientious objection affidavit form via the Internet." However, H.B. 1098, enacted by the Texas state legislature on April 26, 2007, states that HPV immunization is "not required for a person's admission to any elementary or secondary school," and "preempts any contrary order issued by the governor."[29] The bill was filed without the governor's signature and became effective on May 8, 2007.

Of the 22 other states in which legislation mandating HPV vaccination was introduced in 2007, all would have required girls to be vaccinated somewhere between ages 11 and 13 or before entry into sixth grade. Most would have provided for some sort of parental or guardian exemption, whether for religious, moral, medical, cost, or other reasons. However, vaccine mandate bills in California and Maryland were withdrawn.

Bills requiring insurance companies to cover HPV vaccination or allocating state funds for this purpose were enacted in eight states.[30] Eight states also enacted laws aimed at promoting awareness of the HPV vaccine using various mechanisms, such as school-based distribution of educational materials to parents of early adolescent children.[31] Finally, three states established expert bodies to engage in further study of HPV vaccination either instead of or as an adjunct to other educational efforts.[32]

In total, 41 states and D.C. introduced legislation addressing HPV vaccination in some manner during the 2007 legislative session, and 17 of these states enacted laws relating to HPV vaccination.

III. Why Mandating HPV Is Premature

The approval of a vaccine against cancer-causing HPV strains is a significant public health advance. Particularly in developing countries, which lack the health care resources for routine cervical cancer screening, preventing HPV infection has the potential to save millions of lives. In the face of such a dramatic advance, opposing government-mandated HPV vaccination may seem foolhardy, if not heretical. Yet strong legal, ethical, and policy arguments underlie our position that state-mandated HPV vaccination of minor females is premature.

A. Long-Term Safety and Effectiveness of the Vaccine Is Unknown

Although the aim of clinical trials is to generate safety and effectiveness data that can be extrapolated to the general population, it is widely understood that such trials cannot reveal all possible adverse events related to a product. For this reason, post-market adverse event reporting is required for all manufacturers of FDA-approved products, and post-market surveillance (also called "phase IV studies") may be required in certain circumstances. There have been numerous examples in recent years in which unforeseen adverse reactions following product approval led manufacturers to withdraw their product from the market. For example, in August 1998, the FDA approved Rotashield, the first vaccine for the prevention of rotavirus gastroenteritis in infants. About 7,000 children received the vaccine before the FDA granted the manufacturer a license to market the vaccine. Though a few cases of intussusception, or bowel obstruction, were noted during clinical trials, there was no statistical difference between the overall occurrence of intussusception in vaccine compared with placebo recipients. After administration of approximately 1.5 million doses of vaccine, however, 15 cases of intussusception were reported, and were found to be causally related to the vaccine. The manufacturer subsequently withdrew the vaccine from the market in October 1999.[33]

In the case of HPV vaccine, short-term clinical trials in thousands of young women did not reveal serious adverse effects. However, the adverse events reported since the vaccine's approval are, at the very least, a sobering reminder that rare adverse events may surface as the vaccine is administered to millions of girls and young women. Concerns have also been raised that other carcinogenic HPV types not contained in the vaccines will replace HPV types 16 and 18 in the pathological niche.

The duration of HPV vaccine-induced immunity is unclear. The average follow-up period for Gardasil during clinical trials was 15 months after the third dose of the vaccine. Determining long-term efficacy is complicated by the fact that even during naturally occurring HPV infection, HPV antibodies are not detected in many women. Thus, long-term, follow-up post-licensure studies cannot rely solely upon serologic measurement of HPV-induced antibody titers. One study indicates that protection against persistent HPV 16 infection remained at 94 percent 3.5 years after vaccination with HPV 16.[34] A second study showed similar protection for types 16 and 18 after 4.5 years.[35]

The current ACIP recommendation is based on assumptions about duration of immunity and age of sexual debut, among other factors. As the vaccine is used for a longer time period, it may turn out that a different vaccine schedule is more effective. In addition, the effect on co-administration of other vaccines with regard to safety is unknown, as is the vaccines' efficacy with varying dose intervals. Some have also raised concerns about a negative impact of vaccination on cervical cancer screening programs, which are highly effective at reducing cervical cancer mortality. These unknowns must be studied as the vaccine is introduced in the broader population.

At present, therefore, questions remain about the vaccine's safety and the duration of its immunity, which call into question the wisdom of mandated vaccination. Girls receiving the vaccine face some risk of potential adverse events as well as risk that the vaccine will not be completely protective. These risks must be weighed against the state's interest in protecting the public from the harms associated with HPV. As discussed in the next section, the state's interest in protecting the public health does not support mandating HPV vaccination.

B. Historical Justifications for Mandated Vaccination Are Not Met

HPV is different in several respects from the vaccines that first led to state-mandated vaccination. Compulsory vaccination laws originated in the early 1800s and were driven by fears of the centuries-old scourge of smallpox and the advent of the vaccine developed by Edward Jenner in 1796. By the 1900s, the vast majority of states had enacted compulsory smallpox vaccination laws.[36] While such laws were not initially tied to school attendance, the coincidental rise of smallpox outbreaks, growth in the number of public schools, and compulsory school attendance laws provided a rationale for compulsory vaccination to prevent the spread of smallpox among school children as well as a means to enforce the requirement by barring unvaccinated children from school.[37] In 1827, Boston became the first city to require all children entering public school to provide evidence of vaccination.[38] Similar laws were enacted by several states during the latter half of the 19th century.[39]

The theory of herd immunity, in which the protective effect of vaccines extends beyond the vaccinated individual to others in the population, is the driving force behind mass immunization programs. Herd immunity theory proposes that, in diseases passed from person to person, it is difficult to maintain a chain of infection when large numbers of a population are immune. With the increase in number of immune individuals present in a population, the lower the likelihood that a susceptible person will come into contact with an infected individual. There is no threshold value above which herd immunity exists, but as vaccination rates increase, indirect protection also increases until the infection is eliminated.

Courts were soon called on to adjudicate the constitutionality of mandatory vaccination programs. In 1905, the Supreme Court decided the seminal case, *Jacobson v. Massachusetts*,[40] in which it upheld a population-wide smallpox vaccination ordinance challenged by an adult male who refused the vaccine and was fined five dollars. He argued that a compulsory vaccination law was "hostile to the inherent right of every freeman to care for his own body and health in such way as to him seems best." The Court disagreed, adopting a narrower view of individual liberty and emphasizing the duties that citizens have towards each other and to society as a whole. According to the Court, the "liberty secured by the Constitution of the United States . . . does not import an absolute right in each person to be, at all times and in all circumstances, wholly freed from restraint. There are manifold restraints to which every person is necessarily subject for the common good." With respect to compulsory vaccination, the Court stated that "[u]pon the principle of self-defense, of paramount necessity, a community has the right to protect itself against an epidemic of disease which threatens the safety of its members." In the Court's opinion, compulsory vaccination was consistent with a state's traditional police powers, i.e., its power to regulate matters affecting the health, safety, and general welfare of the public.

In reaching its decision, the Court was influenced both by the significant harm posed by smallpox—using the words "epidemic" and "danger" repeatedly—as well as the available scientific evidence demonstrating the efficacy of the vaccine. However, the Court also emphasized that its ruling was applicable only to the case before it, and articulated principles that must be adhered to for such an exercise of police powers to be constitutional. First, there must be a public health necessity. Second, there must be a reasonable relationship between the intervention and public health objective. Third, the intervention may not be arbitrary or oppressive. Finally, the intervention should not pose a health risk to its subject. Thus, while *Jacobson* "stands firmly for the proposition that police powers authorize states to compel vaccination for the public good," it also indicates that "government power must be exercised reasonably to pass constitutional scrutiny."[41] In the 1922 case *Zucht v. King*,[42] the Court reaffirmed its ruling in *Jacobson* in the context of a school-based smallpox vaccination mandate.

The smallpox laws of the 19th century, which were almost without exception upheld by the courts, helped lay the foundation for modern immunization statutes. Many modern-era laws were enacted in response to the transmission of measles in schools in the 1960s and 1970s. In 1977, the federal government launched the Childhood Immunization Initiative, which stressed the importance of strict enforcement of school immunization laws.[43] Currently, all states mandate vaccination as a condition for school entry, and in deciding whether to mandate vaccines, are guided by ACIP recommendations. At present, ACIP recommends vaccination for diphtheria, tetanus, and acellular pertussis (DTaP), Hepatitis B, polio, measles, mumps, and rubella (MMR), varicella (chicken pox), influenza, rotavirus, haemophilus Influenza B (HiB), pneumococcus, Hepatitis A, meningococcus, and, most recently HPV. State mandates differ; for example, whereas all states require DTaP, polio, and measles in order to enter kindergarten, most do not require Hepatitis A.[44]

HPV is different from the vaccines that have previously been mandated by the states. With the exception of tetanus, all of these vaccines fit comfortably within the "public health necessity" principle articulated in *Jacobson* in that the diseases they prevent are highly contagious and are associated with significant morbidity and mortality occurring shortly after exposure. And, while tetanus is not contagious, exposure to *Clostridium tetani* is both virtually unavoidable (particularly by children, given their propensity to both play in the dirt and get scratches), life threatening, and fully preventable only through vaccination. Thus, the public health necessity argument plausibly extends to tetanus, albeit for different reasons.

Jacobson's "reasonable relationship" principle is also clearly met by vaccine mandates for the other ACIP recommended vaccines. School-aged children are most at risk while in school because they are more likely to be in close proximity to each other in that setting. All children who attend school are equally at risk of both transmitting and contracting the diseases. Thus, a clear relationship exists between conditioning school attendance on vaccination and the avoidance of the spread of infectious disease within the school environment. Tetanus, a non-contagious disease, is somewhat different, but school-based vaccination can nevertheless be justified in that children will foreseeably be exposed within the school environment (e.g., on the playground) and, if exposed, face a high risk of mortality.

HPV vaccination, in contrast, does not satisfy these two principles. HPV infection presents no public health necessity, as that term was used in the context of *Jacobson*. While non-sexual transmission routes are theoretically possible, they have not been demonstrated. Like other sexually transmitted diseases which primarily affect adults, it is not immediately life threatening; as such, cervical cancer, if developed, will not manifest for years if not decades. Many women will never be exposed to the cancer-causing strains of HPV; indeed the prevalence of these strains in the U.S. is quite low. Furthermore, many who are exposed will not go on to develop cervical cancer. Thus, conditioning school attendance on HPV vaccination serves only to coerce compliance in the absence of a public health emergency.[45]

The relationship between the government's objective of preventing cervical cancer in women and the means used to achieve it—that is, vaccination of all girls as a condition of school attendance—lacks sufficient rationality. First, given that HPV is transmitted through sexual activity, exposure to HPV is not directly related to school attendance.[46] Second, not all children who attend school are at equal risk of exposure to or transmission of the virus. Those who abstain from sexual conduct are not at risk for transmitting or contracting HPV. Moreover, because HPV screening tests are available, the risk to those who choose to engage in sexual activity is significantly minimized. Because it is questionable how many school-aged children are actually at risk—and for those who are at risk, the risk is not linked to school attendance—there is not a sufficiently rational reason to tie mandatory vaccination to school attendance.

To be sure, the public health objective that proponents of mandatory HPV vaccination seek to achieve is compelling. Vaccinating girls before sexual debut provides an opportunity to provide protection against an adult onset disease. This opportunity is lost once sexual activity begins and exposure to HPV occurs. However, that HPV vaccination may be both medically justified and a prudent public health measure is an insufficient basis for the state to compel children to receive the vaccine as a condition of school attendance.

C. In the Absence of Historical Justification, the Government Risks Public Backlash by Mandating HPV Vaccination

Childhood vaccination rates in the United States are very high; more than half of the states report meeting the Department of Health and Human Services (HHS) Healthy People 2010 initiative's goal of 95 percent vaccination coverage for childhood vaccination.[47] However, from its inception, state mandated vaccination has been accompanied by a small but vocal anti-vaccination movement. Opposition has historically been "fueled by general distrust of government, a rugged sense of individualism, and concerns about the efficacy and safety of vaccines."[48] In recent years, vaccination programs also have been a "victim of their tremendous success,"[49] as dreaded diseases such as measles and polio have largely disappeared in the United States, taking with them the fear that motivated past generations. Some have noted with alarm the rise in the number of parents opting out of vaccination and of resurgence in anti-vaccination rhetoric making scientifically unsupported allegations that vaccination causes adverse events such as autism.[50]

The rash of state legislation to mandate HPV has led to significant public concern that the government is over-reaching its police powers authority. As one conservative columnist has written, "[F]or the government to mandate the expensive vaccine for children would be for Big Brother to reach past the parents and into the home."[51] While some dismiss sentiments such as this one as simply motivated by right wing moral politics, trivializing these concerns is both inappropriate and unwise as a policy matter. Because sexual behavior is involved in transmission, not all children are equally at risk. Thus, it is a reasonable exercise of a parent's judgment to consider his or her child's specific risk and weigh that against the risk of vaccination.

To remove parental autonomy in this case is not warranted and also risks parental rejection of the vaccine because it is perceived as coercive. In contrast, educating the public about the value of the vaccine may be highly effective without risking public backlash. According to one poll, 61 percent of parents with daughters under 18 prefer vaccination, 72 percent would support the inclusion of information about the vaccine in school health classes, and just 45 percent agreed that the vaccine should be included as part of the vaccination routine for all children and adolescents.[52]

Additionally, Merck's aggressive role in lobbying for the passage of state laws mandating HPV has led to some skepticism about whether profit rather than public health has driven the push for state mandates.[53] Even one proponent of state-mandated HPV vaccination acknowledges that Merck "overplayed its hand" by pushing hard for legislation mandating the vaccine.[54] In the face of such criticisms, the company thus ceased its lobbying efforts but indicated it would continue to educate health officials and legislators about the vaccine.[55]

Some argue that liberal opt-out provisions will take care of the coercion and distrust issues. Whether this is true will depend in part on the reasons for which a parent may opt out and the ease of opting out. For example, a parent may not have a religious objection to vaccination in general, but nevertheless may not feel her 11-year-old daughter is at sufficient risk for HPV to warrant vaccination. This sentiment may or may not be captured in a "religious or philosophical" opt-out provision.

Even if opt-out provisions do reduce public distrust issues for HPV, however, liberal opt outs for one vaccine may have a negative impact on other vaccine programs. Currently, with the exception of those who opt out of all vaccines on religious or philosophical grounds, parents must accept all mandated vaccines because no vaccine-by-vaccine selection process exists, which leads to a high rate of vaccine coverage. Switching to an "a la carte" approach, in which parents can consider the risks and benefits of vaccines on a vaccine-by-vaccine basis, would set a dangerous precedent and may lead them to opt out of other vaccines, causing a rise in the transmission of these diseases. In contrast, an "opt in" approach to HPV vaccine would not require a change in the existing paradigm and would still likely lead to a high coverage rate.

D. Mandating HPV for Girls and Not Boys May Violate Constitutional Principles of Equality and Due Process

1. VACCINATION OF MALES MAY PROTECT THEM FROM HPV-RELATED MORBIDITY

The HPV vaccine is the first to be mandated for only one gender. This is likely because the vaccine was approved for girls and not boys. Data demonstrating the safety and immunogenicity of the vaccine are available for males aged 9–15 years. Three phase 1 studies demonstrated that safety, tolerance, and immunogenicity of the HPV vaccine were similar to men and women. The first two studies focused on HPV 16 and 11, respectively, while the third study demonstrated high levels of immunogenicity to prophylactic HPV 6/11/16/18 vaccine in 10–15-year-old males.[56] Phase III clinical trials examining the vaccine's efficacy in men and adolescent boys are currently underway, with results available in the next couple of years.[57]

HPV infection is common among men.[58] One percent of the male population aged 15–49 years has genital warts, with peak incidence in the 20–24-year-old age group.[59] A recent cohort study found the 24-month cumulative incidence of HPV infection among 240 men aged 18–20 years to be 62.4 percent, nearly double the incidence of their female counter-parts.[60] This result may have been due to the increased sensitivity of the new HPV-PCR-based testing procedure used in the study. Nonetheless, the results reaffirm that HPV is common and multifocal in males. Males with genital warts have also been shown to carry the genital type specific HPV virus on their fingertips.[61] While HPV on fingertips may be due to autoinoculation, it may also represent another means of transmission.[62] Men are also at risk for HPV-related anogenital cancers. Up to 76 percent of penile cancers are HPV DNA positive.[63] Fifty-eight percent of anal cancers in heterosexual men and 100 percent among homosexual men are positive for HPV DNA.[64] Therefore, assuming vaccine efficacy is confirmed in males, they also could be protected through HPV vaccination.

2. INCLUDING MALES IN HPV VACCINATION MAY BETTER PROTECT THE PUBLIC THAN FEMALE VACCINATION ALONE

As no clinical trial data on vaccine efficacy in men has been published to date, mathematical models have been used to explore the potential benefits and cost effectiveness of vaccinating boys in addition to girls under various clinical scenarios. Even under the most generous assumption about vaccine efficacy in males and females, cost-effective analyses have found contradictory results. Several studies suggest that if vaccine coverage of women reaches 70–90 percent of the population, then vaccinating males would be of limited value and high cost.[65] Ruanne Barnabas and Geoffrey Garnett found that a multivalent HPV vaccine with 100 percent efficacy targeting males and females 15 years of age with vaccine coverage of at least 66 percent was needed to decrease cervical cancer by 80 percent. They concluded that vaccinating men in addition to women had little incremental benefit in reducing cervical cancer,[66] that vaccine acceptability in males is unknown, and that in a setting with limited resources, the first priority in reducing cervical cancer mortality should be to vaccinate females.

Yet several models argue in favor of vaccinating males. Vaccination not only directly protects through vaccine-derived immunity, but also indirectly through herd immunity, meaning a level of population immunity that is sufficient to protect unvaccinated individuals. If naturally acquired immunity is low and coverage of women is low, then vaccinating men will be of significant benefit. James Hughes et al. found that a female-only monovalent vaccine would be only 60–75 percent as efficient as a strategy that targets both genders.[67] Elamin Elbasha and Erik Dasbach found that while vaccinating 70 percent of females before the age of 12 would reduce genital warts by 83 percent and cervical cancer by 78 percent due to HPV 6/11/16/18, including men and boys in the program would further reduce the incidence of genital warts, CIN, and cervical cancer by 97 percent, 91 percent, and 91 percent, respectively.[68] In all mathematical models, lower female coverage made vaccination of men and adolescent boys more cost effective, as did a shortened duration of natural immunity.

All the models include parameters that are highly inferential and lacking in evidence, such as duration of vaccine protection, reactivation of infections, transmission of infection, and health utilities. The scope of the models is limited to cervical cancer, cancer-in-situ, and genital warts. None of the models accounts for HPV-related anal, head, and neck cancers, or recurrent respiratory papillomatosis. As more data become available, the scope of the models will be broadened and might strengthen the argument in favor of vaccinating males. Given that male vaccination may better protect the public than female vaccination alone, female-specific mandates may be constitutionally suspect, as discussed below.

3. THE GOVERNMENT MUST ADEQUATELY JUSTIFY ITS DECISION TO MANDATE VACCINATION IN FEMALES ONLY

While courts have generally been deferential to state mandate laws, this deference has its limits. In 1900, a federal court struck a San Francisco Board of Health resolution requiring all Chinese residents to be vaccinated with a serum against bubonic plague about which there was little evidence of efficacy. Chinese residents were prohibited from leaving the area unless they were vaccinated. The court struck down the resolution as an unconstitutional violation of the Equal Protection and Due Process clauses. The court found that there was not a defensible scientific rationale for the board's approach and that it was discriminatory in targeting "the Asiatic or Mongolian race as a class." Thus, it was "not within the legitimate police power" of the government.[69]

A sex-based mandate for HPV vaccination could be challenged on two grounds: first, under the Equal Protection Clause because it distinguishes based on gender and second, under the Due Process Clause, because it violates a protected interest in refusing medical treatment. In regard to the Equal Protection concerns, courts review laws that make sex-based distinctions with heightened scrutiny: the government must show that the challenged classification serves an important state interest and that the classification is at least substantially related to serving that interest. To be sure, courts would likely view the goal of preventing cervical cancer as an important public health objective. However, courts would also likely demand that the state justify its decision to burden females with the risks of vaccination, and not males, even though males also contribute to HPV transmission, will benefit from an aggressive vaccination program of females, and also may reduce their own risk of disease through vaccination.

With respect to the Due Process Clause, the Supreme Court has, in the context of right-to-die cases, recognized that individuals have a constitutionally protected liberty interest in refusing unwanted medical treatment.[70] This liberty interest must, however, be balanced against several state interests, including its interest in preserving life. Mandated HPV laws interfere with the right of girls to refuse medical treatment, and therefore could be challenged under the Due Process Clause. Whether the government could demonstrate interests strong enough to outweigh a girl's liberty interest in refusing vaccination would depend on the strength of the government's argument that such vaccination is life-saving and the extent to which opt outs are available and easily exercised in practice.

Even if courts upheld government mandates as consistent with the Due Process and Equal Protection clauses, such mandates remain troubling in light of inequalities imposed by sex-based mandates and the liberty interests that would be compromised by HPV mandates, therefore placing deeply cherished national values at risk.

E. Unresolved Economic Concerns

Mandated HPV vaccination may have negative unintended economic consequences for both state health departments and private physicians, and these consequences should be thoroughly considered before HPV vaccination is mandated. In recent years, state health departments have found themselves increasingly strapped by the rising number of mandated vaccines. Some states that once provided free vaccines to all children have abandoned the practice due to rising costs. Adding HPV could drive more states to abandon funding for other vaccinations and could divert funding from other important public health measures. At the federal level, spending by the federal Vaccines for Children program, which pays for immunizations for Medicaid children and some others, has grown to $2.5 billion, up from $500 million in 2000.[71] Such rapid increases in budgetary expenses affect the program's ability to assist future patients. Thus, before HPV vaccination is mandated, a thorough consideration of its economic consequences for existing vaccine programs and other non-vaccine programs should be undertaken.

The increasing number of vaccines has also has placed a burden on physicians in private practice. Currently, about 85 percent of the nation's children get all or at least some of their inoculations from private physicians' offices.[72] These offices must purchase vaccines and then wait for reimbursement from either government or private insurers. Some physicians have argued that the rising costs of vaccines and the rising number of new mandatory vaccines make it increasingly difficult for them to purchase vaccinations initially and that they net a loss due to insufficient reimbursement from insurers. Adding HPV to the list of mandated vaccines would place further stress on these practices, and could lead them to reduce the amount of vaccines they purchase or require up-front payment for these vaccines. Either of these steps could reduce access not only to HPV but to all childhood vaccines.

Access to HPV is one reason that some proponents favor state mandates. They argue that in the absence of a state mandate, parents will not know to request the vaccine, or will not be able to afford it because it will not be covered by insurance companies or by federal or state programs that pay for vaccines for the uninsured and underinsured. However, mandates are not the only way to increase parental awareness or achieve insurance coverage. In light of the potentially significant economic consequences of state mandates, policymakers should consider other methods of increasing parental awareness and insurance coverage that do not also threaten to reduce access to those who want vaccination.

IV. Conclusion

Based on the current scientific evidence, vaccinating girls against HPV before they are sexually active appears to provide significant protection against cervical cancer.

The vaccine thus represents a significant public health advance. Nevertheless, mandating HPV vaccination at the present time would be premature and ill-advised. The vaccine is relatively new, and long-term safety and effectiveness in the general population is unknown. Vaccination outcomes of those voluntarily vaccinated should be followed for several years before mandates are imposed. Additionally, the HPV vaccine does not represent a public health necessity of the type that has justified previous vaccine mandates. State mandates could therefore lead to a public backlash that will undermine both HPV vaccination efforts and existing vaccination programs. Finally, the economic consequences of mandating HPV are significant and could have a negative impact on financial support for other vaccines as well as other public health programs. These consequences should be considered before HPV is mandated.

The success of childhood vaccination programs makes them a tempting target for the addition of new vaccines that, while beneficial to public health, exceed the original justifications for the development of such programs and impose new financial burdens on both the government, private physicians, and, ultimately, the public. HPV will not be the last disease that state legislatures will attempt to prevent through mandatory vaccination. Thus, legislatures and public health advocates should consider carefully the consequences of altering the current paradigm for mandatory childhood vaccination and should not mandate HPV vaccination in the absence of a new paradigm to justify such an expansion.

Note

The views expressed in this article are those of the authors and do not reflect those of the Genetics and Public Policy Center or its staff.

References

1. D. Saslow et al., "American Cancer Society Guideline for Human Papillomavirus (HPV) Vaccine Use to Prevent Cervical Cancer and Its Precursors," *CA: A Cancer Journal for Clinicians* 57, no. 1 (2007): 7–28.
2. Editorial, "Should HPV Vaccination Be Mandatory for All Adolescents?" *The Lancet* 368, no. 9543 (2006): 1212.
3. U.S. Food and Drug Administration, *FDA Licenses New Vaccine for Prevention of Cervical Cancer and Other Diseases in Females Caused by Human Papillomavirus: Rapid Approval Marks Major Advancement in Public Health*, Press Release, June 8, 2006, *available at* . . . (last visited March 5, 2008).
4. Centers for Disease Control and Prevention, *CDC's Advisory Committee Recommends Human Papillomavirus Virus Vaccination*, Press Release, June 29, 2006, *available at* . . . (last visited March 5, 2008).

5. A. Pollack and S. Saul, "Lobbying for Vaccine to Be Halted," *New York Times,* February 21, 2007, *availiable at . . .* (last visited March 14, 2008).

6. Centers for Disease Control and Prevention, *Childcare and School Immunization Requirements, 2005–2006, August 2006, available at . . .* (last visited March 5, 2008).

7. Centers for Disease Control and Prevention, "A Closer Look at Human Papillomavirus (HPV)," 2000, *available at . . .* (last visited March 5, 2008); Centers for Disease Control and Prevention, "Genital HPV Infection—CDC Fact Sheet," May 2004, *available at . . .* (last visited March 5, 2008).

8. See Saslow et al., *supra* note 1.

9. S. D. Datta et al., "Sentinel Surveillance for Human Papillomavirus among Women in the United States, 2003–2004," in Program and Abstracts of the 16th Biennial Meeting of the International Society for Sexually Transmitted Diseases Research, Amsterdam, The Netherlands, July 10–13, 2005.

10. Centers for Disease Control and Prevention, "Human Papillomavirus (HPV) Infection," July 2, 2007, *available at . . .* (last visited March 5, 2008).

11. J. R. Nichols, "Human Papillomavirus Infection: The Role of Vaccination in Pediatric Patients," *Clinical Pharmacology and Therapeutics* 81, no. 4 (2007) 607–610.

12. See Saslow et al., *supra* note 1.

13. J. M. Walboomers et al., "Human Papillomavirus Is a Necessary Cause of Invasive Cervical Cancer Worldwide," *Journal of Pathology* 189, no. 1 (1999) 12–19.

14. J. K. Chan and J. S. Berek, "Impact of the Human Papilloma Vaccine on Cervical Cancer," *Journal of Clinical Oncology* 25, no. 20 (2007): 2975–2982.

15. See Saslow et al., *supra* note 1.

16. B. Simma et al., "Squamous-Cell Carcinoma Arising in a Non-Irradiated Child with Recurrent Respiratory Papillomatosis," *European Journal of Pediatrics* 152, no. 9 (1993): 776–778.

17. E. F. Dunne et al., "Prevalence of HPV Infection among Females in the United States," *JAMA* 297, no. 8 (2007): 813–819.

18. L. E. Markowitz et al., "Quadrivalent Human Papillomavirus Vaccine: Recommendations of the Advisory Committee on Immunization Practices (ACIP)," *Morbidity and Mortality Weekly Report* 55, no. RR-2 (2007): 1–24.

19. L. A. Koutsky et al., "A Controlled Trial of a Human Papillomavirus Type 16 Vaccine," *New England Journal of Medicine* 347, no. 21 (2002): 1645–1651; D. R. Brown et al., "Early Assessment of the Efficacy of a Human Papillomavirus Type 16L1 Virus-Like Particle Vaccine," *Vaccine* 22, nos. 21–22 (2004): 2936–2942; C. M. Wheeler, "Advances in Primary and Secondary Interventions for Cervical Cancer: Human Papillomavirus Prophylactic Vaccines and Testing," *Nature Clinical Practice Oncology* 4, no. 4 (2007): 224–235; L. L. Villa et al., "Prophylactic Quadrivalent Human Papillomavirus (Types 6, 11, 16, and 18) L1 Virus-Like Particle Vaccine in Young Women: A Randomized Double-Blind Placebo-Controlled Multicentre Phase II Efficacy Trial," *The Lancet Oncology* 6, no. 5 (2005): 271–278; see Saslow, *supra* note 1.

20. *Id.* (Villa).

21. See Wheeler, *supra* note 19.

22. N. B. Miller, *Clinical Review of Biologics License Application for Human Papillomavirus 6, 11, 16, 18 L1 Virus Like Particle Vaccine (S. cerevisiae) (STN 125126 GARDASIL), Manufactured by Merck, Inc.,"* Food and Drug Administration, June 8, 2006, *available at . . .* (last visited March 5, 2008).

23. Centers for Disease Control and Prevention, *HPV Vaccine—Questions and Answers for the Public,* June 28, 2007, *available at . . .* (last visited April 2, 2008).

24. National Conference of State Legislatures, "HPV Vaccine," July 11, 2007, *available at . . .* (last visited March 5, 2008).

25. *Id.*

26. S.B. 1230, 2006 Session, Virginia (2007); H.B. 2035, 2006 Session, Virginia (2007).

27. *HPV Vaccination and Reporting Act of 2007,* B.17–0030, 18th Council, District of Columbia (2007).

28. Governor of the State of Texas, Executive Order RP65, February 2, 2007, *available at . . .* (last visited March 5, 2008).

29. S.B. 438, 80th Legislature, Texas (2007); H.B. 1098, 80th Legislature, Texas (2007).

30. The states are Colorado, Maine, Nevada, New Mexico, New York, North Dakota, Rhode Island, and South Carolina. See National Conference of State Legislatures, *supra* note 24.

31. The states are Colorado, Indiana, Iowa, North Carolina, North Dakota, Texas, Utah, and Washington. *Id.* (National Conference of State Legislatures).

32. The states are Maryland, Minnesota, and New Mexico. *Id.* (National Conference of State Legislatures).

33. Centers for Disease Control and Prevention, *RotaShield (Rotavirus) Vaccine and Intussusception,* 2004, *available at . . .* (last visited March 14, 2008); M. B. Rennels, "The Rotavirus Vaccine Story: A Clinical Investigator's View," *Pediatrics* 106, no. 1 (2000): 123–125.

34. C. Mao et al., "Efficacy of Human Papillomavirus-16 Vaccine to Prevent Cervical Intraepithelial Neoplasia: A Randomized Controlled Trial," *Obstetrics and Gynecology* 107, no. 1 (2006): 18–27.

35. L. L. Villa et al., "Immunologic Responses Following Administration of a Vaccine Targeting Human Papillomavirus Types 6, 11, 16 and 18," *Vaccine* 24, no. 27–28 (2006): 5571–5583; D. M. Harper et al., "Sustained Efficacy Up to

4.5 Years of a Bivalent L1 Virus-Like Particle Vaccine against Human Papillomavirus Types 16 and 18: Follow Up from a Randomized Controlled Trial," *The Lancet* 367, no. 9518 (2006): 1247–1255.

36. J. G. Hodge and L. O. Gostin, "School Vaccination Requirements: Historical, Social, and Legal Perspectives," *Kentucky Law Journal* 90, no. 4 (2001-2002): 831–890.

37. J. Duffy, "School Vaccination: The Precursor to School Medical Inspection," *Journal of the History of Medicine and Allied Sciences* 33, no. 3 (1978): 344–355.

38. See Hodge and Gostin, *supra* note 36.

39. *Id.*

40. *Jacobson v. Commonwealth of Massachusetts,* 197 U.S. 11 (1905).

41. L. O. Gostin and J. G. Hodge, "The Public Health Improvement Process in Alaska: Toward a Model Public Health Law," *Alaska Law Review* 17, no. 1 (2000): 77–125.

42. *Zucht v. King,* 260 U.S. 174 (1922).

43. A. R. Hinman et al., "Childhood Immunization: Laws That Work," *Journal of Law, Medicine & Ethics* 30, no. 3 (2002): 122–127; K. M. Malone and A. R. Hinman, "Vaccination Mandates: The Public Health Imperative and Individual Rights," in R. A. Goodman et al., *Law in Public Health Practice* (New York: Oxford University Press, 2006).

44. See Centers for Disease Control and Prevention, *supra* note 6.

45. B. Lo, "HPV Vaccine and Adolescents' Sexual Activity: It Would Be a Shame if Unresolved Ethical Dilemmas Hampered This Breakthrough," *BMJ* 332, no. 7550 (2006): 1106–1107.

46. R. K. Zimmerman, "Ethical Analysis of HPV Vaccine Policy Options," *Vaccine* 24, no. 22 (2006): 4812–4820.

47. C. Stanwyck et al., "Vaccination Coverage Among Children Entering School—United States, 2005–06 School Year," *JAMA* 296, no. 21 (2006): 2544–2547.

48. See Hodge and Gostin, *supra* note 36.

49. S. P. Calandrillo, "Vanishing Vaccinations: Why Are So Many Americans Opting Out of Vaccinating Their Children?" *University of Michigan Journal of Legal Reform* 37 (2004): 353–440.

50. *Id.*

51. B. Hart, "My Daughter Won't Get HPV Vaccine," *Chicago Sun Times, February* 25, 2007, at B6.

52. J. Cummings, "Seventy Percent of U.S. Adults Support Use of the Human Papillomavirus (HPV) Vaccine: Majority of Parents of Girls under 18 Would Want Daughters to Receive It,"

Wall Street Journal Online 5, no. 13 (2006), *available at . . .* (last visited March 5, 2008).

53. J. Marbella, "Sense of Rush Infects Plan to Require HPV Shots," *Baltimore Sun,* January 30, 2007, *available at . . .* (last visited March 14, 2008).

54. S. Reimer, "Readers Worry about HPV Vaccine: Doctors Say It's Safe," *Baltimore Sun,* April 3, 2007.

55. A. Pollack and S. Saul, "Lobbying for Vaccine to Be Halted," *New York Times,* February 21, 2007, *available at . . .* (last visited March 14, 2008).

56. J. Partridge and L. Koutsky, "Genital Human Papillomavirus in Men," *The Lancet Infectious Diseases* 6, no. 1 (2006): 21–31.

57. See Markowitz et al., *supra* note 18.

58. *Id.*

59. See Partridge and Koutsky, *supra* note 56.

60. J. Partridge, "Genital Human Papillomavirus Infection in Men: Incidence and Risk Factors in a Cohort of University Students," *Journal of Infectious Diseases* 196, no. 15 (2007): 1128–1136. It should be noted that the higher incidence might be due to the increased sensitivity of the HPV-PCR-based testing procedure used in this recent study.

61. *Id.*

62. J. Kim, "Vaccine Policy Analysis Can Benefit from Natural History Studies of Human Papillomavirus in Men," *Journal of Infectious Diseases* 196, no. 8 (2007): 1117–1119.

63. See Partridge and Koutsky, *supra* note 56.

64. *Id.*

65. R. V. Barnabas, P. Laukkanen, and P. Koskela, "Epidemiology of HPV 16 and Cervical Cancer in Finland and the Potential Impact of Vaccination: Mathematical Modeling Analysis," *PLoS Medicine* 3, no. 5 (2006): 624–632.

66. *Id.*

67. J. P. Hughess, G. P. Garnett, and L. Koutsky, "The Theoretical Population Level Impace of a Prophylactic Human Papillomavirus Vaccine," *Epidemiology* 13, no. 6 (2002): 631–639.

68. D. Elbasha, "Model for Assessing Human Papillomavirus Vaccination Strategies," *Emerging Infectious Diseases* 13, no. 1 (January 2007): 28–41. Please note that these researchers are employed by Merck, the producer of Gardasil vaccine.

69. *Wong Wai v. Williamson,* 103 F. 1 (N.D. Cal. 1900).

70. *Vacco v. Quill,* 521 U.S. 793 (1997); *Washington v. Glucksberg,* 521 U.S. 702 (1997).

71. A. Pollack, "Rising Costs Make Doctors Balk at Giving Vaccines," *New York Times,* March 24, 2007.

72. *Id.*

GAIL JAVITT is the law and policy director at the Genetics and Public Policy Center in Washington, D.C. She is also a research scientist in the Berman Institute of Bioethics at Johns Hopkins University in Baltimore, Maryland.

DEENA BERKOWITZ is an assistant professor of pediatrics at George Washington University School of Medicine and Health Sciences in Washington, D.C.

LAWRENCE O. GOSTIN is an associate dean, the Linda D. and Timothy J. O'Neil Professor of Global Health Law, the faculty director of the O'Neil Institute for National and Global Health Law, and the director of the Center for Law and the Public's Health at Georgetown University Law Center in Washington, D.C.

EXPLORING THE ISSUE

Should the Cervical Cancer Vaccine for Girls Be Compulsory?

Critical Thinking and Reflection

1. Discuss why the vaccine is controversial.
2. What are the laws governing vaccinations for school children in the United States?
3. Why is it important to try to prevent and treat cervical cancer, especially among women?

Is There Common Ground?

Currently, all 50 states require children to be vaccinated for a variety of illnesses before enrolling in school. Exemptions apply for children whose parents' religious beliefs prohibit vaccinations. Some children are exempt for medical reasons, which must be certified by their doctors. However, almost all children are vaccinated by the time they enter school. The recent development of Gardasil could add another shot to what many children receive by age 5. Should all states make it mandatory for school attendance?

There is considerable opposition to the HPV vaccination due partly to the increasing trend among some parents to refuse to have their children vaccinated. These parents believe, erroneously, that many vaccines are more dangerous than the diseases they prevent. The HPV vaccine adds the additional element of parents' beliefs that their children will remain abstinent until marriage. Abstinence provides effective and absolute protection against this sexually transmitted infection. Unfortunately, by age 19, nearly 70 percent of American girls are sexually active. Another concern among parents is that the vaccine will actually increase sexual activity among teens by removing the threat of HPV infection.

Some additional arguments against the HPV vaccine maintain that cervical cancer is different from measles or polio, diseases that are spread through casual contact. While cervical cancer kills approximately 3,700 women each year in the United States, and nearly 10,000 cases are diagnosed, the disease has a high survival rate though treatment can leave women infertile. In addition, cervical cancer deaths have dropped 75 percent from 1955 to 1992 and the numbers continue to decrease due to the widespread use of the Pap smear. Most women diagnosed with cervical cancer today either have never had a Pap smear or did not have one on a regular basis. Would it make more sense to use public funds to ensure all women have access to Pap smears? Also, not all viral strains are prevented through the use of the vaccine and women would still need to have routine Pap smears. Also, what if the vaccine causes health issues later in life? To determine the safety of Gardasil, researchers conducted a systematic review and meta-analysis to determine the effectiveness and safety of vaccines against cervical cancer. They concluded that the HPV vaccines are safe, well tolerated, and highly effective in preventing infections and cervical diseases among young females. The authors determined, however, that long-term efficacy and safety need to be addressed in future trials. See "Efficacy and Safety of Prophylactic Vaccines Against Cervical HPV Infection and Diseases among Women: A Systematic Review & Meta-Analysis," *BMC Infectious Diseases* (2011).

The American Cancer Society continues to endorse mandatory vaccination for HPV for all girls before entering school. They contend that since not all women get regular Pap smears, the vaccine would be a way to effectively prevent cervical cancer among American women. Attorney R. Alta Charo supports mandatory vaccination with Gardasil and is concerned that "cancer prevention has fallen victim to the culture wars."

Create Central

www.mhhe.com/createcentral

Additional Resources

Clayton, J. (2012). Clinical approval: Trials of an anticancer jab. *Nature, 488*(7413), S4–S6.

Collins, T. P. (2010). Is Gardasil good medicine? *National Catholic Bioethics Quarterly, 10*(3), 459–469.

Dooren, J. (2012, October 2). Study finds HPV vaccine Gardasil safe. *Wall Street Journal—Eastern Edition*, p. D2.

Jenson, H. B. (2012). Community (herd) immunity follows HPV vaccination. (Cover story). *Infectious Disease Alert, 31*(12), 133–134.

Tomljenovic, L. & Shaw, C. A. (2012). Too fast or not too fast: The FDA's approval of Merck's HPV vaccine Gardasil. *Journal Of Law, Medicine & Ethics, 40*(3), 673–681.

Internet References . . .

American Cancer Society

www.cancer.org

HPV—Centers for Disease Control and Prevention

www.cdc.gov/vaccines/pubs/vis/downloads/vis-hpv-gardasil.pdf

U.S. National Institutes of Health (NIH)

www.nih.gov

U.S. National Library of Medicine

www.nlm.nih.gov

World Health Organization

www.who.int/en

Selected, Edited, and with Issue Framing Material by:
Eileen Daniel, *SUNY College at Brockport*

ISSUE

Do Ultrathin Models and Actresses Influence the Onset of Eating Disorders?

YES: Janet L. Treasure, Elizabeth R. Wack, and Marion E. Roberts, from "Models as a High-Risk Group: The Health Implications of a Size Zero Culture," *The British Journal of Psychiatry* (April 2008)

NO: Fred Schwarz, from "Not Our Stars but Ourselves: Skinny Actresses and Models Do Not Make Girls Anorexic," *The National Review* (February 23, 2009)

Learning Outcomes
After reading this issue, you should be able to:
• Discuss the risk factors associated with eating disorders.
• Assess the influence of models and actresses on the onset of eating disorders.
• Understand the physical effects of eating disorders.
• Discuss eating disorders from a historical perspective.

ISSUE SUMMARY

YES: Physician Janet L. Treasure and psychologists Elizabeth R. Wack and Marion E. Roberts maintain that the promotion of an ultrathin ideal produces an environment that favors eating disorders.

NO: Journalist Fred Schwarz disagrees and contends that skinny models and actresses do not make girls and women anorexic since the disease predates the era of an ultrathin beauty standard.

Eating disorders are conditions characterized by abnormal eating habits that may involve either too little or excessive food intake, which can harm an individual's mental and physical health. Anorexia nervosa and bulimia are the most common types of eating disorders in the United States. Anorexia is characterized by refusal to maintain a healthy body weight and an obsessive fear of gaining weight. Anorexia can cause menstruation to stop, often leads to bone loss, and stresses the heart, increasing the risk of heart attacks and related heart problems. The risk of dying is significantly increased in individuals with this condition. Bulimia nervosa is typified by regular binge eating followed by purging, which includes self-induced vomiting and/or excessive use of laxatives and/or diuretics.

An estimated 5–10 million girls and women are affected in the United States, although eating disorders affect males as well. Currently, approximately 1 million men and boys have an eating disorder. Although the prevalence of eating disorders is rising globally among both men and women, there is evidence to suggest that it is women in the developed world who are at the highest risk of an eating disorder diagnosis. The exact cause of

these conditions is not completely known or understood, although there is evidence that it may be linked to other physical and mental health conditions. For instance, there are data that indicate girls with attention deficit hyperactive disorder (ADHD) have a greater chance of getting an eating disorder than those not affected by ADHD. Some researchers also think that peer pressure and idealized ultrathin body types seen in the media are also important risk factors. However, research shows that for some people there may be genetic reasons why they are prone to developing an eating disorder. Overall, however, the disease is believed to be due to a combination of biological, psychological, and/or environmental abnormalities. This may indicate that some people might be born with a predisposition to developing an eating disorder, triggered by the environment and reactions to it. Many men and women with eating disorders may also suffer from body dysmorphic disorder, which alters the way a person sees himself or herself. In general, although there are many theories, the exact causes of eating disorders are unclear and not well understood.

Although genetics may play a role, in various studies, peer pressure was shown to be a major contributor to body image concerns and attitudes toward eating, especially among girls and young women in their teens and early 20s. Researchers from the University of Miami studied 236 teen girls from public high schools in southeast Florida. They found that teenage girls who were focused on their weight, how they appear to others, and their perceptions that their peers want them to be thin are more likely to have eating issues. According to one study, 40 percent of 9- and 10-year-old girls are already on diets. This dieting is linked to influence from peers, and many individuals on a diet report that their friends also were trying to lose weight. The number of friends dieting and the number of friends who pressured them to diet also played a significant role in their own choices.

There is also a cultural focus on ultrathinness, which is especially persistent in Western culture. There is an unrealistic stereotype of what comprises beauty and the ideal body type as depicted by the media, fashion, and entertainment industries. The societal pressure on men and women to meet this unrealistic ideal may be an important predisposing factor for the rise in eating disorders. In the YES and NO selections, physician Janet L. Treasure and psychologists Elizabeth R. Wack and Marion E. Roberts claim that the promotion of an ultrathin ideal produces an environment that favors eating disorders. Journalist Fred Schwarz disagrees and contends that skinny models and actresses do not make girls and women anorexic since the disease predates the era of an ultrathin beauty standard.

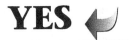

**Janet L. Treasure, Elizabeth R. Wack,
and Marion E. Roberts**

Models as a High-Risk Group: The Health Implications of a Size Zero Culture

There has been widespread concern that the fashion industry, by promulgating ever-diminishing extremes of thinness, is creating a 'toxic' environment in which eating disorders flourish. The Academy of Eating Disorders has written a position statement for the attention of the fashion industry outlining several recommendations to improve both the health of the public and that of models (www.aedweb.org/media/fashion.cfm).

The aim of this editorial is to consider the implications of the fashion industry's expectation of extreme leanness on the models' own health and also to set this into the context of public health. The direct risks for the models are twofold. First, starvation has a general effect upon all organs in the body, including the brain, and the impact may be profound if the deprivation occurs during development. Second, the demand for, and overvaluation of, extreme thinness within a culture of scrutiny and judgement about weight, shape and eating, increases the risk of developing an eating disorder.

The Health Consequences of Low Weight

There are many health consequences of being underweight. We briefly consider the impact on reproduction, bones and the brain.

Leptin decreases as body weight falls. Without adequate levels of leptin the cascade of hormonal events that controls ovulation and implantation becomes disrupted. Menstruation becomes irregular or absent and fertility is diminished. The Dutch famine in 1944 and the Chinese famine of 1959–1961 were associated with a fall in fertility. In addition, children *in utero* and beyond had an increased risk of metabolic and reproductive problems and mental illness later in life.[1] Poor nutrition stunts bone development (in the growth phase) and reduces bone turnover and repair, leading to osteoporosis (the impact on bones in eating disorders is a clear exemplar of these effects). Even minor disturbance in eating behaviour during adolescence is associated with adverse health outcomes later in life.[2]

In humans, the brain accounts for 20% of an individual's energy expenditure and plays a key role in nutritional homoeostasis. The brain itself shrinks in anorexia nervosa and there is uncertainty as to whether this is fully reversible. The response to starvation includes adjustment of metabolic and physiological processes and changes in drive, thoughts, feelings and behaviour. Starved individuals become preoccupied with food. Keys *et al* described in great detail subjective and objective reactions to a short period of experimental starvation in men.[3]

Binge Priming

Animal models explain how environmental changes might produce eating disorders. For example, if after a period of food restriction animals are intermittently exposed to highly palatable food, they will significantly overeat. This pattern continues when their weight is restored.[4] This tendency to overconsume, or 'binge', when exposed to palatable foods remains several months after the period of 'binge priming.' Not only do these animals overeat palatable food but they are also more prone to show addictive behaviours to the more typical substances of misuse, such as alcohol and cocaine. Underpinning these behavioural changes is an imbalance in chemical transmitters in the reward network, for example, dopamine, acetylcholine, endogenous opiates and cannabinoids. The persistent priming of reward circuits by palatable foods resembles the phenomenon of reward sensitisation produced by drug misuse.

Translating into the human situation, we would predict that binge priming caused by irregular dieting and/or extreme food restriction, interspersed with intermittent consumption of snacks and other highly palatable food, might lead to permanent changes in the reward system. Several hypotheses follow from this:

(a) if binge priming occurs in adolescence, when the developing brain is more susceptible to reward, persistent eating problems may follow;
(b) people exposed to binge priming will be more prone to develop substance misuse.

Some empirical evidence supports the first hypothesis in that there are developmental continuities between eating patterns in early life and the later development of eating disorders. For example, people with eating disorders report a higher consumption of high-palatability foods (fast foods and snack foods) and less regular meal times in childhood. Binge eating is persistent, with binge eating disorder present on average for 14 years, and bulimia nervosa for 5.8 years.[5] Abnormal eating behaviours in early adolescence precede substance misuse[6] and alcohol use disorders commonly supersede clinical bulimic disorders,[7] confirming the second hypothesis.

Models and the Risk of Eating Disorders

Eating patterns that an individual may have found to be integral in the maintenance of a particular shape during her modelling career may lead to deleterious health consequences and maladaptive eating behaviours that affect her far beyond the typically rather short years of such a career. Furthermore, binge priming might also explain why models have such a high rate of substance misuse.[8]

In addition to the biological factors described above, social factors contribute to the unhealthy lifestyle common among those pursuing a modelling career. Constant exposure to media images depicting thin women reduces body-related self-esteem. A meta-analysis of data from 25 studies found that this effect was most pronounced in adolescents and in participants who valued thinness.[9] Body-related self-esteem is particularly pertinent in young models as it relates to their career success. Criticism, teasing and bullying focused on food, weight and shape issues increase the risk of developing an eating disorder. Fashion models are frequently judged and evaluated on these domains and critical and hostile comments, under the guise of professional development, will increase the risk of developing eating disorders.

Successful Intervention in Other Domains

Prevention and regulation of toxic environments is not impossible. Progress has been made in sport and dance. High-performance athletes are also at risk of eating disorders especially in those areas in which excess weight is a handicap or where aesthetic factors are judged. Concerted efforts have been made in the UK to set forth guidelines for high-performance athletes and their coaches in an attempt to reduce the prevalence of eating disorders, unhealthy weight loss and maintenance practices. The UK Sport guidelines[10] are based on practical strategies that consider the demands of the sport and the long-term health consequences often resulting from those demands.

Following this template, similar approaches to standardisation of care and health for fashion models could be introduced. Unfortunately, such initiatives are yet to be embraced by the fashion industry, as evidenced by the recent inconclusive outcomes from the UK Model Health Inquiry.[11] As models are embedded within the fashion industry, which holds responsibility for the idealisation of emaciation, it is hoped that the drive for ever more extreme thinness could be stemmed at the source, resulting in benefits for all of society.

The Future

The current fashion for extreme thinness among models unnecessarily puts their physical and psychological health in jeopardy. Starvation disrupts growth and reproductive function and can have profound and persistent effects on brain development. These risks are particularly profound in young women who, in a binge-priming environment, may be more prone to develop other addictive behaviours. Along with an increased risk of substance and alcohol use and misuse, the risk of developing an eating disorder will also be increased. The longer-term health implications on models' bone and reproductive health are unknown but evidence suggests the outcomes are not promising. The recent guidelines from the British Fashion Council, proposing not to include children under 16 years of age as models, is a welcome first step. Might this be taken further (e.g. legislation on age limit for competitive gymnastics)?

Beyond the catwalk, there are wider public health implications. The promotion of the thin ideal, in conjunction with the ready access of highly palatable foods, produces a binge-priming environment. This might explain the exponential increase in eating disorders seen in women born in the last half of the 20th century and in part also contributes to the increase in obesity.

Public health initiatives can be integrated to tackle both of these problems. The fashion and beauty industry can play a key role in preventing the development of unhealthy lifestyles in young people. Indeed, Body Talk, a prevention programme focused on self-esteem developed by Dove in partnership with the UK eating disorder charity beat (http://www.b-eat.co.uk) takes steps to modify the unrealistic 'ideal form' both as displayed in the flesh by fashion models and through the use of digitally enhanced photography. More focus on these issues will decrease unhealthy forms of dieting, dysregulated eating behaviours and body dissatisfaction among young people. Although it may take time to change such an ideal we should not be faint hearted but remember what has similarly been achieved in relationship to cigarette smoking. People are now starting to listen to the abundance of scientific evidence concerning the harm that such images hold not only for those paid to portray it, but for those who pay to emulate it.

References

1. Altschuler EL. Schizophrenia and the Chinese famine of 1959–1961. *JAMA* 2005; **294**: 2968.
2. Johnson JG, Cohen P, Kasen S, Brook JS. Eating disorders during adolescence and the risk for physical and mental disorders during early adulthood. *Arch Gen Psychiatry* 2002; **59**: 545–52.
3. Keys A, Brozek J, Henschel A. *The Biology of Human Starvation.* University of Minnesota Press, 1950.

4. Corwin RL. Bingeing rats: a model of intermittent excessive behavior? *Appetite* 2006; **46**: 11–15.

5. Pope HG Jr, Lalonde JK, Pindyck LJ, Walsh T, Bulik CM, Crow SJ, McElroy SL, Rosenthal N, Hudson JI. Binge eating disorder: a stable syndrome. *Am J Psychiatry* 2006; **163**: 2181–3.

6. Measelle JR, Stice E, Hogansen JM. Developmental trajectories of cooccurring depressive, eating, antisocial, and substance abuse problems in female adolescents. *J Abnorm Psychol* 2006; **115**: 524–38.

7. Bulik CM, Klump KL, Thornton L, Kaplan AS, Devlin B, Fichter MM, Halmi KA, Strober M, Woodside DB, Crow S, Mitchell JE, Rotondo A, Mauri M, Cassano GB, Keel PK, Berrettini WH, Kaye WH. Alcohol use disorder comorbidity in eating disorders: a multicenter study. *J Clin Psychiatry* 2004; **65**: 1000–6.

8. Santonastaso P, Mondini S, Favaro A. Are fashion models a group at risk for eating disorders and substance abuse? *Psychother Psychosom* 2002; **71**: 168–72.

9. Groesz LM, Levine MP, Murnen SK. The effect of experimental presentation of thin media images on body satisfaction: a meta-analytic review. *Int J Eat Disord* 2002; **31**: 1–16.

10. UK Sport. *Eating Disorders in Sport: A Guideline Framework for Practitioners Working with High Performance Athletes*. UK Sport, 2007 (http://www.uksport.gov.uk/pages/uk_sport_publications/).

11. Model Health Inquiry. *Fashioning a Healthy Future: the Report of the Model Health Inquiry, September 2007*. Model Health Inquiry, 2007 (http://www.modelhealthinquiry.com/docs/The%20Report%20of%20the%20Model%20Health%20Inquiry,%20September%202007.pdf).

JANET L. TREASURE is a physician with the Institute of Psychiatry, Department of Psychological Medicine and Psychiatry, Section of Eating Disorders, King's College, London, UK.

ELIZABETH R. WACK is a psychologist with the Institute of Psychiatry, Department of Psychological Medicine and Psychiatry, Section of Eating Disorders, King's College, London, UK.

MARION E. ROBERTS is a psychologist with the Institute of Psychiatry, Department of Psychological Medicine and Psychiatry, Section of Eating Disorders, King's College, London, UK.

Fred Schwarz

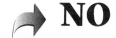
NO

Not Our Stars but Ourselves: Skinny Actresses and Models Do Not Make Girls Anorexic

What causes anorexia nervosa, the terrible mental illness whose victims (mostly young women) starve themselves, sometimes to death? To many observers, the answer is clear: Hollywood, Madison Avenue, and Seventh Avenue. Film and television actresses are impossibly thin; advertisers hawk an endless profusion of diet products and banish average-looking people from their commercials; the fashion industry recruits tall, scrawny teenagers as its models and tosses them aside if they become too womanly. When girls and young women are constantly bombarded with thin-is-beautiful messages, is it any wonder that some of them overreact?

Christy Greenleaf, assistant professor of kinesiology, health promotion, and recreation at the University of North Texas, doesn't think so. She has written: "Girls and women, in our society, are socialized to value physical appearance and an ultra-thin beauty that rarely occurs naturally and to pursue that ultra-thin physique at any cost. Research demonstrates that poor body image and disordered eating attitudes are associated with internalizing the mediated (i.e., commodified, airbrushed) bodies that dominate the fashion industry." The narrative is a plausible one, and it fits a familiar template: Big business uses mass media to destroy consumers' health by creating harmful desires. Yet there are large parts of it that don't hold up.

In the first place, anorexia is not in any way an artifact of our modern, weight-obsessed society. Thomas Hobbes wrote about it in the 1680s. A 1987 study showed that anorexia in the United States increased throughout the 19th century and peaked around 1900, when chorus girls were voluptuous and the boyish flapper look was still two decades away. A similar historical pattern has been found for eating disorders in France. Some interplay of genetic and environmental factors may be at work in these cases, or they may have resulted from the common pattern in medicine of certain diagnoses' rising and falling in popularity. But it's clear that none of these outbreaks can be attributed to the late-20th- and early-21st-century emphasis on skinniness.

There are plenty of other examples. The medical historian I. S. L. Loudon has identified chlorosis, the 19th-century "virgin's disease," with anorexia and shown that diagnoses of it reached "epidemic proportions" in Victorian England before disappearing completely between 1900 and 1920. A pair of Dutch historians have traced the practice of severe self-starvation all the way back to the early Christians and described the various explanations that were offered for it over the centuries (holiness, witchcraft, demonic possession, miracles, various nervous or emotional disturbances) before a newly scientific medical profession defined it as an illness in the mid-19th century.

All these statistics must be taken as rough indications only. Eating-disorder rates, like those for most psychiatric illnesses, are notoriously slippery, since the conditions are so hard to pin down. Journalists sometimes say that anorexia rates have been increasing for decades, as Americans' lives have become more media-saturated; one source reports that anorexia in young adult females has tripled over the past 40 years. This is a case of the common phenomenon in which growing awareness of a condition leads to increased diagnosis of it, even when there is no real increase in its prevalence. Researchers who have carefully studied the data conclude that there has been no significant change in the rate of anorexia in America since at least the mid-20th century.

Moreover, while it's tempting to blame America's appearance-obsessed culture for the plight of its self-starving daughters, anorexia is a global phenomenon. A 2001 article reviewed the extensive literature on eating disorders among residents of Europe, Asia, Africa, the Middle East, and Australia. In some regions, the reported rates of anorexia were several times that of the United States (though, as above, such figures must be taken with caution). In a case of political correctness attacking itself, one researcher says those who attribute anorexia to media sexism are being ethnocentric: "The biomedical definition of anorexia nervosa emphasizes fat-phobia. . . . However, evidence exists that suggests anorexia nervosa can exist without the Western fear of fatness and that this culturally biased view of anorexia nervosa may obscure health care professionals' understanding of a patient's own cultural reasons for self-starvation."

If it isn't skinny models, what's the cause? In the last dozen years or so, scientists have linked anorexia to many different physiological conditions: high levels of estrogen in the womb; low levels of serotonin in the brain; a genetic mutation; overactivity by dopamine receptors; a general tendency toward anxiety and obsessionality; high age at menarche; elevated amounts of a mysterious peptide called CART; autism (which is underdiagnosed in girls, perhaps because it sometimes manifests itself in the form of eating disorders); premature birth or other birth complications; irregular activity in the insular cortex of the brain; post-traumatic stress disorder; an autoimmune disorder affecting the hypothalamus and pituitary gland; variations in the structure of the anterior ventral striatum (the brain region responsible for emotional responses); and even being born in June (seriously—one theory is that a winter-type disease in the mother at a certain vulnerable point during the pregnancy is responsible). Some of these causes may overlap with one another, but biomedical researchers are virtually unanimous that anorexia has physical roots, though the mechanism remains poorly understood.

Might these physiological factors be what makes one *susceptible* to anorexia, but cultural images are what sets it off? Walter Kaye, a psychiatry professor at UC–San Diego, has suggested such a mechanism: "Less than half of 1 percent of all women develop anorexia nervosa, which indicates to us that societal pressure alone isn't enough to cause someone to develop this disease. Our research has found that genes seem to play a substantial role in determining who is vulnerable to developing an eating disorder. However, the societal pressure isn't irrelevant; it may be the environmental trigger that releases a person's genetic risk."

Maybe, but probably not. As noted above, anorexia has flourished in many times and places with no mass media and no ideal of thinness. Anorexia could be just another manifestation of self-destructiveness, like slashing one's wrists. It could stem from some cause unrelated to body image, such as disgust with the processes of digestion and elimination (as well as menstruation, which often ceases in long-term anorexics). Psychiatrists believe that many anorexic women want to reverse the effects of puberty, such as breasts and hips, and while most of today's film and television sex symbols are indeed slender, they rarely lack for breasts and hips.

Despite the uncertain connection, some observers still think the media need to change their act. Professor Greenleaf has suggested: "A potentially healthier approach is to include [in advertising] a variety of body shapes and sizes (as opposed to idealizing only one physique). Healthy bodies come in all shapes and sizes—and health is what should be valued, which may not fit with the fashion industry's emphasis on ultra-thin beauty."

The suggestion is not outlandish. Many advertisers and fashion magazines have, in fact, tried using "a variety of body shapes and sizes" among their models—once. It makes a decent publicity gimmick, but there's a reason they always go back to slender models: Clothes look better on them. (Also, it usually isn't practical to custom-sew garments for individual models, so clothing samples are made for a standard size 6.) And for some reason, viewers of films and television, male and female, tend to like beautiful actresses rather than healthy ones—not to mention the common observation that "the camera adds ten pounds."

If increasing the labor pool for models and actresses by including heftier ones yielded equally good results, the industries in question would have done it long ago. Why deal with a bunch of stuck-up teenagers if you don't have to? If media and fashion conglomerates really do dictate our image of the ideal female, why don't they manipulate us into going crazy for plumpish housewives instead? And even if it's true that media images make some people weight-conscious, the benefits must easily exceed the costs, since obesity is a much greater problem in America than anorexia.

Nonetheless, some lawmakers are calling for bans on skinny models. Madrid and Milan have prohibited those with a body-mass index lower than 18 from their fashion shows. (Body-mass index is the weight in kilograms divided by the square of the height in meters. A BMI of 18 is considered the low end of the normal range, but you wouldn't expect models as a group to have "normal" physiques, any more than you would expect it from football players.) Similar bans have been proposed in Quebec, London, New York City, New York State, and France's national assembly. The main goal of these bills, which began to be introduced after several models starved themselves to death, is supposedly to reduce anorexia within the industry, though proponents always invoke the baleful effects that waif-like models have on society as a whole. Yet this assumes that self-starvation is a willful choice that anorexics will abandon if given the proper incentive, when in fact it is a mental illness that for centuries has proven stubbornly impervious to rational arguments.

Anorexia is a dreadful disease, and still poorly understood. If the growing scientific knowledge about it can be pieced together, we may eventually learn to identify, prevent, treat, and possibly cure it. But political activists do not help its sufferers when they oversimplify a complicated condition and blame it on their stock assortment of evil forces in American society.

Fred Schwarz is a journalist who writes for the *National Review*.

EXPLORING THE ISSUE

Do Ultrathin Models and Actresses Influence the Onset of Eating Disorders?

Critical Thinking and Reflection

1. Why are women much more likely to suffer from eating disorders?
2. Describe the psychological profiles of someone suffering from an eating disorder.
3. What are the most serious physical consequences related to eating disorders?
4. What role does the media play in the development of eating disorders?

Is There Common Ground?

It is estimated that of the several million people in the United States who are suffering from an eating disorder approximately 10 percent are men and boys. Researchers believe that the number of males with the condition is actually much higher, but because of the incorrect belief that this illness affects only females, few men present for treatment. When males do seek help, there is evidence that clinicians may be less likely to diagnose either bulimia or anorexia. Men are more likely to be diagnosed as suffering from depression with associated eating changes than to receive a primary diagnosis of an eating disorder.

Males who are involved in weight-oriented sports such as wrestling, gymnastics, and track are at an increased risk of developing an eating disorder such as anorexia or bulimia nervosa. The pressure to win, to excel, and to be competitive combined with any nonathletic pressures in their lives can contribute to the development of eating disorders. Men who suffer with an eating disorder may also experience problems with alcohol and/or substance abuse concurrently. In addition, as with women, there may also be a correlation between ADHD with male sufferers of anorexia and bulimia nervosa. More research is needed in this area.

For both males and females who suffer from an eating disorder, there are many possible concurrent psychological illnesses that can be present including anxiety, depression, substance abuse, and obsessive compulsive disorder. Most of the underlying psychological factors that lead to an eating disorder are similar for both males and females and include low self-esteem, a need to be accepted, depression and anxiety, and other existing psychological conditions. All of the physical risks and complications associated with eating disorders are the same for both males and females.

The primary difference is the greater number of female sufferers.

Create Central

www.mhhe.com/createcentral

Additional Resources

Bair, C. E., Kelly, N. R., Serdar, K. L., & Mazzeo, S. E. (2012). Does the Internet function like magazines? An exploration of image-focused media, eating pathology, and body dissatisfaction. *Eating Behaviors, 13*(4), 398–401.

Darcy, A. M., Doyle, A., Lock, J., Peebles, R., Doyle, P., & Le Grange, D. (2012). The eating disorders examination in adolescent males with anorexia nervosa: How does it compare to adolescent females? *International Journal of Eating Disorders, 45*(1), 110–114.

Levine, M. P. & Murner, S. K. (2009). "Everybody knows that mass media are/are not [pick one] a cause of eating disorders": A critical review of evidence for a causal link between media, negative body image, and disordered eating in females. *Journal of Social & Clinical Psychology, 28*(1), 9–42.

Slevec, J. & Tiggemann, M. (2011). Media exposure, body dissatisfaction, and disordered eating in middle-aged women: A test of the sociocultural model of disordered eating. *Psychology of Women Quarterly, 35*(4), 617–627.

Trujillo, A. E. (2012). Adolescents and eating disorders. *Insights to A Changing World Journal, 3*, 126–140.

Internet References . . .

American Psychological Association

Information and resources on anorexia nervosa, bulimia nervosa, and binge eating.

www.apa.org

Mayo Clinic Eating disorders

Eating disorders—Comprehensive overview covers symptoms, complications, and treatment of these potentially life-threatening conditions.

www.mayoclinic.com/health/eating-disorders

National Eating Disorders Association

The site supplies information about the National Eating Disorders Association (NEDA), a nonprofit organization dedicated to supporting individuals and families affected by eating disorders. There is information on prevention, improved access to quality treatment, and increased research funding.

www.nationaleatingdisorders.org/

National Institute of Mental Health (NIMH) Eating Disorders

A detailed booklet that describes the symptoms, causes, and treatments of eating disorders.

www.nimh.nih.gov/health/.../eating-disorders/ complete-index.shtml

Selected, Edited, and with Issue Framing Material by:
Eileen Daniel, *SUNY College at Brockport*

ISSUE

Is There a Valid Reason for Routine Infant Male Circumcision?

YES: Hanna Rosin, from "The Case Against the Case Against Circumcision; Why One Mother Heard All of the Opposing Arguments, Then Circumcised Her Sons Anyway," *New York Magazine* (October 26, 2009)

NO: Michael Idov, from "Would You Circumcise This Baby? Why a Growing Number of Parents, Especially in New York and Other Cities, Are Saying No to the Procedure" *New York Magazine* (October 26, 2009)

Learning Outcomes
After reading this issue, you should be able to:
• Discuss the health risks associated with infant male circumcision.
• Distinguish the difference between routine circumcision and religious rituals.
• Understand the health benefits associated with male circumcision.

ISSUE SUMMARY

YES: Writer Hanna Rosin argues that male circumcision decreases the risk of disease transmission and that people who oppose the operation are filled with anger that transcends the actual outcome.

NO: Michael Idov, author and contributing editor of *New York Magazine*, counters that newborns feel pain and that there is no valid medical reason to perform the surgery.

Male circumcision is the removal of the foreskin (prepuce) from the penis, and in the United States it is typically performed shortly after birth. In the Jewish religion, male circumcision is considered a commandment from God. It is also a common practice among Muslims. Worldwide, about 30 percent of males are circumcised and of those, about two-thirds are Muslim. About 55–65 percent of all newborn boys are circumcised in the United States each year, although this rate varies by region (western states have the lowest rates and the north central region has the highest). Up to 20 percent of men who are not circumcised during the newborn periods will be circumcised sometime later in life. Circumcision is much more common in the United States, Canada, and the Middle East than in other parts of the world. Currently, the United States is the only country in the developed world where the majority of male infants are circumcised for nonreligious reasons.

Circumcision is an elective procedure that has both pros and cons. As a benefit, circumcised infants are less likely to develop urinary tract infections (UTIs), especially in the first year of life. UTIs are about 10 times more common in uncircumcised infants compared with circumcised ones. However, even with this increased risk of UTIs, only

1 percent or less of uncircumcised baby boys are typically affected. Circumcised men may also be at lower risk for penile cancer, although the disease is uncommon in both circumcised and uncircumcised males. Some studies indicate that circumcision might also help protect against sexually transmitted diseases including AIDS/HIV. Irritation, inflammation, infection, and other problems of the penis occur more frequently among uncircumcised males since it is easier to keep a circumcised penis clean. There are also claims that circumcision affects the sensitivity of the tip of the penis, decreasing or increasing sexual pleasure later in life.

While circumcision appears to offer some medical benefits, it also carries potential risks since it is a surgical procedure. Complications of newborn circumcision are rare, occurring in between 0.2 and 3 percent of cases. Of these, the most frequent are treatable minor bleeding and local infection. Anesthesia is used more frequently now than in the past to prevent the newborn from feeling pain.

There are also negative outcomes of a psychological nature that have been anecdotally reported. These include sexual dysfunction of various forms and degrees, including impotence; awareness of a loss of normal protective, sensory, and mechanical functioning; anger; resentment;

feelings of parental betrayal; feeling (awareness) of being mutilated; feelings of one's right to a normal intact body having been violated and removed; feelings of not being whole and natural; addictions or dependencies; sense of anatomical and sexual inferiority to genitally intact (noncircumcised) men; foreskin (or intact penis) envy. The quality and quantity of long-term psychologically negative effects of infant circumcision on men, however, have never been scientifically investigated.

Medical practice has long respected an adult's right to self-determination in health care decision making through the practice of informed consent. This process requires the physician to explain any procedure or treatment and to address the risks, benefits, and alternatives for the patient to make an informed choice. Since infants or small children lack the ability to decide for themselves, parents must make these choices. However, it is often uncertain as to what is in the best interest of any individual patient. In cases such as the decision to perform a circumcision shortly after birth when there are potential

benefits and risks and the procedure is not essential to the child's current well-being, it is the parents who determine what is in the best interest of the child. In the United States, it is valid for the parents to take into account cultural, religious, and ethnic traditions, in addition to medical factors, when making this choice.

Overall, infant male circumcision is neither essential nor harmful to a boy's health. The American Academy of Pediatrics (AAP) and the American Academy of Family Physicians (AAFP) do not endorse the procedure as a way to prevent any of the medical conditions mentioned previously. The AAP also does not find sufficient evidence to medically recommend circumcision or argue against it.

In the YES and NO selections, Hanna Rosin argues that male circumcision decreases the risk of disease transmission and that people who oppose the operation are filled with anger that transcends the actual outcome. Author and contributing editor of *New York Magazine* Michael Idov counters that newborns feel pain and that there is no valid medical reason to perform the surgery.

YES ↵

Hanna Rosin

The Case Against the Case Against Circumcision; Why One Mother Heard All of the Opposing Arguments, Then Circumcised Her Sons Anyway

Anyone with a heart would agree that the Jewish bris is a barbaric event. Grown-ups sit chatting politely, wiping the cream cheese off their lips, while some religious guy with minimal medical training prepares to slice up a newborn's penis. The helpless thing wakes up from a womb-slumber howling with pain. I felt near hysterical at both of my sons' brisses. Pumped up with new-mother hormones, I dug my nails into my palms to keep from clawing the rabbi. For a few days afterward, I cursed my God and everyone else for creating the bloody mess in the diaper. But then the penis healed and assumed its familiar heart shape and I promptly forgot about the whole trauma. Apparently some people never do.

I am Jewish enough that I never considered not circumcising my sons. I did not search the web or call a panel of doctors to fact-check the health benefits, as a growing number of wary Americans now do. Despite my momentary panic, the words "genital mutilation" did not enter my head. But now that I have done my homework, I'm sure I would do it again—even if I were not Jewish, didn't believe in ritual, and judged only by cold, secular science.

Every year, it seems, a new study confirms that the foreskin is pretty much like the appendix or the wisdom tooth—it is an evolutionary footnote that serves no purpose other than to incubate infections. There's no single overwhelming health reason to remove it, but there are a lot of smaller health reasons that add up. It's not critical that any individual boy get circumcised. For the growing number of people who feel hysterical at the thought, just don't do it. But don't ruin it for the rest of us. It's perfectly clear that on a grand public-health level, the more boys who get circumcised, the better it is for everyone.

Twenty years ago, this would have been a boring, obvious thing to say, like feed your baby rice cereal before bananas, or don't smoke while pregnant. These days, in certain newly enlightened circles on the East and West Coasts, it puts you in league with Josef Mengele. Late this summer, when *The New York Times* reported that the U.S. Centers for Disease Control might consider promoting routine circumcision as a tool in the fight against AIDS, the vicious comments that ensued included references to mass genocide.

There's no use arguing with the anti-circ activists, who only got through the headline of this story before hunting down my e-mail and offering to pay for me to be genitally mutilated. But for those in the nervous middle, here is my best case for why you should do it. Biologists think the foreskin plays a critical role in the womb, protecting the penis as it is growing during the third month of gestation. Outside the womb, the best guess is that it once kept the penis safe from, say, low-hanging thorny branches. Nowadays, we have pants for that.

Circumcision dates back some 6,000 years and was mostly associated with religious rituals, especially for Jews and Muslims. In the nineteenth century, moralists concocted some unfortunate theories about the connection between the foreskin and masturbation and other such degenerate impulses. The genuinely useful medical rationales came later. During the World War II campaign in North Africa, tens of thousands of American GIs fell short on their hygiene routines. Many of them came down with a host of painful and annoying infections, such as phimosis, where the foreskin gets too tight to retract over the glans. Doctors already knew about the connection to sexually transmitted diseases and began recommending routine circumcision.

In the late eighties, researchers began to suspect a relationship between circumcision and transmission of HIV, the virus that causes AIDS. One researcher wondered why certain Kenyan men who see prostitutes get infected and others don't. The answer, it turned out, was that the ones who don't were circumcised. Three separate trials in Uganda, Kenya, and South Africa involving over 10,000 men turned up the same finding again and again. Circumcision, it turns out, could reduce the risk of HIV transmission by at least 60 percent, which, in Africa, adds up to 3 million lives saved over the next twenty years. The governments of Uganda and Kenya recently started mass-circumcision campaigns.

These studies are not entirely relevant to the U.S. They apply only to female-to-male transmission, which is relatively rare here. But the results are so dramatic that people who work in AIDS prevention can't ignore them. Daniel Halperin, an AIDS expert at the Harvard School of

Public Health, has compared various countries, and the patterns are obvious. In a study of 28 nations, he found that low circumcision rates (fewer than 20 percent) match up with high HIV rates, and vice versa. Similar patterns are turning up in the U.S. as well. A team of researchers from the CDC and Johns Hopkins analyzed records of over 26,000 heterosexual African-American men who showed up at a Baltimore clinic for HIV testing and denied any drug use or homosexual contact. Among those with known HIV exposure, the ones who did turn out to be HIV-positive were twice as likely to be uncircumcised. There's no causal relationship here; foreskin does not cause HIV transmission. But researchers guess that foreskins are more susceptible to sores, and also have a high concentration of certain immune cells that are the main portals for HIV infection.

Then there are a host of other diseases that range from rare and deadly to ruin your life to annoying. Australian physicians give a decent summary: "STIs such as carcinogenic types of human papillomavirus (HPV), genital herpes, HIV, syphilis and chancroid, thrush, cancer of the penis, and most likely cancer of the prostate, phimosis, paraphimosis, inflammatory skin conditions such as balanoposthitis, inferior hygiene, sexual problems, especially with age and diabetes, and, in the female partners, HPV, cervical cancer, HSV-2, and chlamydia, which is an important cause of infertility." The percentages vary in each case, but it's clear that the foreskin is a public-health menace.

Edgar Schoen, now a professor emeritus of pediatrics at the University of California San Francisco, has been pushing the pro-circumcision case since 1989, when he chaired an American Academy of Pediatrics Task Force on the practice. The committee later found insufficient evidence to recommend routine circumcision, but to Schoen, this is the "narrow thinking of neonatologists" who sit on the panels. All they see is a screaming baby, not a lifetime of complications. In the meantime, sixteen states have eliminated Medicaid coverage for circumcision, causing the rates among Hispanics, for one, to plummet. For Schoen and Halperin and others, this issue has become primarily a question of "health-care parity for the poor." The people whom circumcision could help the most are now the least likely to get it.

This mundane march of health statistics has a hard time competing with the opposite side, which is fighting for something they see as fundamental: a right not to be messed with, a freedom from control, and a general sense of wholeness. For many circumcision opponents, preventive surgery is a bizarre, dystopian disruption. I can only say that in public health, preventive surgery is pretty common—appendix and wisdom teeth, for example. "If we could remove the appendix in a three- or four-minute operation without cutting into the abdomen, we would," says Schoen. Anesthesia is routine now, so the infants don't suffer the way they used to. My babies didn't seem to howl more than they did in their early vaccines, particularly the one where they "milk" the heel for blood.

Sexual pleasure comes up a lot. Opponents of circumcision often mention studies of "penile sensitivity regions," showing the foreskin to be the most sensitive. But erotic experience is a rich and complicated affair, and surely can't be summed up by nerve endings or friction or "sensitivity regions." More-nuanced studies have shown that men who were circumcised as adults report a decrease in sexual satisfaction when they were forced into it, because of an illness, and an increase when they did it of their own will. In a study of Kenyan men who volunteered for circumcision, 64 percent reported their penis to be "much more sensitive" and their ease of reaching orgasm much greater two years after the operation. In a similar study, Ugandan women reported a 40 percent increase in sexual satisfaction after their partners were circumcised. Go figure. Surely this is more psychology than science.

People who oppose circumcision are animated by a kind of rage and longing that seems larger than the thing itself. Websites are filled with testimonies from men who believe their lives were ruined by the operation they had as an infant. I can only conclude that it wasn't the cutting alone that did the ruining. An East Bay doctor who came out for circumcision recently wrote about having visions of tiny foreskins rising up in revenge at him, clogging the freeways. I see what he means. The foreskin is the new fetus—the object that has been imbued with magical powers to halt a merciless, violent world—a world that is particularly callous to children. The notion resonates in a moment when parents are especially overprotective, and fantasy death panels loom. It's all very visual and compelling—like the sight of your own newborn son with the scalpel looming over him. But it isn't the whole truth.

HANNA ROSIN is a senior editor for *The Atlantic* magazine.

Michael Idov

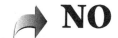 **NO**

Would You Circumcise This Baby? Why a Growing Number of Parents, Especially in New York and Other Cities, Are Saying No to the Procedure

To cut or not to cut. The choice loomed the moment New Yorkers Rob and Deanna Morea found out, three months into Deanna's pregnancy, that their first child was going to be a boy. Both had grown up with the view of circumcision as something automatic, like severing the umbilical cord. To Rob—white, Catholic, and circumcised—an intact foreskin seemed vaguely un-American. Deanna, African-American and also Catholic, dismissed the parents who don't circumcise their children as a "granola-eating, Birkenstock-wearing type of crowd." But that was before they knew they were having a son.

Circumcision is still, as it has been for decades, one of the most routinely performed surgical procedures in the United States—a million of the operations are performed every year. Yet more Americans are beginning to ask themselves the same question the Moreas did: Why, exactly, are we doing this? Having peaked at a staggering 85 percent in the sixties and seventies, the U.S. newborn-circumcision rate dropped to 65 percent in 1999 and to 56 percent in 2006. Give or take a hiccup here and there, the trend is remarkably clear: Over the past 30 years, the circumcision rate has fallen 30 percent. All evidence suggests that we are nearing the moment (2014?) when the year's crop of circumcised newborns will be in the minority.

Opposition to circumcision isn't new, of course. What is new are the opponents. What was once mostly a fringe movement has been flowing steadily into the mainstream. Today's anti-circumcision crowd are people like the Moreas—people whose religious and ideological passions don't run high either way and who arrive at their decision through a kind of personal cost-benefit analysis involving health concerns, pain, and other factors. At the same time, new evidence that circumcision can help prevent the spread of AIDS, coupled with centuries-old sentiments supporting the practice, are touching off a backlash to the backlash. Lately, arguments pro and con have grown fierce, flaring with the contentious intensity of our time.

The idea of separating the prepuce from the penis is older than the Old Testament. The first depiction of the procedure exists on the walls of an Egyptian tomb built in 2400 B.C.—a relief complete with hieroglyphics that read, "Hold him and do not allow him to faint." The notion appears to have occurred to several disparate cultures, for reasons unknown. "It is far easier to imagine the impulse behind Neolithic cave painting than to guess what inspired the ancients to cut their genitals," writes David L. Gollaher in his definitive tome *Circumcision: A History of the World's Most Controversial Surgery.* One theory suggests that the ritual's original goal was to simply draw blood from the sexual organ—to serve as the male equivalent of menstruation, in other words, and thus a rite of passage into adulthood. The Jews took their enslavers' practice and turned it into a sign of their own covenant with God; 2,000 years later, Muslims followed suit.

Medical concerns didn't enter the picture until the late-nineteenth century, when science began competing with religious belief. America took its first step toward universal secular circumcision, writes Gollaher, on "the rainy morning of February 9, 1870." Lewis Sayre, a leading Manhattan surgeon, was treating an anemic 5-year-old boy with partially paralyzed leg muscles when he noticed that the boy's penis was encased in an unusually tight foreskin, causing chronic pain. Going on intuition, Sayre drove the boy to Bellevue and circumcised him, improvising on the spot with scissors and his fingernails. The boy felt better almost immediately and fully recovered the use of his legs within weeks. Sayre began to perform circumcisions to treat paralysis—and, in at least five cases, his strange inspiration worked. When Sayre published the results in the *Transactions of the American Medical Association,* the floodgates swung open. Before long, surgeons were using circumcision to treat all manner of ailments.

There was another, half-hidden appeal to the procedure. Ever since the twelfth-century Jewish scholar and physician Maimonides, doctors realized that circumcision dulls the sensation in the glans, supposedly discouraging promiscuity. The idea was especially attractive to the Victorians, famously obsessed with the perils of masturbation. From therapeutic circumcision as a cure for insomnia there was only a short step toward circumcision as a way to dull the "out of control" libido.

In the thirties, another argument for routine circumcision presented itself. Research suggested a link between circumcision and reduced risk of penile and cervical cancer. In addition to the obvious health implications, the finding strengthened the idea of the foreskin as unclean. On par with deodorant and a daily shower, circumcision became a means of assimilating the immigrant and urbanizing the country bumpkin—a civilizing cut. And so at the century's midpoint, just as the rest of the English-speaking world began souring on the practice (the British National Health Service stopped covering it in 1949), the U.S. settled into its status as the planet's one bastion of routine neonatal circumcision—second only to Israel.

That belief held sway for decades. Men had it done to their sons because it was done to them. Generations of women came to think of the uncircumcised penis as odd. To leave your son uncircumcised was to expose him to ostracism in the locker room and the bedroom. No amount of debunking seemed to alter that. As far back as 1971, the American Academy of Pediatrics declared that there were "no valid medical indications for circumcision in the neonatal period." The following year, some 80 percent of Americans circumcised their newborns.

What changed? The shift away from circumcision is driven by a mass of converging trends. For one, we live in an age of child-centric parenting. New research suggests that the babies feel and process more than previously thought, including physical pain (see "How Much Does It Hurt?"). In a survey conducted for this story, every respondent who decided against circumcision cited "unwillingness to inflict pain on the baby" as the main reason. The movement toward healthier living is another factor. Just as people have grown increasingly wary of the impact of artificial foods in their diets and chemical products in the environment, so too have they become more suspicious of the routine use of preventive medical procedures. We've already rejected tonsillectomy and appendectomy as bad ideas. The new holistically minded consensus seems to be that if something is there, it's there for a reason: Leave it alone. Globalization plays a part too. As more U.S. women have sex with foreign-born men, the American perception of the uncut penis as exotic has begun to fade. The decline in the number of practicing Jews contributes as well. Perhaps as a reflection of all of these typically urban-minded ideas, circumcision

rates are dropping in big coastal cities at a faster rate than in the heartland. In 2006, for example, a minority of male New York City newborns were circumcised—43.4 percent. In Minnesota, the rate was 70 percent. Circumcision, you could say, is becoming a blue-state-red-state issue.

The Moreas considered all of this and more, having imbibed more information about both the pros and cons of circumcision during the last four months of Deanna's pregnancy than they care to recall. They still hadn't decided what to do until the day after their son, Anderson, was born. Then, when a nurse came to take the boy to be circumcised, the decision came clear to them. "We didn't want to put him through that—we didn't want to cut him," says Deanna. "It's mutilation. They do it to girls in Africa. No matter how accepted it is, it's mutilation."

And yet, the pendulum is already swinging back. Earlier this year, *The New York Times* published a front-page story noting that the Centers for Disease Control was considering recommending routine circumcision to help stop the spread of AIDS. The idea was based largely on studies done in Africa indicating that circumcised heterosexual men were at least 60 percent less susceptible to HIV than uncircumcised ones. The story promptly touched off a firestorm, with pro- and anti-circumcision commenters exchanging angry barbs. The CDC will now say only that it's in the process of determining a recommendation.

Caught at the crossroads of religion and science, circumcision has proved to be a free-floating symbol, attaching itself to whatever orthodoxy captures a society's imagination. Its history is driven by wildly shifting rationales: from tribal rite of passage to covenant with God to chastity guarantor to paralysis cure to cancer guard to unnecessary, painful surgery to a Hail Mary pass in the struggle with the AIDS pandemic. There's no reason to think a new rationale won't come down the pike when we least expect it. Our millennia-long quest to justify one of civilization's most curious habits continues.

Michael Idov is a contributing editor at *New York Magazine* and the author of the novel *Ground Up*.

EXPLORING THE ISSUE

Is There a Valid Reason for Routine Infant Male Circumcision?

Critical Thinking and Reflection

1. What are the medical benefits of male circumcision?
2. What role does the procedure have in religious rites? Which religions promote circumcision?
3. Describe why some individuals believe that circumcision violates a boy's body.

Is There Common Ground?

In southern Africa, the small country of Swaziland is experiencing one of the highest rates of HIV in the world. Slightly less than 20 percent of Swaziland's 1 million people are HIV positive, an epidemic linked to poverty, a lack of medical resources, and a culture in which having multiple sex partners is common. Nearly half of women ages 25–29 and men 35–39 are infected. During recent times, the average life expectancy has dropped from about 61 years to 47 due to the AIDS epidemic. To help fight the disease and prevent new cases, Swaziland has been preparing its male citizens for mass circumcision since 2006. This is in response to a 2005 study conducted in South Africa, which determined that circumcised men are as much as 60 percent less likely to contract HIV through heterosexual sex. Researchers do not fully understand why the disease rate was so much lower, but the study was so convincing that it was halted after 18 months, because preventing the uncircumcised control group from getting the procedure would not have been ethical. According to a recent article in the *Atlantic Monthly* ("The Kindest Cut," January/February 2011), there was a nationwide campaign in Swaziland to circumcise 160,000 HIV-negative males by the end of 2011. While Swaziland is in the process of circumcising thousands of men, not all researchers are convinced of the benefits of the procedure as a means to combat AIDS. In "Circumcision" (*Journal of Pediatrics & Child Health*, January/February 2011) author David Isaacs argues that there is insufficient proof of the health benefits of the procedure. However, the article "Role of the Foreskin in Male Circumcision: An Evidence-Based Review" (*Journal of Reproductive Immunology*, March 2011) presents evidence that shows HIV transmission is reduced when a man is circumcised. Similar results were found in the study published in *Preventive Medicine* in March 2011

("Male Circumcision as an HIV Prevention Intervention in the US: Influence of Health Care Providers and Potential for Risk Compensation"), which also found male circumcision was an HIV-prevention intervention and reduced the potential for disease transmission. While it's clear that researchers don't always agree, many studies argue that circumcision may help prevent diseases among males. Overall, the procedure remains controversial and many experts disagree on the risks and benefits.

Create Central

www.mhhe.com/createcentral

Additional Resources

Carbery, B., Zhu, J., Gust, D. A., Chen, R. T., Kretsinger, K., & Kilmarx, P. H. (2012). Need for physician education on the benefits and risks of male circumcision in the United States. *AIDS Education & Prevention, 24*(4), 377–387.

Earp, B. D. (2012). Can Religious beliefs justify circumcision? *Attorneys for the Rights of the Child Newsletter, 9* (3), 1–13.

Fox, M. & Thomson, M. (2012). The new politics of male circumcision: HIV/AIDS, health law and social justice. *Legal Studies. 32*(2), 255–281.

Morris, B. J., Bailey, R. C., Klausner, J. D., et al. (2012). Review: A critical evaluation of arguments opposing male circumcision for HIV prevention in developed countries. *AIDS Care, 24*(12), 1565–1575.

Schultheiss, C. E. (2010). The ethics of nontherapeutic neonatal male circumcision. *Penn Bioethics Journal, 6*(2), 21–24.

Internet References . . .

Cleveland Clinic Fact Sheet—Circumcision

Offers information about the procedure and the health risks and benefits.

http://my.clevelandclinic.org/services/circumcision/hic_circumcision.aspx

Mayo Clinic Circumcision Fact Sheet

Offers information about the procedure.

www.mayoclinic.com/health/circumcision/MY01023

Medline Plus: National Institutes of Health

Offers a fact sheet with numerous links on the topic.

www.nlm.nih.gov/medlineplus/circumcision.html

National Circumcision Resource Center

The site is a source of male circumcision information for parents and children's advocates; childbirth educators and allied professionals; medical, mental health, and academic people; Jews; and others.

www.circumcision.org/

Unit 5

UNIT

Public Health Issues

*T*here are many health issues that concern the public and are affected by public policy and public health laws. The focus of public health intervention is to improve the health and quality of life of populations. This is accomplished through the prevention and treatment of disease and other physical and mental health conditions, surveillance of disease cases, enactment of public health laws (i.e., smoking bans in public), and the promotion of healthy behaviors. An important component of public health policy is the balance between protecting public health and the maintenance of individual freedoms.

Selected, Edited, and with Issue Framing Material by:
Eileen Daniel, *SUNY College at Brockport*

ISSUE

Is There a Link Between Vaccination and Autism?

YES: **Robert F. Kennedy Jr.**, from "Deadly Immunity," *Rolling Stone* (June 30–July 14, 2005)

NO: **Matthew Normand and Jesse Dallery**, from "Mercury Rising: Exposing the Vaccine-Autism Myth," *Skeptic* (vol. 13, no. 3, 2007)

Learning Outcomes

After reading this issue, you should be able to:

- Discuss the risk factors associated with the development of autism.
- Distinguish the various conditions associated with the autism spectrum.
- Understand the reasons for the increase in children being diagnosed with autism.
- Assess the relationship between autism and vaccination.

ISSUE SUMMARY

YES: Environmentalist and attorney Robert F. Kennedy Jr. argues that childhood vaccines containing thimerosal are linked to autism and that the government has colluded with pharmaceutical companies to cover up this information.

NO: Psychology professors Matthew Normand and Jesse Dallery contend that studies have failed to uncover any specific link between autism and mercury-containing thimerosal vaccines.

The brain development disorder known as autism is characterized by impaired communication and interpersonal interactions and restricted and repetitive behavior. These symptoms tend to begin before a child is three years old. The autism spectrum disorders (ASD) also include related conditions such as Asperger syndrome that have milder signs and symptoms.

Overall, males are affected more often than females by about 4:1. It appears that 4–10 individuals per 10,000 children are affected, though recent surveys have shown a much higher prevalence of 40–60 cases/10,000 people. While there has been much publicity over the increased numbers of autism cases identified over the past 20–30 years, there is limited evidence that the actual number of new cases has risen over this time frame. Changes in the way autism is diagnosed have been suggested as a reason for the increased rates. Researchers studied population groups in California and documented a rise in the number of children diagnosed with autism and a decrease in the number diagnosed with mental retardation. This may suggest that a change in diagnosis from mental retardation to autism may be responsible for the increase in the incidence of autism. It is clear that further research is needed to determine if the actual number of cases of autism is truly increasing.

Scientists aren't clear about what causes autism, but it's likely that both genetics and environment play a role. Researchers have identified a number of genes associated with the disorder. Research involving individuals with autism has found abnormalities in multiple regions of the brain. Other studies indicate that people with autism have unusual levels of serotonin or other neurotransmitters in the brain. These irregularities imply that autism may develop from the disruption of normal brain growth early in fetal development. These irregularities are caused by defects in genes that control brain growth and that regulate how neurons communicate with each other. While these findings are interesting, they are preliminary and require additional research.

Vaccination against infectious diseases such as measles, polio, and mumps has been a very successful preventive agent. However, because of this success, many people have forgotten how dreadful these diseases were and can be. Most of the concerns about the role of vaccines in autism have focused on the measles, mumps, and rubella (MMR) vaccine and on thimerosal, the mercury-based preservative used in some vaccines before 2001. In 1998, researcher Andrew Wakefield published a paper in the British medical journal, *Lancet*. It reported on 12 children who had autism spectrum disorder as well as bowel symptoms. In eight of these children, the parents or the child's doctor linked the MMR vaccination with the onset of the behavioral symptoms. The paper was seized upon by the media and parents' groups, creating a furor that led to a significant drop in the number of British children who were vaccinated, leading to a return of mumps and measles cases in England. Interestingly, in February 2009 a special federal court ruled that there was no proven link between certain early childhood vaccines such as MMR and autism that developed in three children.

Though a special federal court ruled that there was no proven link between the MMR vaccine and autism, many parents and their doctors believe otherwise. In the YES and NO selections, attorney and environmentalist Robert F. Kennedy Jr. argues that the mercury-based thiomersal used as a preservative is linked to autism and that the government is in collusion with pharmaceutical companies. Psychology professors Matthew Normand and Jesse Dallery disagree and contend that studies have failed to uncover any specific link between autism and mercury-containing thimerosal vaccines.

YES ↵

Robert F. Kennedy Jr.

Deadly Immunity

In June 2000, a group of top government scientists and health officials gathered for a meeting at the isolated Simpsonwood conference center in Norcross, Georgia. Convened by the Centers for Disease Control and Prevention, the meeting was held at this Methodist retreat center, nestled in wooded farmland next to the Chattahoochee River, to ensure complete secrecy. The agency had issued no public announcement of the session—only private invitations to fifty-two attendees. There were high-level officials from the CDC and the Food and Drug Administration, the top vaccine specialist from the World Health Organization in Geneva and representatives of every major vaccine manufacturer, including GlaxoSmithKline, Merck, Wyeth and Aventis Pasteur. All of the scientific data under discussion, CDC officials repeatedly reminded the participants, was strictly "embargoed." There would be no making photocopies of documents, no taking papers with them when they left.

The federal officials and industry representatives had assembled to discuss a disturbing new study that raised alarming questions about the safety of a host of common childhood vaccines administered to infants and young children. According to a CDC epidemiologist named Tom Verstraeten, who had analyzed the agency's massive database containing the medical records of 100,000 children, a mercury-based preservative in the vaccines—thimerosal—appeared to be responsible for a dramatic increase in autism and a host of other neurological disorders among children. "I was actually stunned by what I saw," Verstraeten told those assembled at Simpsonwood, citing the staggering number of earlier studies that indicate a link between thimerosal and speech delays, attention-deficit disorder, hyperactivity and autism. Since 1991, when the CDC and the FDA had recommended that three additional vaccines laced with the preservative be given to extremely young infants—in one case, within hours of birth—the estimated number of cases of autism had increased fifteenfold, from one in every 2,500 children to one in 166 children.

Even for scientists and doctors accustomed to confronting issues of life and death, the findings were frightening. "You can play with this all you want," Dr. Bill Weil, a consultant for the American Academy of Pediatrics, told the group. The results "are statistically significant." Dr. Richard Johnston, an immunologist and pediatrician from the University of Colorado whose grandson had been born early on the morning of the meeting's first day, was even more alarmed. "My gut feeling?" he said. "Forgive this personal comment—I do not want my grandson to get a thimerosal-containing vaccine until we know better what is going on."

But instead of taking immediate steps to alert the public and rid the vaccine supply of thimerosal, the officials and executives at Simpsonwood spent most of the next two days discussing how to cover up the damaging data. According to transcripts obtained under the Freedom of Information Act, many at the meeting were concerned about how the damaging revelations about thimerosal would affect the vaccine industry's bottom line. "We are in a bad position from the standpoint of defending any lawsuits," said Dr. Robert Brent, a pediatrician at the Alfred I. duPont Hospital for Children in Delaware. "This will be a resource to our very busy plaintiff attorneys in this country." Dr. Bob Chen, head of vaccine safety for the CDC, expressed relief that "given the sensitivity of the information, we have been able to keep it out of the hands of, let's say, less responsible hands." Dr. John Clements, vaccines adviser at the World Health Organization, declared flatly that the study "should not have been done at all" and warned that the results "will be taken by others and will be used in ways beyond the control of this group. The research results have to be *handled*."

In fact, the government has proved to be far more adept at handling the damage than at protecting children's health. The CDC paid the Institute of Medicine to conduct a new study to whitewash the risks of thimerosal, ordering researchers to "rule out" the chemical's link to autism. It withheld Verstraeten's findings, even though they had been slated for immediate publication, and told other scientists that his original data had been "lost" and could not be replicated. And to thwart the Freedom of Information Act, it handed its giant database of vaccine records over to a private company, declaring it off-limits to researchers. By the time Verstraeten finally published his study in 2003, he had gone to work for GlaxoSmithKline and reworked his data to bury the link between thimerosal and autism.

Vaccine manufacturers had already begun to phase thimerosal out of injections given to American infants—but they continued to sell off their mercury-based supplies of vaccines until last year. The CDC and FDA gave them a hand, buying up the tainted vaccines for export to developing countries and allowing drug companies to continue using the preservative in some American vaccines—including several pediatric flu shots as well as tetanus boosters routinely given to eleven-year-olds.

The drug companies are also getting help from powerful lawmakers in Washington. Senate Majority Leader Bill Frist, who has received $873,000 in contributions from the pharmaceutical industry, has been working to immunize vaccine makers from liability in 4,200 lawsuits that have been filed by the parents of injured children. On five separate occasions, Frist has tried to seal all of the government's vaccine-related documents—including the Simpsonwood transcripts—and shield Eli Lilly, the developer of thimerosal, from subpoenas. In 2002, the day after Frist quietly slipped a rider known as the "Eli Lilly Protection Act" into a homeland security bill, the company contributed $10,000 to his campaign and bought 5,000 copies of his book on bioterrorism. The measure was repealed by Congress in 2003—but earlier this year, Frist slipped another provision into an anti-terrorism bill that would deny compensation to children suffering from vaccine-related brain disorders. "The lawsuits are of such magnitude that they could put vaccine producers out of business and limit our capacity to deal with a biological attack by terrorists," says Andy Olsen, a legislative assistant to Frist.

Even many conservatives are shocked by the government's effort to cover up the dangers of thimerosal. Rep. Dan Burton, a Republican from Indiana, oversaw a three-year investigation of thimerosal after his grandson was diagnosed with autism. "Thimerosal used as a preservative in vaccines is directly related to the autism epidemic," his House Government Reform Committee concluded in its final report. "This epidemic in all probability may have been prevented or curtailed had the FDA not been asleep at the switch regarding a lack of safety data regarding

injected thimerosal, a known neurotoxin." The FDA and other public-health agencies failed to act, the committee added, out of "institutional malfeasance for self protection" and "misplaced protectionism of the pharmaceutical industry."

The story of how government health agencies colluded with Big Pharma to hide the risks of thimerosal from the public is a chilling case study of institutional arrogance, power and greed. I was drawn into the controversy only reluctantly. As an attorney and environmentalist who has spent years working on issues of mercury toxicity, I frequently met mothers of autistic children who were absolutely convinced that their kids had been injured by vaccines. Privately, I was skeptical. I doubted that autism could be blamed on a single source, and I certainly understood the government's need to reassure parents that vaccinations are safe; the eradication of deadly childhood diseases depends on it. I tended to agree with skeptics like Rep. Henry Waxman, a Democrat from California, who criticized his colleagues on the House Government Reform Committee for leaping to conclusions about autism and vaccinations. "Why should we scare people about immunization," Waxman pointed out at one hearing, "until we know the facts?"

It was only after reading the Simpsonwood transcripts, studying the leading scientific research and talking with many of the nation's pre-eminent authorities on mercury that I became convinced that the link between thimerosal and the epidemic of childhood neurological disorders is real. Five of my own children are members of the Thimerosal Generation—those born between 1989 and 2003—who received heavy doses of mercury from

Figure 1

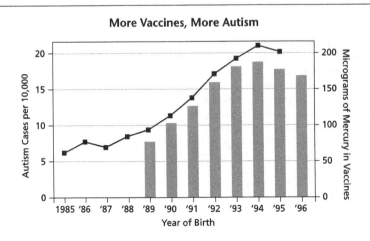

After the CDC began recommending additional vaccinations in 1989, the number of autism cases nationwide spiked sharply. Figures for California show the link to the increasing "mercury load" in vaccines, as surveyed two years after birth.

vaccines. "The elementary grades are overwhelmed with children who have symptoms of neurological or immune-system damage," Patti White, a school nurse, told the House Government Reform Committee in 1999. "Vaccines are supposed to be making us healthier; however, in twenty-five years of nursing I have never seen so many damaged, sick kids. Something very, very wrong is happening to our children."

More than 500,000 kids currently suffer from autism, and pediatricians diagnose more than 40,000 new cases every year. The disease was unknown until 1943, when it was identified and diagnosed among eleven children born in the months after thimerosal was first added to baby vaccines in 1931.

Some skeptics dispute that the rise in autism is caused by thimerosal-tainted vaccinations. They argue that the increase is a result of better diagnosis—a theory that seems questionable at best, given that most of the new cases of autism are clustered within a single generation of children. "If the epidemic is truly an artifact of poor diagnosis," scoffs Dr. Boyd Haley, one of the world's authorities on mercury toxicity, "then where are all the twenty-year-old autistics?" Other researchers point out that Americans are exposed to a greater cumulative "load" of mercury than ever before, from contaminated fish to dental fillings, and suggest that thimerosal in vaccines may be only part of a much larger problem. It's a concern that certainly deserves far more attention than it has received—but it overlooks the fact that the mercury concentrations in vaccines dwarf other sources of exposure to our children.

What is most striking is the lengths to which many of the leading detectives have gone to ignore—and cover up—the evidence against thimerosal. From the very beginning, the scientific case against the mercury additive has been overwhelming. The preservative, which is used to stem fungi and bacterial growth in vaccines, contains ethylmercury, a potent neurotoxin. Truckloads of studies have shown that mercury tends to accumulate in the brains of primates and other animals after they are injected with vaccines—and that the developing brains of infants are particularly susceptible. In 1977, a Russian study found that adults exposed to much lower concentrations of ethylmercury than those given to American children still suffered brain damage years later. Russia banned thimerosal from children's vaccines twenty years ago, and Denmark, Austria, Japan, Great Britain and all the Scandinavian countries have since followed suit.

"You couldn't even construct a study that shows thimerosal is safe," says Haley, who heads the chemistry department at the University of Kentucky. "It's just too darn toxic. If you inject thimerosal into an animal, its brain will sicken. If you apply it to living tissue, the cells die. If you put it in a petri dish, the culture dies. Knowing these things, it would be shocking if one could inject it into an infant without causing damage."

Internal documents reveal that Eli Lilly, which first developed thimerosal, knew from the start that its product could cause damage—and even death—in both animals and humans. In 1930, the company tested thimerosal by administering it to twenty-two patients with terminal meningitis, all of whom died within weeks of being injected—a fact Lilly didn't bother to report in its study declaring thimerosal safe. In 1935, researchers at another vaccine manufacturer, Pittman-Moore, warned Lilly that its claims about thimerosal's safety "did not check with ours." Half the dogs Pittman injected with thimerosal-based vaccines became sick, leading researchers there to declare the preservative "unsatisfactory as a serum intended for use on dogs."

In the decades that followed, the evidence against thimerosal continued to mount. During the Second World War, when the Department of Defense used the preservative in vaccines on soldiers, it required Lilly to label it "poison." In 1967, a study in *Applied Microbiology* found that thimerosal killed mice when added to injected vaccines. Four years later, Lilly's own studies discerned that thimerosal was "toxic to tissue cells" in concentrations as low as one part per million—100 times weaker than the concentration in a typical vaccine. Even so, the company continued to promote thimerosal as "nontoxic" and also incorporated it into topical disinfectants. In 1977, ten babies at a Toronto hospital died when an antiseptic preserved with thimerosal was dabbed onto their umbilical cords.

In 1982, the FDA proposed a ban on over-the-counter products that contained thimerosal, and in 1991 the agency considered banning it from animal vaccines. But tragically, that same year, the CDC recommended that infants be injected with a series of mercury-laced vaccines. Newborns would be vaccinated for hepatitis B within twenty-four hours of birth, and two-month-old infants would be immunized for haemophilus influenzae B and diphtheria-tetanus-pertussis.

The drug industry knew the additional vaccines posed a danger. The same year that the CDC approved the new vaccines, Dr. Maurice Hilleman, one of the fathers of Merck's vaccine programs, warned the company that six-month-olds who were administered the shots would suffer dangerous exposure to mercury. He recommended that thimerosal be discontinued, "especially when used on infants and children," noting that the industry knew of nontoxic alternatives. "The best way to go," he added, "is to switch to dispensing the actual vaccines without adding preservatives."

For Merck and other drug companies, however, the obstacle was money. Thimerosal enables the pharmaceutical industry to package vaccines in vials that contain multiple doses, which require additional protection because they are more easily contaminated by multiple needle entries. The larger vials cost half as much to produce as smaller, single-dose vials, making it cheaper for international agencies to distribute them to impoverished regions at risk of epidemics. Faced with this "cost consideration," Merck ignored Hilleman's warnings, and government

Figure 2

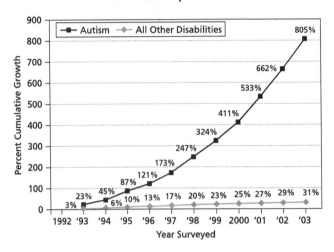

The Autism Epidemic

Skeptics insist that the nationwide rise in autism is the result of better diagnosis. But as Department of Education figures show, the disease increased much more rapidly between 1992 and 2003 than other disabilities among six- to twenty-two-year-olds.

officials continued to push more and more thimerosal-based vaccines for children. Before 1989, American pre-schoolers received only three vaccinations—for polio, diphtheria-tetanus-pertussis and measles-mumps-rubella. A decade later, thanks to federal recommendations, children were receiving a total of twenty-two immunizations by the time they reached first grade.

❧

As the number of vaccines increased, the rate of autism among children exploded. During the 1990s, 40 million children were injected with thimerosal-based vaccines, receiving unprecedented levels of mercury during a period critical for brain development. Despite the well-documented dangers of thimerosal, it appears that no one bothered to add up the cumulative dose of mercury that children would receive from the mandated vaccines. "What took the FDA so long to do the calculations?" Peter Patriarca, director of viral products for the agency, asked in an e-mail to the CDC in 1999. "Why didn't CDC and the advisory bodies do these calculations when they rapidly expanded the childhood immunization schedule?"

But by that time, the damage was done. Infants who received all their vaccines, plus boosters, by the age of six months were being injected with levels of ethylmercury 187 times greater than the EPA's limit for daily exposure to methylmercury, a related neurotoxin. Although the vaccine industry insists that ethylmercury poses little danger because it breaks down rapidly and is removed by the body, several studies—including one published in April by

the National Institutes of Health—suggest that ethylmercury is actually *more* toxic to developing brains and stays in the brain *longer* than methylmercury.

Officials responsible for childhood immunizations insist that the additional vaccines were necessary to protect infants from disease and that thimerosal is still essential in developing nations, which, they often claim, cannot afford the single-dose vials that don't require a preservative. Dr. Paul Offit, one of CDC's top vaccine advisers, told me, "I think if we really have an influenza pandemic—and certainly we will in the next twenty years, because we always do—there's no way on God's earth that we immunize 280 million people with single-dose vials. There has to be multidose vials."

But while public-health officials may have been well-intentioned, many of those on the CDC advisory committee who backed the additional vaccines had close ties to the industry. Dr. Sam Katz, the committee's chair, was a paid consultant for most of the major vaccine makers and shares a patent on a measles vaccine with Merck, which also manufactures the hepatitis B vaccine. Dr. Neal Halsey, another committee member, worked as a researcher for the vaccine companies and received honoraria from Abbott Labs for his research on the hepatitis B vaccine.

Indeed, in the tight circle of scientists who work on vaccines, such conflicts of interest are common. Rep. Burton says that the CDC "routinely allows scientists with blatant conflicts of interest to serve on intellectual advisory committees that make recommendations on new vaccines," even though they have "interests in the products and companies for which they are supposed to be providing unbiased oversight." The House Government Reform Committee discovered that four of the eight CDC advisers who approved guidelines for a rotavirus vaccine laced with thimerosal "had financial ties to the pharmaceutical companies that were developing different versions of the vaccine."

Offit, who shares a patent on the vaccine, acknowledged to me that he "would make money" if his vote to approve it eventually leads to a marketable product. But he dismissed my suggestion that a scientist's direct financial stake in CDC approval might bias his judgment. "It provides no conflict for me," he insists. "I have simply been informed by the process, not corrupted by it. When I sat around that table, my sole intent was trying to make recommendations that best benefited the children in this country. It's offensive to say that physicians and public-health people are in the pocket of industry and thus are making decisions that they know are unsafe for children. It's just not the way it works."

Other vaccine scientists and regulators gave me similar assurances. Like Offit, they view themselves as enlightened guardians of children's health, proud of their "partnerships" with pharmaceutical companies, immune to the seductions of personal profit, besieged by irrational activists whose anti-vaccine campaigns are endangering children's health. They are often resentful of questioning. "Science," says Offit, "is best left to scientists."

Still, some government officials were alarmed by the apparent conflicts of interest. In his e-mail to CDC administrators in 1999, Paul Patriarca of the FDA blasted federal regulators for failing to adequately scrutinize the danger posed by the added baby vaccines. "I'm not sure there will be an easy way out of the potential perception that the FDA, CDC and immunization-policy bodies may have been asleep at the switch re: thimerosal until now," Patriarca wrote. The close ties between regulatory officials and the pharmaceutical industry, he added, "will also raise questions about various advisory bodies regarding aggressive recommendations for use" of thimerosal in child vaccines.

⚫

If federal regulators and government scientists failed to grasp the potential risks of thimerosal over the years, no one could claim ignorance after the secret meeting at Simpsonwood. But rather than conduct more studies to test the link to autism and other forms of brain damage, the CDC placed politics over science. The agency turned its database on childhood vaccines—which had been developed largely at taxpayer expense—over to a private agency, America's Health Insurance Plans, ensuring that it could not be used for additional research. It also instructed the Institute of Medicine, an advisory organization that is part of the National Academy of Sciences, to produce a study debunking the link between thimerosal and brain disorders. The CDC "wants us to declare, well,

that these things are pretty safe," Dr. Marie McCormick, who chaired the IOM's Immunization Safety Review Committee, told her fellow researchers when they first met in January 2001. "We are not ever going to come down that [autism] is a true side effect" of thimerosal exposure. According to transcripts of the meeting, the committee's chief staffer, Kathleen Stratton, predicted that the IOM would conclude that the evidence was "inadequate to accept or reject a causal relation" between thimerosal and autism. That, she added, was the result "Walt wants"—a reference to Dr. Walter Orenstein, director of the National Immunization Program for the CDC.

For those who had devoted their lives to promoting vaccination, the revelations about thimerosal threatened to undermine everything they had worked for. "We've got a dragon by the tail here," said Dr. Michael Kaback, another committee member. "The more negative that [our] presentation is, the less likely people are to use vaccination, immunization—and we know what the results of that will be. We are kind of caught in a trap. How we work our way out of the trap, I think is the charge."

Even in public, federal officials made it clear that their primary goal in studying thimerosal was to dispel doubts about vaccines. "Four current studies are taking place to rule out the proposed link between autism and thimerosal," Dr. Gordon Douglas, then-director of strategic planning for vaccine research at the National Institutes of Health, assured a Princeton University gathering in May 2001. "In order to undo the harmful effects of research claiming to link the [measles] vaccine to an elevated risk of autism, we need to conduct and publicize additional studies to assure parents of safety." Douglas formerly served as president of vaccinations for Merck, where he ignored warnings about thimerosal's risks.

In May of last year, the Institute of Medicine issued its final report. Its conclusion: There is no proven link between autism and thimerosal in vaccines. Rather than reviewing the large body of literature describing the toxicity of thimerosal, the report relied on four disastrously flawed epidemiological studies examining European countries, where children received much smaller doses of thimerosal than American kids. It also cited a new version of the Verstraeten study, published in the journal *Pediatrics,* that had been reworked to reduce the link between thimerosal and autism. The new study included children too young to have been diagnosed with autism and overlooked others who showed signs of the disease. The IOM declared the case closed and—in a startling position for a scientific body—recommended that no further research be conducted.

The report may have satisfied the CDC, but it convinced no one. Rep. David Weldon, a Republican physician from Florida who serves on the House Government Reform Committee, attacked the Institute of Medicine, saying it relied on a handful of studies that were "fatally flawed" by "poor design" and failed to represent "all the available scientific and medical research." CDC officials are not interested in an honest search for the truth, Weldon told me, because "an association between vaccines and autism would force them to admit that their policies irreparably damaged thousands of children. Who would want to make that conclusion about themselves?"

⋅⊙⋅

Under pressure from Congress, parents and a few of its own panel members, the Institute of Medicine reluctantly convened a second panel to review the findings of the first. In February, the new panel, composed of different scientists, criticized the earlier panel for its lack of transparency and urged the CDC to make its vaccine database available to the public.

So far, though, only two scientists have managed to gain access. Dr. Mark Geier, president of the Genetics Center of America, and his son, David, spent a year battling to obtain the medical records from the CDC. Since August 2002, when members of Congress pressured the agency to turn over the data, the Geiers have completed six studies that demonstrate a powerful correlation between thimerosal and neurological damage in children. One study, which compares the cumulative dose of mercury received by children born between 1981 and 1985 with those born between 1990 and 1996, found a "very significant relationship" between autism and vaccines. Another study of educational performance found that kids who received higher doses of thimerosal in vaccines were nearly three times as likely to be diagnosed with autism and more than three times as likely to suffer from speech disorders and mental retardation. Another soon-to-be published study shows that autism rates are in decline following the recent elimination of thimerosal from most vaccines.

As the federal government worked to prevent scientists from studying vaccines, others have stepped in to study the link to autism. In April, reporter Dan Olmsted of UPI undertook one of the more interesting studies himself. Searching for children who had not been exposed to mercury in vaccines—the kind of population that scientists typically use as a "control" in experiments—Olmsted scoured the Amish of Lancaster County, Pennsylvania, who refuse to immunize their infants. Given the national rate of autism, Olmsted calculated that there should be 130 autistics among the Amish. He found only four. One had been exposed to high levels of mercury from a power plant. The other three—including one child adopted from outside the Amish community—had received their vaccines.

At the state level, many officials have also conducted in-depth reviews of thimerosal. While the Institute of Medicine was busy whitewashing the risks, the Iowa legislature was carefully combing through all of the available scientific and biological data. "After three years of review, I became convinced there was sufficient credible research to show a link between mercury and the increased incidences in autism," says state Sen. Ken Veenstra, a Republican who oversaw the investigation. "The fact that Iowa's 700 percent increase in autism began in the 1990s, right after more and more vaccines were added to the children's vaccine schedules, is solid evidence alone." Last year, Iowa became the first state to ban mercury in vaccines, followed by California. Similar bans are now under consideration in thirty-two other states.

But instead of following suit, the FDA continues to allow manufacturers to include thimerosal in scores of over-the-counter medications as well as steroids and injected collagen. Even more alarming, the government continues to ship vaccines preserved with thimerosal to developing countries—some of which are now experiencing a sudden explosion in autism rates. In China, where the disease was virtually unknown prior to the introduction of thimerosal by U.S. drug manufacturers in 1999, news reports indicate that there are now more than 1.8 million autistics. Although reliable numbers are hard to come by, autistic disorders also appear to be soaring in India, Argentina, Nicaragua and other developing countries that are now using thimerosal-laced vaccines. The World Health Organization continues to insist thimerosal is safe, but it promises to keep the possibility that it is linked to neurological disorders "under review."

I devoted time to study this issue because I believe that this is a moral crisis that must be addressed. If, as the evidence suggests, our public-health authorities knowingly allowed the pharmaceutical industry to poison an entire generation of American children, their actions arguably constitute one of the biggest scandals in the annals of American medicine. "The CDC is guilty of incompetence and gross negligence," says Mark Blaxill, vice president of Safe Minds, a nonprofit organization concerned about the role of mercury in medicines. "The damage caused by vaccine exposure is massive. It's bigger than asbestos, bigger than tobacco, bigger than anything you've ever seen."

It's hard to calculate the damage to our country—and to the international efforts to eradicate epidemic diseases—if Third World nations come to believe that America's most heralded foreign-aid initiative is poisoning their children. It's not difficult to predict how this scenario will be interpreted by America's enemies abroad. The scientists and researchers—many of them sincere, even idealistic—who are participating in efforts to hide the science on thimerosal claim that they are trying to advance the lofty goal of protecting children in developing nations from disease pandemics. They are badly misguided. Their failure to come clean on thimerosal will come back horribly to haunt our country and the world's poorest populations.

ROBERT F. KENNEDY JR., an environmentalist, is the president of Waterkeeper Alliance.

Matthew Normand and Jesse Dallery

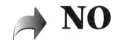 **NO**

Mercury Rising: Exposing the Vaccine-Autism Myth

On June 11, 2007, nearly 5,000 parents of autistic children filed a lawsuit against the federal government, claiming that childhood vaccines (specifically the mercury-containing thimerosal in the vaccines) caused their children's autism. The previous year the *New York Times* ran a column that was skeptical of the alleged link between autism and vaccines. It generated the following comment on an Internet message board, typical of the anecdotal analyses that perpetuate the claim:

> You say, "There is no proven link" between mercury and autism. There also is "no proven link" between going outside in the rain and cold without a hat or coat and getting the sniffles. Look at the data: the epidemic of autism mirrors the administration of vaccines with mercury. Now that they are off the shelves (more or less), the cases are going down.

Here we see how the writer dismisses scientific evidence that fails to support a link between cold and illness and vaccines and autism in favor of her personal experiences. And the vaccine-autism controversy is not constrained to a small fringe group of parents or advocates. Increasingly, people of position and power are leaping into the fray, spurred on by vocal groups demanding action. For example, an article by Robert F. Kennedy, Jr. appeared in a June 2005 issue of *Rolling Stone* magazine[1] that alleged thimerosal-containing vaccines were at the heart of the autism epidemic and, moreover, that the government was aware of this and actively engaged in a cover-up.

This article makes five points concerning the relation between thimerosal-containing vaccines and autism: (1) the dangers of mercury are well established, but this does not lead inexorably to a relationship between vaccines containing thimerosal and autism; (2) a number of well controlled studies have failed to uncover any correlation between the delivery of the vaccines and the onset of autism; (3) even if some correlation existed there are a number of alternative explanations for the correlation that do not assume any causal relationship between the vaccine and autism; (4) much attention has been given to a possible government cover up, which is certainly of concern if true but is otherwise independent of the problems with claims of a link between thimerosal and autism; and (5) the type of public hysteria manifested in the current controversy is not new and we would be well served to learn from similar controversies of recent times.

Mercury, Thimerosal, and the Potential for Harm

Science has told us unequivocally that mercury is bad for our bodies. In sufficient doses, mercury kills cells that it contacts, causes neurological damage in humans and other animals, and generally wreaks havoc on living things. Yet since the 1930s, thimerosal has been used as a preservative in vaccines.[2] One of the breakdown products of thimerosal is ethylmercury, which is an organic compound of mercury. Public concern about thimerosal is certainly understandable, but does this mean that concern about a link between vaccines and autism is justified as well? In a word, no. Mercury might do a number of nasty things to the human body, and concern about it is therefore justified, but that does not mean it causes autism.

Ethylmercury is not the same thing as its cousin, methylmercury. Cumulative and high doses of methylmercury can produce renal and neurologic damage. It can build up in the brain and stay in the body for a long time. Ethylmercury is more, well, mercurial. It is expelled rapidly from the body and it does not accumulate. Nevertheless, guidelines for the ingestion of ethylmercury were based on those for methylmercury. Around the same time these guidelines were formalized, children were receiving more vaccines that contained thimerosal. For example, in the early 1990s the Haemophilus influenzae b and hepatitis B became staple features of the vaccine schedule for infants, which already included another thimerosal-containing vaccine (diphtheria tetanus and variants). Based on the very conservative guidelines established by the Environmental Protection Agency (EPA), it was concluded that by age two some children might be receiving excessive levels of ethylmercury when considered in the context of known risks of methylmercury exposure.[3]

Against this backdrop enter skyrocketing rates of autism diagnoses. In California, the Department of Developmental Services reported a 273% increase from 1987 to 1998 in the number of individuals served under the category of autism.[4] Surely this increase in rates was caused by an environmental source, right? In 2001, the Institute of Medicine (IOM) Immunization Safety Review Committee held a public meeting to address the link between one environmental source—thimerosal—and autism. At the meeting, Mark Blaxill, a board member of a nonprofit organization dedicated to investigating the risks of mercury exposure, presented a graph showing the *estimated* cumulative dose of thimerosal to the *estimated* prevalence of autism in California.[5] The increasing trend lines during the early 1990s were right on top of each other, about as close as you can get to perfect correlation in ecological data. Such orderly correlations are all that it takes to convince the uncritical eye.

Even before the IOM meeting, thimerosal was removed as a preservative in vaccines in the U.S., based on a request from the Food and Drug Administration (FDA) (it remains in some influenza vaccines and in some vaccines outside of the U.S.). The request was made as a precautionary measure, and not because there was evidence to accept or reject a causal relationship between thimerosal and autism. (Thimerosal is still used during manufacture of some vaccines to ensure sterility, but the trace amounts remaining are 50 times lower than when thimerosal is used as a preservative.) Since the FDA decision, a number of research reports published in some of the most esteemed peer-reviewed journals in the world have failed to find any relation between thimerosal and autism. Despite these negative findings and the removal of thimerosal from vaccines, parents, politicians and health professionals remain alarmed that children are at risk.

Much is at stake in this debate. Based on the assumption that metals such as mercury are causing autism, some parents are avoiding vaccinations altogether. Others have sought treatments like chelation therapy, which uses special chemicals to rid the body of heavy metals following acute poisoning. However, chelation is not a risk-free procedure and should not be undertaken lightly. In August of 2005, a Pittsburgh, PA area newspaper reported that a 5-year old boy with autism died following chelation therapy. Finally, there are ongoing class action lawsuits against the manufacturers of vaccines. These lawsuits could potentially endanger the production and distribution of effective vaccines according to well-established protocols, putting scores of young children at risk.

Evidence of Harm

Let's begin with the hypothesis that thimerosal is one of the causes of autism and that it is the main culprit in the increased incidence of autism during the 1990s. This is a plausible hypothesis, but as Karl Popper taught us, a good scientific hypothesis must be falsifiable. That is, it must be possible to conceive of evidence that would prove it wrong. What evidence might suggest that the thimerosal hypothesis is false? For obvious ethical reasons, we can't perform the kind of gold-standard experiment—a randomized double-blind study—which would most convincingly indicate the lack of a causal relation. We must rely on natural experiments. One such experiment was occasioned by the removal of thimerosal in Denmark in 1992. If the thimerosal hypothesis were false, we would not expect to see changes in the rates of autism following the removal of thimerosal. In fact, the results were more robust: despite the removal of thimerosal, the rates of autism continued to climb. And not only in Denmark but in Sweden, too, where thimerosal was removed at about the same time.[6]

Another way the thimerosal hypothesis could be falsified is if it could be shown that there is no link between the amount of thimerosal exposure and the likelihood of autism. That is, we would ask if there is a dose-response relation between thimerosal exposure and developmental problems. Several studies have confirmed that there is no convincing evidence of a dose-response relation.[7] In fact, one study suggested a beneficial effect of thimerosal! For example, exposure at three months was inversely related to problems of hyperactivity, conduct, and motor development months or years later.[8] Now, these results do not imply causation, nor do they pertain to autism *per se*, but they do question the general validity of the thimerosal hypothesis.

So what of the data favoring the thimerosal hypothesis? Indeed, we must consider all sources of evidence in evaluating the truth of a claim—we must be comprehensive. Recently, some researchers have suggested that the incidence rate of autism has been on the decline since thimerosal was officially removed from vaccines in the US. If true, this would be evidence of a possible causal relationship between thimerosal and autism, and such data has been reported by one team of researchers, Mark and David Geier. Unfortunately, the study that proposed such a relationship used the Vaccine Adverse Event Reporting System (VAERS) database to make the claim.[9] The VAERS is a passive reporting system that is subject to reporting biases and errors. A health-care professional, parent, or even someone trying to prove a point[10] can enter data into the VAERS. There is no way to verify diagnoses, identify mistakes in filing, or substantiate causal hypotheses.

The irreparably flawed studies by the Geiers prompted a strong rebuke from the Centers for Disease Control (CDC) and by the American Academy of Pediatrics.[11] Simply put, the VAERS data may be useful to raise some potential questions about a phenomenon, but it certainly cannot be used to prove a hypothesis. Studies that use methods consistent with well-established scientific standards have failed to find any association between thimerosal and autism. In 2004, the Institute of Medicine concluded, "Given the lack of direct evidence for a biological mechanism and the fact that all well-designed epidemiological studies provide evidence of no association between thimerosal and autism, the committee recommends that cost-benefit assessments regarding the use of thimerosal-containing versus thimerosal-free vaccines and other biological or pharmaceutical products, whether in the United States or other countries, should not include autism as a potential risk."[12]

But what if it were determined that a strong correlation existed between the administration of thimerosal-containing vaccines and the onset of autism? Much would still be left unanswered. Consider that the average age for many vaccinations is between 12 and 18 months. Now consider that many of the "symptoms" of autism—such as social withdrawal and delayed language—aren't readily detectable until this same age or just a bit later. It could very well be that any relationship between vaccination and diagnosis is purely coincidental. If these vaccinations were not commonly given until age four, perhaps no correlation would be observed. Not to mention that the vast majority of children receive these vaccinations without incident.[13]

The bottom line is that *correlation is not causation*.

Autism Epidemic or Statistical Artifact?

Another problem for the purported vaccine-autism link is that there is good reason to be suspicious of claims of an autism epidemic. A number of factors can account for the dramatic increase in numbers, including the expansion of diagnostic criteria in 1994, and changes in criteria for inclusion in child-count data for children with autism. Remember that 273% increase over a decade in autism spectrum disorders in California? Consider, as did the authors of a recent paper published in *Current Directions in Psychological Science*,[14] that this increase could be due to an expanded diagnostic definition of autism. The authors found that a similar expansion in the definition of "tall"—from 74.5 inches to 72 inches—generated a 273% increase if these two criteria were applied a decade apart in one county in Texas.

More important, autism is not even a "thing" that can be clearly correlated with any other thing. Unlike cancer or a broken bone, there are no discrete physical, biological, or genetic markers on which to base a diagnosis. Instead, autism is a diagnostic label based on the presence of a number of behavioral excesses and deficits. The diagnosis is subjective and subject to great variability. When you consider that many resources are made available only to those children with some formal diagnosis, it is easy to see why some diagnoses might be made with scant supporting evidence. The physician or psychologist notices some obvious learning delays and behavior problems in a patient and recognizes the need for intensive services, but the only way the family can obtain those services is if the child fits a certain diagnostic category.

Correlations are tenuous things under the best conditions. Degrade one of the variables, and you are in serious trouble. Such is the case with the autism-vaccine correlation.

A Vast Government Conspiracy?

So what do vaccine opponents make of the evidence against the vaccine-autism hypothesis? Mostly, they assert a vast conspiracy propagated by government and industry. It is proposed that government agencies such as the Centers for Disease Control and Prevention, in conjunction with scientists with varying ties to the pharmaceutical industry, have gone to great lengths to suppress evidence supporting a link between vaccines and autism. Indeed, this was the main point of Robert Kennedy Jr.'s *Rolling Stone* article. He and others claim that a conspiracy does exist and was formally discussed at a top-secret meeting in Simpsonwood, GA in 2000.

One hotly discussed result of this meeting is the purported doctoring of data by Thomas Verstraeten who, according to the vaccine opponents, presented data supporting the autism-vaccine link but later altered the data to support the opposite conclusion because he was, by then, employed by a large pharmaceutical company. Verstraeten has denied such manipulation and the data he reports support the conclusions reached by a number of other independent researchers.[15] The problem is that the only evidence of doctored data sets, dubious activity at the Simpsonwood meeting, and assorted cover-ups seems to come from a small number of zealous vaccine opponents who can offer no corroborating evidence to support the hearsay.

Now let us return to the research team purporting to have data supporting the autism-vaccine hypothesis. In addition to the flawed methods on which their conclusions are based, there are conflicts of interest that should cause one to question their motives. As it turns out, David Geier is the president of MedCon, Inc., a legal firm that seeks compensation for people claiming to have been harmed by vaccines. He also has filed, with his father Mark Geier, two patents related to a treatment for autism involving a combination of drugs and chelation. Chelation therapy is, of course, predicated on the assumption of excessive amounts of heavy metals in the blood stream of children with autism. The Geiers are clearly in a position to benefit if claims concerning a vaccine-autism link are accepted by the public.

History Repeating

A revealing aspect of this controversy is how closely it resembles past controversies, pitting science against vaccine-induced autism claims, spurred on by desperate parents, media support, and various servants of the public interest. Not so long ago, science was up against a similar set of public crusaders pushing a different cause: carcinogenic power lines. In 1979, a small, poorly controlled and poorly conducted sampling of leukemia patients in Denver, CO supposedly revealed a correlation between the patients and the proximity of their homes to high-power lines.[16] The published report of these suspect findings was largely ignored by the scientific community because of the many fatal flaws evident in the methodology. Enter Paul Brodeur, a journalist with a track record of sensationalism (in the 1960s he wrote *The Zapping of America,* a book "exposing the dangers" of microwave ovens), now warned the world of the dangers posed by power lines in his book *Currents of Death.*

No amount of scientific evidence to the contrary could persuade the journalists, advocacy groups, and legal teams demanding accountability. Of course, the million-dollar question was, "Accountability for what?" Ultimately, after numerous well-controlled studies failed to find any correlation between power-lines and cancer, the story grew cold and the public outrage slowly faded away. But not before tens of millions of dollars in research funding, decreased property values, and lawsuits were lost because the matter was pursued long after science had delivered a verdict. Are we doomed to repeat this history with the vaccine controversy?

Clarifying Claims

Claims of a causal link between the administration of thimerosal-containing vaccines and the onset of autism are unfounded. The controversy has been driven more by public fervor than it has by science. This is not to suggest that the advocates and parents fueling the fire are malicious or intentionally misleading the public. The reality is that too many families face the unimaginable hardship of learning that their child has been diagnosed with autism and must encounter the subsequent trials and tribulations of providing the best possible care and education for their child. These parents are in desperate need of both assistance and answers. Compounding the difficulty is that many must navigate the waters of emerging science without having received the necessary training to do so. Clarifying misguided claims of causative factors can help redirect necessary resources to more promising treatments, and perhaps reveal a better understanding of the real factors that cause autism.

References

1. Kennedy, R. F., Jr. 2005. "Deadly Immunity." *Rolling Stone, 977/978,* June–July, 57–61.

2. U.S. Food and Drug Administration. n.d. *Thimerosal in Vaccines.* Accessed on March 23, 2007 from . . .

3. U.S. Food and Drug Administration. n.d.

4. Gernsbacher, M. A., Dawson, M., Goldsmith, H. H. 2005. "Three Reasons Not to Believe in an Autism Epidemic." *Current Directions in Psychological Science, 14,* 55–58.

5. Blaxill, M. 2001. "The Rising Incidence of Autism: Associations with Thimerosal." Accessed on March 23, 2007 from . . .

6. Stehr-Green P., Tull P., Stellfeld M., Mortenson P. B., Simpson D. 2003. Autism and Thimerosal-Containing Vaccines: Lack of Consistent Evidence for an Association. *American Journal of Preventive Medicine, 25,* 101–106.

7. Hvild A., Stellfeld M., Wohlfahrt J., Melbye M. 2003. "Association Between Thimerosal-Containing Vaccines and Autism." *Journal of the American Medical Association, 290,* 1763–1766.

8. Heron J., Golding J.; ALSPAC Study Team. "Thimerosal Exposure in Infants and Developmental Disorders: A Prospective Cohort Study in the United Kingdom Does Not Support a Causal Association." *Pediatrics, 114,* 577–583.

9. Geier, M. R., Geier, D. A., 2003. "Thimerosal in Childhood Vaccines, Neurodevelopment Disorders and Heart Disease in the United States." *Journal of American Physicians and Surgeons, 8,* 6–11.

10. Such a system cannot be used to prove a hypothesis. Consider that Dr. James Laidler allegedly reported that the influenza virus turned him into the Incredible Hulk, and the VAERS system accepted his report! Dr. Laidler reports that a representative of the CDC did contact him after noticing the report and, ultimately, it was deleted from the VAERS system, but only because Dr. Laidler granted permission. According to Laidler, had his permission not been granted, the report would have remained in the VAERS system. Others have reported submitting spurious reports to the VAERS system—for example that a vaccine turned someone into Wonder Woman—with similar success.

11. American Academy of Pediatrics. n.d. "Study Fails to Show a Connection Between Thimerosal and Autism." Accessed on March 23, 2007 from . . .

12. Institute of Medicine. Accessed on March 28, 2007 from . . .

13. Of course, this does not exclude the possibility that thimerosal might differentially affect an especially sensitive subset of children. Recently, researchers have reported that the neurotoxic effects of thimerosal exposure are related to autoimmune disease-sensitivity in mice. It is unclear whether these results will hold true for humans and whether such neurotoxicity has any relationship to autism, but it is an important area for further research. Unfortunately, because the "differential sensitivity" hypothesis is not yet well researched, there is no way to identify and protect those that might be at risk if it proves true. However, we know without question the dangers of disease and risks of avoiding vaccination. No matter the suspicions, the most prudent course of action is to go the vaccine route until there is real evidence to do otherwise. Also, we should note that existing evidence already casts doubt on the differential sensitivity hypothesis. If the

rates of sensitivity to thimerosal remained constant before and after thimerosal was removed from vaccines, we would still expect a decrease in rates of autism. As reviewed above, this was not the case.

14. Gernsbacher, M. A., Dawson, M., Goldsmith, H. H. 2005. "Three Reasons Not to Believe in an Autism Epidemic." *Current Directions in Psychological Science, 14,* 55–58.

15. Stehr-Green et al., 2003.

16. Park, R. 2000. *Voodoo Science: The Road from Foolishness to Fraud.* Oxford: University Press.

Matthew Normand is an assistant professor of psychology at the University of the Pacific.

Jesse Dallery is an associate professor in the behavior analysis program, Department of Psychology, the University of Florida, Gainesville.

EXPLORING THE ISSUE

Is There a Link Between Vaccination and Autism?

Critical Thinking and Reflection

1. Do parents have the right to withhold certain vaccinations from their children? On what grounds?
2. Is the government doing enough to make sure that vaccinations are safe? Explain your answer.
3. To what do you attribute the rise in diagnoses for autism? When can you say that autism started to "appear on the scene"?

Is There Common Ground?

Nine-year-old Hannah Poling had an uneventful birth and appeared to be developing normally. And then, right after receiving several routine vaccines, she became ill. Hannah recovered from her acute illness but lost her speech and eye contact and, in a matter of months, began displaying the repetitive behaviors and social withdrawal that indicate autism. Her parents reported that after her vaccinations, she just deteriorated and never came back.

Parents of children with autism have been blaming vaccines—and, especially, the mercury-based vaccine preservative thimerosal—as a cause of autism for over a decade, but researchers have repeatedly failed to identify a connection.

What is unusual about Hannah's case is that for the first time federal authorities agreed there was a connection between her autistic symptoms and the vaccines she received, though the relationship is by no means clear. A panel of medical evaluators at the Department of Health and Human Services determined that Hannah had been injured by vaccines and recommended that her family be compensated for the injuries. The panel said that Hannah had an underlying cellular disorder that was aggravated by the vaccines, causing brain damage with features of autism spectrum disorder.

The Poling case is also causing concern among public health officials, who are anxious to reassure parents that immunizations are safe and valuable. In a recent public statement, Dr. Julie Gerberding, director of the Centers for Disease Control and Prevention (CDC), insisted that "the government has made absolutely no statement about indicating that vaccines are the cause of autism, as this would be a complete mischaracterization of any of the science that we have at our disposal today." Dr. Gerberding and other health authorities point out that the benefits of vaccines far exceed their risks. They also note that thimerosal was eliminated from routinely administered childhood vaccines manufactured after 2001, and yet autism rates have not dropped. The current CDC estimate is that 1 of 150 American children has an autism spectrum disorder.

But there are circumstances that take Hannah's case out of the ordinary. For one thing, she received an unusually large number of vaccines in 2000 (when thimerosal was still in use). Because of a series of ear infections, Hannah had lagged behind in the vaccine schedule, so in one day she was given five immunizations to prevent a total of nine diseases: measles, mumps, rubella, polio, varicella, diphtheria, pertussis, tetanus, and *Haemophilus influenzae*. A second issue in Hannah's situation is that she suffers from a mitochondrial disorder, a dysfunction in basic cell metabolism. In Hannah's case, the vaccine court determined that the underlying dysfunction of her mitochondria put her at an increased risk of injury from vaccines.

Experts on autism spectrum disorders believe that most cases are caused by a combination of genetic vulnerabilities and environmental factors. There may be hundreds of routes to autism, involving multiple combinations of genes and external variables. While it is possible thimerosal or some other aspect of vaccines is one of these factors, it has not been definitively proven and further research is needed. It's challenging to draw any clear conclusions from the case of Hannah Poling, other than the need for more research. One plausible conclusion is that pediatricians should avoid giving small children a large number of vaccines at once, even if they are thimerosal-free.

Dr. Andrew Wakefield's research, which linked autism to vaccination, has generally been discredited. In "How the Case Against the MMR Vaccine Was Fixed" (*British Medical Journal*, August 1, 2011), the authors offer a look at the controversies raised by the paper written by Andrew Wakefield and colleagues linking autism with measles, mumps, rubella (MMR) vaccine. The authors address details of how the discrepancies and fraudulent data in the paper were discovered. "Study Linking Vaccine to Autism Is Called Fraud" (*New York Times*, June 1, 2011) reported on the fraudulent first study to link a vaccination to autism. The research was based on doctored information about the children involved, according to a new report on the widely discredited research. The conclusions of the 1998 paper by Dr. Andrew Wakefield and his colleagues were renounced by 10 of its 13 authors and later retracted by the medical journal *The Lancet*, where it was originally published. Still, the suggestion that the combined measles, mumps, and rubella vaccine was connected to autism scared parents worldwide and vaccination rates for the MMR shot plummeted. Despite overwhelming evidence to the contrary, approximately 20 percent of Americans still believe that vaccines cause autism, a disturbing fact that will probably continue to hold true even after the early 2011 publication of a *British Medical Journal* report thoroughly debunking the 1998 paper that began the vaccine–autism scare.

Create Central

www.mhhe.com/createcentral

Additional Resources

DeLong, G. (2011). A positive association found between autism prevalence and childhood vaccination uptake across the U.S. population. *Journal*

of Toxicology & Environmental Health: Part A, 74(14), 903–916.

Dietert, R. R., Dietert, J. M., & DeWitt, J. C. (2011). Environmental risk factors for autism. *Emerging Health Threats, 4,* 1–11.

Holton, A., Weberling, B., Clarke, C. E., & Smith, M. J. (2012). The blame frame: Media attribution of culpability about the MMR–autism vaccination scare. *Health Communication, 27*(7), 690–701.

Miller, L. & Reynolds, J. (2009). Autism and vaccination—the current evidence. *Journal for Specialists in Pediatric Nursing, 14*(3), 166–172.

Offit, P. A. (2008, May 15). Vaccines and autism revisited—The Hannah Poling case. *New England Journal of Medicine, 359*(6), 2089–2091.

Internet References . . .

Environmental Protection Agency

Use this site to find environmental health information provided by various EPA agencies.

www.epa.gov

Autism Society

The site provides information on treatment, diagnosis, causes, and symptoms of autism. It also has a national directory of autism services.

www.autism-society.org/

Centers for Disease Control: Vaccines & Immunizations

This site offers information on all types of vaccinations.

www.cdc.gov/vaccines/

National Institutes of Health/Autism

This site offers information on the following: causes–symptoms–tests–treatment–prognosis–complications.

www.ncbi.nlm.nih.gov

Selected, Edited, and with Issue Framing Material by:
Eileen Daniel, *SUNY College at Brockport*

ISSUE

Do Cell Phones Cause Cancer?

YES: Ronald B. Herberman, from "Tumors and Cell Phone Use: What the Science Says" (September 25, 2008) http://cellphones.procon.org/sourcefiles/Herberman_Testimony.pdf

NO: Bernard Leikind, from "Do Cell Phones Cause Cancer?" *Skeptic* (2010)

Learning Outcomes

After reading this issue, you should be able to:

- Discuss the possible mechanisms in which cell phones may trigger cancers.
- Assess other health risks associated with cell phone usage including traffic safety.
- Discuss why the long-term health implications of cell phones are unclear.
- Discuss why some countries, including France, have warned about the use of cell phones.

ISSUE SUMMARY

YES: Physician and director of the Pittsburgh Cancer Institute Ronald B. Herberman maintains that radio frequency radiation associated with cell phones is a potential health risk factor for users, especially children.

NO: Physicist Bernard Leikind argues that there is no plausible mechanism by which cell phone radiation can cause cancer.

A cell phone is a device used to make mobile telephone calls across a wide geographic area. It can make and receive telephone calls to and from the public telephone network, which includes other mobile and landline phones throughout the world. Cell phones work by connecting to a mobile network managed by a cellular phone company. In addition to operating as a telephone, mobile phones usually offer additional services including text messaging, e-mail, and Internet access along with a variety of business and gaming applications, and photography. They are extremely popular both in the United States and throughout the world. Currently, there are nearly 4.5 billion cell phones used globally.

Although cell phones have many communication advantages and are extensively used, they are also associated with health and safety risks. Cell phone use while driving is widespread, but controversial. Distractions like texting or talking on a cell phone while driving a car or other motor vehicle have been shown to increase the risk of accidents. Because of this, many areas prohibit the use of cell phones while driving and several states ban handheld cell phone use only, while allowing hands-free calling. Texting while driving is also illegal in some states.

In addition to the links between cell phone use and motor vehicle accidents, there may be a relationship between mobile phones and long-term health risks includ-

ing certain cancers. Some countries, including France, have warned against the use of cell phones, especially by minors, due to health risk uncertainties. Groups of scientists claim that because mobile phone use is employing relatively new technology, long-term conclusive evidence has been impossible to determine and that the use should be restricted, or monitored closely, to be on the safe side.

Cell phones use radiation in the microwave range, which some scientists believe may be harmful to human health. In epidemiological and animal and human research, the majority show no definite causal relationship between cell phone exposure and harmful biological effects in humans. Overall, most evidence shows no harm to humans is caused by cell phones, although a significant number of individual studies do suggest such a relationship, or are inconclusive. Based upon the majority view of scientific and medical communities, the World Health Organization (WHO) has asserted that cancer is unlikely to be caused by cellular phones or their base stations and that studies have found no convincing evidence for other health problems. Some national radiation scientists have recommended measures to minimize exposure only as a precautionary approach.

While most research investigations have found no relationship between cell phones and tumor growth, at least some recent studies have found an association between cell phone use and certain kinds of brain and salivary gland cancers. A major meta-analysis of 11 studies from peer-reviewed journals concluded that cell phone usage for at least 10 years may double the risk of being diagnosed with a brain tumor on the same side of the head that is most often used for cell phone conversations.

Clearly, there is no definitive answer on the potential safety issues associated with cell phone use. In the YES selection, Ronald B. Herberman, a physician and director of the Pittsburgh Cancer Institute, maintains that radio frequency radiation associated with cell phones is a potential health risk factor for users, especially children. In the NO selection, physicist Bernard Leikind argues that there is no plausible mechanism by which cell phone radiation can cause cancer.

YES ↵

Ronald B. Herberman

Tumors and Cell Phone Use:
What the Science Says

Thank you for inviting me to speak with you today about the important matter of cell phones and our health. I have served as the Founding Director of the University of Pittsburgh Cancer Institute (UPCI) since 1985, and as the Founding Director of University of Pittsburgh Medical Center (UPMC) Cancer Centers since 2001. The organizations that I lead employ more than 660 oncologists, other cancer experts and research faculty and more than 2,000 other staff members. In addition to the cutting edge cancer research performed at UPCI, our cancer centers, located throughout western Pennsylvania and adjacent states, annually treat more than 27,000 new cancer patients each year.

The UPCI is a National Cancer Institute (NCI)-designated comprehensive cancer center, and is one of the top ranked cancer research facilities in the nation. In fact, in 2007, UPCI was ranked 10th nationally in its level of NCI funding for cancer research. During the past two decades, UPCI has recruited some of the world's top scientists.

At UPCI, I am the Hillman Professor of Oncology, Professor of Medicine and Associate Vice Chancellor for Cancer Research at the University of Pittsburgh. I also was the founding Chairman of the Board of Directors, and I currently am the President, of the Pennsylvania Cancer Control Consortium, a state-wide cancer control organization. I am a longstanding member and Chairman of the Research and Clinical Trials Team, of C-Change, a national cancer organization, that has President George H.W. Bush, First Lady Barbara Bush, and Sen. Dianne Feinstein as the honorary co-chairs. For the past few years, C-Change has focused mainly on innovative strategies to reduce smoking and other personal risk factors for cancer, and to facilitate medical interventions to protect people at increased risk for cancer.

I also served from 1999–2001 as the President of the Association of American Cancer Institutes, an organization that includes almost all of the major academic cancer centers in the US. All of the organizations that I am associated with are focused on eliminating cancer as a public health problem, a commitment that I take very seriously.

As a cancer researcher, I have published more than 700 peer-reviewed articles in major biomedical journals, and for two decades my scientific publications placed me as among the 100 most cited biomedical scientists. In addition, I have served as an associate editor on more than 10 major, peer-reviewed journals, including Cancer Research, the Journal of the National Cancer Institute (JNCI), and the Journal of Immunology, and I have been a peer reviewer for over 1,000 manuscripts submitted for publication. For nearly two decades before I was recruited to Pittsburgh to found the UPCI, I led research teams at the NCI that focused mainly on characterizing the cellular basis for human anti-tumor immunity and utilizing the insights derived from those studies to develop innovative approaches to use immunotherapy to improve the treatment of cancer. The work of my research team at NCI resulted in the initial identification and then extensive characterization of natural killer (NK) cells. Research by my team at NCI and then at UPCI, along with other leading researchers around the world, have shown that NK cells are a key component of our natural defense against the development and metastatic spread of cancer.

In addition to world class studies in cancer immunology and immunotherapy at UPCI, other programs at our institute are developing prognostic indicators of response to treatment. UPCI also includes experts working on strategies for cancer prevention, early detection, and treatment and approaches for cancer control. Through our innovative Center for Environmental Oncology, we are carrying out studies to better define the role of environmental exposures on cancer risk, coupled with measures to reduce cancer risk by reducing exposure to environmental carcinogens, or using nutritional and other interventions to protect people who have been exposed to environmental hazards.

As part of our overall efforts, we are also working to identify important policy changes that should be developed to reduce the burden of cancer. After years of protracted delays, our nation has finally made progress against smoking by getting individuals to stop smoking. But, smoking control policies proved difficult to implement for many years, because of complex strategies to manipulate information on its dangers. Analogous efforts to identify and then effectively implement actions for other controllable causes of cancer have been fairly limited.

Now, to turn to the issues of direct interest to this committee, I first want to point out that, in contrast to several of the other speakers at this important hearing, who are longstanding experts on some aspects of radio-frequency (RF) radiation associated with cell phones or on the design and implementation of population-based

Herberman, Ronald B. From statement before the Domestic Policy Subcommittee of the Oversight and Government Reform Committee, U.S. House of Representatives, September 25, 2008.

studies, I have only recently become involved in the issue of the possible health risks of cell phones, by issuing a precautionary message to the faculty and staff of the UPCI and the UPMC Cancer Centers. For you to understand why a non-expert in the field took this action, I believe it is important to explain the process that led up to the issuance of the advisory to reduce direct cell phone exposures to the head and body.

Last year, as she was finalizing her well-researched book, The Secret History of the War on Cancer, my colleague, Dr. Devra Davis, Director of the UPCI's Center for Environmental Oncology and an internationally acclaimed expert in environmentally-induced health risks, shared with me the growing scientific literature on the possible association between extensive cell phone and increased risk of malignant and benign brain tumors. My attention was directed to a large body of evidence, including expert analyses showing absorption of RF into the brain and the comprehensive Bioinitiative Report, review of experimental and public health studies pointing to potential adverse biologic effects of RF signals, including brain tumors, associated with long-term and frequent use of cell phones held to the ear. I also learned of a recent series of similar precautionary advisories from international experts and various governments in Europe and Canada. I reacted to this information in the same fashion as I do with other reports of claims of biologically and/or clinically important findings, namely I first carefully reviewed the reports and consulted with a variety of relevant experts.

My evaluation of the scientific and technical information indicating the potential hazards of cell phones was built on the foundation of my extensive experience in cancer research and critical evaluations of reports being submitted for peer-reviewed publications. I recognized that there was sufficient evidence to justify the precautionary advisories that had been issued in other countries, to alert people about the possibility of harm from long-term, frequent cell phone use, especially by young children. Then, Dr. Davis and I consulted with international experts in the biology of radiofrequency (RF) effects and the epidemiology of brain tumors, and with experts in neurology, oncology and neurosurgery at UPCI. Without exception, all of the experts contacted confirmed my impression that there was a sound basis to make the case for precaution, especially since there are simple and practical measures that can be taken, to be able to continue to use cell phones while substantially reducing the potential hazards.

Another factor influencing my decision was my growing conviction that substantially more attention should be devoted to promoting a range of strategies to reduce the future burden of cancer. Of course, I appreciate the tremendous progress that the US has made in treating cancer, some of which was achieved by studies at the University of Pittsburgh, on melanoma, breast, brain, and colorectal cancer. I also recognize that approaches that aim to prevent new cases from occurring are the most likely ways to more effectively and efficiently reduce the overall burden

of cancer. Accordingly, I decided to act, consistent with my responsibilities as the leader of a major US cancer institute, by informing my colleagues about my concerns that cell phone use may be a substantial risk to public health. I also wanted to stimulate broader awareness and discussion of the evidence that I came to be familiar with, and to encourage changes in the behavior of some of my colleagues and by extension, also their families and friends.

Summary of Review of the Published Scientific Evidence for an Association Between Cell Phone Use and Brain Tumors

Obviously, scientific research plays a central role in identifying exposures that may affect our health. In public health research, scientists generally rely on two major types of evidence to evaluate potential risks. First, a combination of laboratory-based experimental studies using animals, cell cultures, and computer models can be used to examine mechanisms, identify biological effects and predict the potential impact for humans. Then, population-based human studies can also be used to determine if observed patterns of disease can be correlated with specific exposures, and other more detailed studies of people with a particular disease in comparison with healthy controls, so-called case-control studies, can be carried out to determine if there are different health patterns in those with and without certain exposures.

Although in some cases a clear association between an exposure and health effect can be demonstrated, often methodological differences among studies can introduce subtle differences in the way data are evaluated, and in some cases can lead to very different conclusions. This is especially true for human population-based cancer epidemiology studies where it is sometimes very difficult to select non-exposed controls, where the critical timing of exposure is not precisely known, where the mechanism by which an exposure might cause cancer is not well defined or understood, or where the characteristics of the exposure change over time. A critical review of the literature on the biological effects of cell phones exemplifies this point. Despite the lack of consistency in outcomes in all the cell phone publications, there are several well-designed studies that suggest that long-term (10 years or more) use of wireless phone devices is associated with a significant increase in risk for glioblastoma (glioma), a very aggressive and fatal brain tumor, and acoustic neuroma, a benign tumor of the auditory nerve that is responsible for our hearing.

For more than eight years, the World Health Organization has been conducting a combined effort to study cell phones and brain cancer in thirteen countries, called the Interphone study. No results synthesizing this overall effort have been published yet. But, several reports from countries participating in the Interphone study have appeared. Some analyses have found no increased risk of cell phones, while others, from countries where study participants used cell phones for a decade or longer, have found increased risks for brain tumors. But, even in these negative studies, when the subset of long-term users are examined separately, there is evidence of increased risk of brain tumors.

Clearly, not all of the published cell phone studies have reached the same conclusion. What are some of the characteristics of study design that can explain the differences among cell phone use studies generally and between the Interphone-related studies and the independent, non-Interphone-related studies?

To address this question, in 2008, Dr. Lennart Hardell, a distinguished oncologist and senior author on several cell phone studies in Sweden that have shown increases in brain tumor risk with long-term use, published a combined analysis (also called a meta-analysis) of published case-control studies that evaluated the effects of cell phone use on brain tumor risk. For gliomas, a malignant tumor of the supporting tissue of the brain, he and his colleagues found 10 studies; 7 were part of the Interphone Study, one was partly based on Interphone participation and partly independent, and 2 were not part of Interphone (one was a Swedish study from Hardell's team, and the second was a Finnish study). In contrast to the Interphone-related studies which found no increased risk for glioma, both of the independent studies found an increased risk of 40–50%. Since 8 of these 10 studies were Interphone-related, and these studies all showed no effect of cell phone use on glioma risk, the combined data result (meta-analysis) also showed no effect. It should be noted, however, that most of these studies included as cell phone users those who only made a single phone call a week and did so over a limited duration.

In contrast, focusing on those who had used cell phones for a decade provided a different story. Of these 10 studies, 6 evaluated long-term exposure effects, resulting from 10 or more years of cell phone use. Of these 6 studies, all showed an increase risk for developing a glioma on the same side of the head where the phone was used, and this increased risk ranged from a low of 20% increased risk for low grade (less aggressive) glioma to more than 400% increase risk of high grade (very aggressive) glioma. The meta-analysis for the combined data indicated that those who regularly used cell phones had twice the risk of malignant brain tumors overall, and four times the risk if they were high users of phones.

For acoustic neuroma, 9 case-control studies have been published that have compared the reported history of cell phone use of persons with and without this benign tumor on the hearing nerve. Eight of these studies are Interphone study-related and one, by Hardell's group, was independent. Whereas six of the 7 Interphone studies showed that no increased risk with regular cell phone use, Hardell found that regular cell phone users had a 70% greater risk. What struck me as especially relevant, and to possibly account for the divergent reports, is one simple fact: all three studies that looked at cell phone users for at least a decade, found a significantly increased risk. In long term users, acoustic neuromas are twice as frequent in regular, long-term users.

Within the last month, as also noted by Dr. David Carpenter in this hearing, Dr. Hardell reported at a meeting of the Royal Society of London that very frequent and long term users of cell phones by teenagers that started before age 20, resulted in a five times higher rate of brain cancer by the age of 29, when compared with non-cell phone users.

Brain cancer, which is one of the health effects of very serious concern, is believed to develop in adults over a period of at least one decade and in some cases, up to several decades. Among the known causes of brain cancer is ionizing radiation, such as x-rays. RF radiation is not ionizing, but it is absorbed into the brain, according to modeling studies that have been produced by the cell phone industry, in particular by French Telecom. There is no debate that radiation emitted by cell phones is absorbed into the brain—dramatically more so in children than in adults.

In summary, my review of the literature suggests that most studies claiming that there is no link between cell phones and brain tumors are outdated, had methodological concerns, and did not include sufficient numbers of long-term cell phone users to find an effect, since most of these negative studies primarily examined people with only a few years of phone use and did not inquire about cordless phone use. In addition, many studies defined regular cell phone use as "once a week."

One major negative study, published by the Danish Cancer Society and supported by the cell phone industry, started with nearly three quarters of a million cell phone users during the period between 1982 and 1995. This study excluded more than 200,000 business users, who were most likely to be the most frequent users during that time period. Recall bias was a problem with all of these studies as solid data such as cell phone records were not used to document usage and people were simply asked, often the day after surgery, whether or not they had used a cell phone and for how long.

Scientists appreciate that diseases like brain cancer can take decades to develop. This means that even well conducted studies of those who have used phones for only a few years, as most of us have, cannot tell us whether or not there are hazards from long-term use.

In contrast, some recent studies in Nordic countries, where phones have been used longest, find that persons who have used cell phones for at least a decade have 30% to more than 200% more brain tumors than do those without such use, and only on the side of the head where the user holds his or her phone. To put these numbers in context, this is at least as high an increase as the added risk of breast cancer that women face from long-term use of hormone replacement therapy. Based on these findings and the increased absorption into the brains of the young, the

French Ministry of Health advised that children should be discouraged from using cell phones, a position also taken by British, German and other authorities.

Precautionary Advisory Based on Review of the Published Reports and Consideration of the Precautionary Advisories from Several Countries in Europe and Elsewhere

While those issues are being debated and resolved, and as we eagerly await the results, my review of the available published evidence suggesting some increased brain tumor risk following long-term cell phone use, combined with the current near ubiquity of exposure to cell phones and cordless phone RF fields (more than 90% of the population in the Western European countries and about 90% of the population in the USA use cellular phones), led me to work with both international experts and experts at UPCI to develop a set of prudent and simple precautions that I felt could reduce potential risk, while awaiting more definitive evidence. Certainly, if it turns out that long-term use of cell phones does increase brain tumor risk, the public health implications of *not* taking action are obvious.

On July 21, 2008, I issued the advisory on the safe use of cell phones to the physicians, researchers and staff at UPCI and UPMC Cancer Centers. Before its issuance, this document was reviewed by UPCI experts in neuro-oncology, epidemiology, environmental oncology, and neurosurgery as well as national and international scientific and engineering experts. A copy can be found at the end of my testimony. My sole goal in issuing the cell phone advisory was to suggest simple precautions that would reduce exposure to cell phone electromagnetic radiation. The advisory clearly indicated that the human evidence on the potential hazard of cell phones is still evolving, but it pointed out that there are some studies using experimental and population-based approaches that suggest an association between long-term cell phone use and development of brain tumors. It also pointed out that modeling studies suggest the possibility that there may be additional differences in susceptibility between young children and adults. Based on my review of the data, I felt that there was sufficient evidence for possible human health risks, to warrant providing precautionary advice on cell phone use, especially by children.

What are the main points of the advisory? Adults can reduce direct exposure of the head and bone marrow to radiofrequency radiation by using ear pieces or the speaker phone mode whenever possible. Cell phone use by children should be restricted. Here we advised, as do a number of governments, that cell phone use by children be limited to emergency calls and for older children, text messaging. In circulating this warning, I joined with an international expert panel of pathologists, oncologists and public health specialists, who recently declared that RF radiation

emitted by cell phones should be considered a potential human health risk.[1] In fact, shortly before I sent my precautionary message to faculty and staff at UPCI and UPMC Cancer Centers, a number of countries including France, Germany and India, and the province of Ontario, Canada, issued similar advice, suggesting that exposure to RF radiation from cell phones be limited. Very soon after the UPCI advisory was issued, Israel's Health Ministry endorsed my recommendations, and Toronto's Department of Public Health advised that teenagers and young children limit their use of cell phones, to avoid potential health risks.

I appreciate the interest of this committee in exploring the current state of the scientific evidence on the potential hazards of cell phones. I have provided appendices that include links and references to reviews and advisories that have been issued within the past few years by other authorities. In addition, the web site for UPCI's Center for Environmental Oncology (www.preventingcancernow.org) includes the actual papers as pdf files for all major studies published over the past two years. In addition, the Bioinitatives Report (www.bioinitiativereport.org) provides comprehensive, critical review, that includes references to the more than 4,000 relevant studies that have been published to date on this subject.

Most people throughout the developed world are using cell phones. Cell phones save lives and have revolutionized our world in many positive ways. Without doubt, the most immediate danger from the use of cell phones is that of traffic crashes. But, the longer term spectre of harm cannot easily be dismissed at this point. The absence of definitive positive studies should not be confused with proof that there is no association. Rather, it reflects the difficulties of assembling definitive proof and the absence of well-conducted, large-scale independent studies on the problem.

Throughout my career I have witnessed the tremendously important discoveries that have improved cancer care. I also recognize that cancer professionals and physicians in general have failed to pay adequate attention to the need to identify and then promptly and effectively control avoidable causes of cancer. Nowhere is our failure more evident than in the protracted and prolonged debate that played out over the hazards of tobacco. By all accounts, we have also missed the boat with respect to our national policies on known workplace cancer causes such as exposure to asbestos, and we waited far too long before acting to reduce dangers associated with hormone replacement therapy.

It is worth noting that in the case of tobacco and lung cancer, debates over whether there was a true increase in lung cancer associated with smoking raged far longer than they should have, fomented by an active disinformation campaign of which this Congress is well aware. The dilemma of public policy when it comes to controlling and identifying the causes of cancer is profound. If we insist we must be certain of human harm and wait for definitive evidence of such damage, we are effectively saying that we can only act to prevent future cancers, once past ones have become evident. Recalling the 70 years that it took to remove lead from paint and gasoline and the 50 years that it took to convincingly establish the link between smoking and lung cancer, I argue that we must learn from our past to do a better job of interpreting evidence of potential risk. In failing to act quickly, we subject ourselves, our children and our grandchildren to the possibility of grave harm and to living with the knowledge that with more rapid action that harm could have been averted.

I do not envy policy makers and regulators as they do not always have adequate solid data on which to base standards. In the present case, the link between cell phones and health effects is suggestive but not solidly established. From my careful review of the evidence, I cannot tell you conclusively that phones cause cancer or other diseases. But, I can tell you that there are published peer reviewed studies that have led me to suspect that long term cell phone use may cause cancer. It should be noted in this regard that worldwide, there are three billion regular cell phone users, including a rapidly growing number of children. If we wait until the human evidence is irrefutable and then act, an extraordinarily large number of people will have been exposed to a technology that has never really been shown to be safe. In my opinion, for public health, when there is some evidence of harm and the exposed group is very large, it makes sense to urge caution. This is why I issued advice to our faculty and staff, especially to take precautions to reduce cell phone RF exposures to children.

Now that the issue of a possible association of long-term cell phone with increased brain tumor risk has reached national and international attention, the central question is where we go from here. Should we simply wait and watch? Or, should we take some actions now? I am not sufficiently expert to comment on possible new regulations to affect cell phone usage. Rather, from my perspective as a scientist and cancer center director, I want to do all that I can to see that the matter of cell phones and our health is resolved. I believe that we should undertake additional, more definitive research that will tell the whole story. Many of my colleagues at UPCI, Rutgers University, University of California, San Francisco and a number of senior faculty at M.D. Anderson Cancer Institute are joining with me in calling for an independent scientific investigation, avoiding as many of the limitations of the prior studies as possible, to determine if long-term, frequent use of cell phones and cordless phones increases brain tumor risk. We will urge that these studies engage both university and NIH experts and also the full cooperation of the cell phone industry, which will be asked to provide solid usage data in the form of access to billing records and substantial contribution to the funding of the study but without any direct review or control of the results, in order to clearly settle this issue in the not too distant future.

In the meantime, while we continue to conduct progressively better research on this question, I believe it makes sense to urge caution: it's better to be safe than sorry.

Note

1. *The Case for Precaution in the Use of Cell Phones Advice from University of Pittsburgh Cancer Institute Based on Advice from an International Expert Panel,* available at www.preventingcancernow.org

---

RONALD B. HERBERMAN is a physician and the director of the Pittsburgh Cancer Institute, Pittsburgh, Pennsylvania.

Bernard Leikind

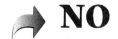 **NO**

Do Cell Phones Cause Cancer?

News reports threaten that our cell phones may cause cancer—brain cancer, eye cancer, and others. We are told that fragile children's developing brains are at risk. Concerned epidemiologists collect their data and warn that they cannot rule out the possibility of harm from cell phone radiation and that they must do more research. Medical professionals assert, as a precaution and in the absence of definitive data, that we should place our phones at arm's length. News accounts fill us with alarm. Danger lurks.

Fears that cell phones cause cancer are groundless. There is not a shred of evidence that the electromagnetic radiation from your cell phones causes harm, much less that from the wiring in the walls of your house, your hair dryer, electric blanket, or the power distribution wires nearby.

We know exactly what happens to energy from any of these sources when it meets the atoms and molecules in your body, and that energy cannot cause cancer. There is no known way that this energy can cause any cancer, nor is there any unknown way that this energy can cause any cancer.

There is a link between some forms of electromagnetic radiation and some cancers. These forms of electromagnetic radiation are ultraviolet radiation, X-rays, and gamma rays. They are dangerous because they may break covalent chemical bonds in your body. Breakage of certain covalent bonds in key molecules leads to an increased cancer risk. For example, there is a link between ultraviolet light from the sun and skin cancers.

All other forms of electromagnetic radiation other than these may add to molecules' or atoms' thermal agitation, but can do nothing else. Visible light has sufficient energy to affect chemical bonds. When light strikes the cones and rods in our retinas rhodopsin bends from its resting state to another, but it does not break. When visible light strikes the chlorophyll molecules in plants, electrons shift about but the chlorophyll does not break. Visible light does not cause cancer.

Electromagnetic radiation transfers its energy to atoms and molecules in chunks called *photons*. The energy of single photon is proportional to the photon's frequency. The photons of high frequency radiation, such as ultraviolet light, X-rays, and gamma rays, carry relatively large amounts of energy compared to those of lower frequency radiation. That is why high-energy photons can break covalent chemical bonds while the photon energy of all other forms of electromagnetic radiation, including visible light, infrared light, microwave, TV and radio waves, and AC power cannot.

Figure 1 shows a range of energy that is important for life and for the science of biochemistry. The figure displays an energy scale to help you place relevant energy states or processes in context. Horizontal positions indicate the energy range.

Look at the area covered by the long bracket in the middle. It shows the general energy range of the major strong chemical bonds—covalent bonds— which are significant for all of life's molecules. Below to the right you can see where the energy of an important organic covalent bond—that which occurs between two carbon atoms— falls on the scale. Further up the scale, on the upper right, is the energy range of carcinogenic electromagnetic radiation. Notice where the call out for green light falls on this scale. Visible light does not cause cancer.

Notice that the energy of cell phone radiation and AC power radiation in this scale is very low. Cell phone radiation cannot break, damage, or weaken any covalent bond.

Figure 2 shows the lowest energy part of Figure 1's energy scale. Figure 1 ranges from 0 kJ/mole to 600 kJ/mole. Figure 2 ranges from 0 kJ/mole to 30 kJ/mole.

Notice the bracket that shows the range of weak bonds in each figure. These are hydrogen bonds, van der Waals bonds, electrostatic bonds, and various other effects, such as hydrophobic or hydrophilic forces. In the complex molecules of life, these bonds play critical roles holding strands together and creating the three-dimensional shapes of molecules.

Covalent bonds hold together the single strands of DNA. Hydrogen bonds connect one strand to its mate. Enzymes fold and twist to create the forms they require as they perform their role as catalysts. The various weak bonds maintain the shapes of these folds and twists.

Drawn in both figures is a graph that suggests the energy of molecular thermal motions at body temperature. Everything in our bodies partakes in these thermal motions. The molecules jostle one another. They twist and vibrate. The thick gray line on the graph shows how energy distributes itself among these various motions. The motion's average energy is about 2.5 kJ/mole. Some molecules, but not many, have much more energy.

If energy transfers of 2.5 kJ/mole, more or less, were sufficient to damage life's molecules, life would

Figure 1

The units of this scale are familiar to chemists. Chemists like to think about test-tube-sized quantities of stuff. A mole is a unit that measures how much stuff you have. It is a count of objects: atoms, molecules, photons, chemical bonds. One mole of any object contains 6.023×10^{23} of those objects. Physicists prefer to state the energy in one bond or in one photon. A physicist would divide all the numbers in this figure by the number of objects in a mole to show the energy in Joules in a single object. An (old) physicist might prefer to express this energy in units of electron volts. Measured in electron volts, the energy in one green light photon is about 2.5 electron volts. The energy in one banana is 150 to 200 Calories, which corresponds to 600 or 800 kJ/banana; that is, one banana, not a mole of bananas.

Biochemistry's Energy World

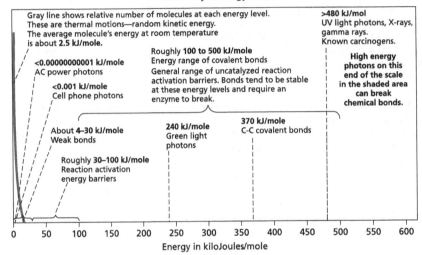

Figure 2

Biochemistry's Low Energy World

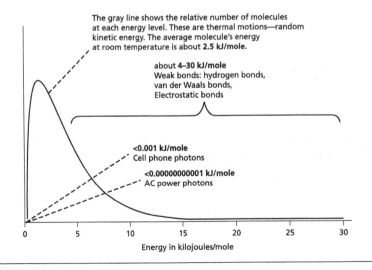

be impossible because random thermal motions would quickly break most of them. Fortunately, covalent bonds require ten to fifty times this amount of energy transfer before they break. Thermal jostling does not interfere with them. Weak biochemical bonds, however, live within the upper range of thermal bonds and shakes. That is why they do not enter into life's structure as single bonds, but always as groups. In the long double helices of DNA, the hydrogen bonds are like the individual teeth of a long zipper. Together they withstand what any single one of them could not.

These collisions are electromagnetic interactions. The molecules' outer electrons sense the presence of their neighbors though electromagnetic forces. These electrons resist oncoming neighbors, pushing them away, and pushing upon their own molecules as well. Electromagnetic forces transmit these pushes. All of the molecules of biology must be able to withstand these electromagnetic forces to maintain their shapes and their functions. The forces that electromagnetic fields from cell phones exert on life's molecules are no different from any of these molecular pushes, except that they are much, much smaller.

Cancer is a disease of the heredity of individual cells. Something must cause a cell to begin transferring mistakes to its progeny. One cell goes haywire, replicating wildly, transmitting the mistaken instructions—the damaged DNA—to each of its daughters. If the damage is too great, the cell will die. If the damage is not sufficient, it is not cancer. The damaged cell and its damaged progeny must continue to function in their crippled, uncontrolled states. Cancer generally requires more than one mutation in a single cell.

It is worth understanding how chemical changes occur, why life's molecules are stable in the cytoplasm, and how life controls its chemical reactions, turning them on or off. Consider Figure 3.

This famous diagram appears in all biochemistry books. It is a schematic representation of a reaction. Consider this reaction A + B → C + D, where A and B are reactants and C and D are products. In the diagram and the equation, the reaction begins on the left and moves to the right. The vertical scale is energy. Don't worry about the technical details. Begin with the upper solid black line with the label *Reaction Energy Barrier without an Enzyme*. For this reaction, the molecules A and B must assemble sufficient energy to carry them over the hill. This energy may come from the incessant thermal collisions, from some other molecule's internal energy, from an incoming photon of electromagnetic radiation, or other sources. The total energy of the entire system, including the surroundings, is a constant.

Through the continual random exchange of energy between the molecules A and B and their surroundings, if A and B happen to meet when they have sufficient energy to make it over the top of the hill, then they will react, forming C and D. These products appear on the diagram's right.

This diagram is illustrative. The actual diagram of even a simple reaction might have several dimensions in place of the single horizontal axis. The hills would be

Figure 3

The symbol E_a is the activation energy, the amount of energy the reactants must have to react. This energy is available to the products on the right. The reactants collect energy E_a from their surroundings. The products have returned it and a little extra ΔE to the surroundings. The surroundings, in this case, are warmer than before the reaction.

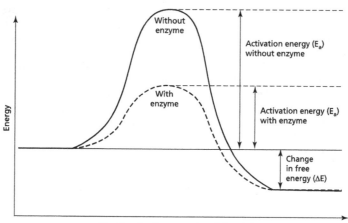

Reaction energy barrier with and without an enzyme

complicated surfaces with mountains and valleys. The diagram would have to take into account factors such as the orientation of the reactant molecules, and much else. It is the case, however, that all of life's stable molecules live in a well—a valley—similar to the left side of the diagram. They will require an injection of energy from their surroundings to escape. Biological molecules have many possible reactions in which they might take part. Remove an atom and replace it with another. Switch any molecular piece with another molecular piece. Natural selection has designed all of the molecules of life so that they are stable in chemical composition, form, and function. High activation energy barriers in all directions make all possible reactions rare. If this were not the case, then the molecules of life would not be stable.

When life requires a particular reaction to take place, there will be an enzyme to facilitate it. An enzyme is a biological catalyst. Consider the lower dashed line in Figure 3. This line has the label *Reaction Energy Barrier with an Enzyme*. This depicts the same reaction A + B → C + D, but this time there is an enzyme to facilitate the reaction. Without going into the remarkable details of enzymatic function, we can say that the enzyme has the effect of lowering the activation energy barrier for the reaction. With lower activation energy, the thermal jostling or other sources of reaction energy have a much easier time pushing the reactants over the hill. The reaction rate goes from nearly zero to some reasonable value.

There are no enzymes for unwanted reactions. Enzymes have and maintain the proper constitution and form to work correctly. For a mutation to occur or an enzyme to change, the energy for the chemical reaction must come from some place. An X-ray photon—from a cosmic ray, from the earth's radioactivity, or from an X-ray machine—may provide the required energy. Photons from any other form of electromagnetic radiation cannot.

Glance at Figure 1 again. All of those chemical bonds across the middle of the diagram are stable. They do not break and reform, unless there is an enzyme to do it. On the left of the diagram is the graph showing the energy available from ordinary thermal motions to break these bonds. Also on the left is a bracket showing the range of typical activation energies. Thermal motions are insufficient to take molecules over the activation energy barrier for any reaction. Far to the right, however, you can see the photons of ultraviolet light, X-rays, and gamma rays. These photons may break bonds. They may cause mutations directly. They may damage individual enzyme molecules. Even green visible light photons in the middle of this range do not have enough energy to break bonds and take molecules over any activation energy barrier.

Now find the photons of cell phone radiation and of AC power. They are at the far left of this diagram. No photon from a cell phone can ever break a chemical bond.

Making the radiation more intense does not make the photons stronger. It just means that there are more of them. The photons cannot gang up. Lots of them cannot do what one of them cannot.

When those weak photons disappear into a molecule, the molecule shifts and quivers a tiny bit. Its energy is a bit larger and the photon is gone. The molecule adjusts itself to its new slightly higher energy, and in subsequent collisions with its neighbors, it may transfer some of that energy to them. The temperature of the biological soup—the cytoplasm—is then a bit higher. The amount of heating due to cell phone radiation is small compared to your microwave, or standing in the sunshine, or wearing a scarf around your neck. This small increase in temperature does not cause cancer.

If cell phone photons or AC power photons, far to the left of Figure 1, were able to cause cancer by any mechanism, known or unknown, then those thermal vibrations also shown to the left side of the diagram would also cause cancer. So would all the forms of electromagnetic radiation that have more energetic photons than cell phone radiation.

Some of the concern over cell phone radiation may have originated from the normal statistical fluctuations that occur when studies are conducted. In recent years, epidemiologists have found significant environmental hazards, such as smoking and asbestos. They are now searching for hazards among much weaker effects. Some studies of a supposed hazard will show a small risk. Other studies of the same hazard will show no risk. In fact, some studies of the same potential hazard will show a benefit. This is the sign that there is no hazard, only statistical fluctuations. But only the studies that suggest risks, even small risks, will make news.

We can all be confident that any epidemiological study that purports to show that cell phone radiation causes any cancer must have at least one mistake. We can be certain because there is no plausible—or even implausible—mechanism by which cell phone radiation can cause any cancer.

When asked for a physicist's advice about cell phone safety, I explain that the radiation cannot cause cancer by any mechanism, known or unknown. If I am further pressed for comment I respond, "don't text while you drive, and don't eat your cell phone."

Acknowledgment: I thank physicists Dr. Arthur West and Dr. Craig Bohren, and biochemists Dr. Joseph H. Guth and Dr. Jill Ferguson, for their careful review of this paper and for their suggestions.

Bernard Leikind is a physicist and board member of *Skeptic* magazine.

EXPLORING THE ISSUE

Do Cell Phones Cause Cancer?

Critical Thinking and Reflection

1. Why do you think so many studies investigating health risks of cell phones are inconclusive and contradictory?
2. Describe some of the reasons researchers believe cell phone pose a risk.
3. What are health concerns related to cell phone use other than cancer?
4. Describe the type of radiation used by cell phones.

Is There Common Ground?

In May 2010, the largest cell phone cancer study, the Interphone Study, conducted by the World Health Organization, proved to be inconclusive (*International Journal of Epidemiology*, May 2010). Over 6,000 people with brain tumors and a similar number of healthy people were asked about their cell phone usage. The hypothesis was that cell phones increase the risk of brain tumors and there would be greater use in the cancer group compared with the healthy population. The study found the opposite to be true initially. However, when the researchers contacted healthy people who declined to take part in the initial investigation, they found that these individuals were less likely to regularly use cell phones than the healthy people who took part in the study. This indicates that the "benefit" that cell phones seemed to offer could be based on an over-representation of individuals who were healthy and regular mobile phone users. It might also mean that any negative effects might have been hidden. The researchers then compared frequent mobile phone users with infrequent ones and found that the level of use seemed to increase the risk of two different types of brain tumors by 40 and 15 percent, respectively.

While the results of the study are intriguing, it is certainly not conclusive. The study relied on peoples' memories regarding their cell phone use. It may be that people with brain tumors tend to have different memories of cell usage than those who are healthy. Several other studies are in progress, and the final verdict is not yet out. In "Jury Still Out on Cell Phone-Cancer Connection" (*Cancer*, January 5, 2010), author Michael Thun indicates that further research is needed. Since cell phones are a fairly recent phenomenon, it may be several years before any conclusive evidence surfaces relative to their safety.

Create Central

www.mhhe.com/createcentral

Additional Resources

Anderson, S. (2011). Are cell phones safe until the FCC tells us they are not? A preemption analysis in the context of cell phone radiation emissions standards. *Journal of Technology Law & Policy, 16*(2), 307–341.

Boice, J. D. & Tarone, R. E. (2011). Cell phones, cancer, and children. *JNCI: Journal of The National Cancer Institute, 103*(16), 1211–1213.

Feychting, M. (2011). Mobile phones, radiofrequency fields, and health effects in children—Epidemiological studies. *Progress in Biophysics & Molecular Biology, 107*(3), 343–348.

Gultekin, D. H. & Moeller, L. (2013). NMR imaging of cell phone radiation absorption in brain tissue. *Proceedings of the National Academy of Sciences of the United States of America, 110*(1), 58–63.

Holland, C. & Rathod, V. (2013). Influence of personal mobile phone ringing and usual intention to answer on driver error. *Accident Analysis & Prevention, 50*, 793–800.

Mortazavi, S. J., Mahbudi, A. A., Atefi, M. M., Bagheri, S. H., Bahaedini, N. N., & Besharati, A. A. (2011). An old issue and a new look: Electromagnetic hypersensitivity caused by radiations emitted by GSM mobile phones. *Technology & Health Care, 19*(6), 435–443.

Internet References . . .

American Cancer Society—Cell Phones and Cancer

Extensive references and information about a possible cell phone and cancer connection.

www.cancer.org/Cancer/CancerCauses/OtherCarcinogens/AtHome/cellular-phones

Environmental Protection Agency

This site includes educational resources, information about environmental concerns, FAQs, environmental laws, news releases, air quality by state, and links to additional resources.

www.epa.gov

Federal Communications Commission (FCC)

The Federal Communications Commission (FCC) site offers information on regulations, interstate and international communications by radio, television, wire, satellite, and cable.

www.fcc.gov/

Selected, Edited, and with Issue Framing Material by:
Eileen Daniel, *SUNY College at Brockport*

ISSUE

Will Hydraulic Fracturing (Fracking) Negatively Affect Human Health and the Environment?

YES: John Rumpler, from "Fracking: Pro and Con," *Tufts Now* (May 30, 2013) http://now.tufts.edu/articles/fracking-pro-and-con

NO: Bruce McKenzie Everett, from "Fracking: Pro and Con," *Tufts Now* (May 30, 2013) http://now.tufts.edu/articles/fracking-pro-and-con

---

Learning Outcomes

After reading this issue, you should be able to:

- Understand the environmental impact of fracking.
- Discuss the health concerns of fracking.
- Discuss the impact that fracking has on the economy and oil dependence.

ISSUE SUMMARY

YES: Environmentalist and senior attorney for Environment America, John Rumpler argues that fracking is not worth the damage to health and the environment.

NO: Energy researcher and Adjunct Professor Bruce McKenzie Everett claims fracking provides substantial economic benefits and its health and environmental problems are relatively small.

Hydraulic fracturing, or fracking, is a process that extracts natural gas from rock beneath the earth's surface. Many rocks such as shale, sandstones, and limestone deep in the ground contain natural gas, which was formed as dead organisms in the rock decomposed. This gas can be released and captured at the surface for energy use, when the rocks in which it is trapped are drilled. To enhance the flow of released gas, the rocks are broken apart, or fractured. In the past, drillers often detonated small explosions in the wells to increase flow. Starting about 70 years ago, oil and gas drilling companies began fracking rock by pumping pressurized water into it.

Since the 1940s, about 1 million American wells have been fracked. The majority of these are vertical wells that tap into porous sandstone or limestone. During the past 20 years, however, energy companies have had the ability to capture the gas still stuck in the original shale source. Fracking shale is achieved by drilling level wells that expand from their vertical well shafts along thin, horizontal shale layers. Drilling of this nature has allowed engineers to insert millions of gallons of high-pressure water directly into layers of shale to generate the fractures that release the gas. Chemicals added to the water dissolve minerals, destroy bacteria that might block the well, and add sand to hold open the fractures.

While the process offers inexpensive energy options, there are many opponents of the process. The majority of these opponents concentrate on possible local environmental outcomes. Some of these consequences are specific to the more recent fracking technology, while others are more relevant to the overall processes of natural gas extraction. The mixture of chemicals used in fracking processes includes acids, detergents, and toxins that are not controlled by federal laws but can cause problems if they leak into drinking water. Since the 1990s, the fracking process has employed increased amounts of chemical-laden water, injected at higher pressures. This causes the escape of methane gas into the environment out of gas wells, producing the real, though slight, chance of hazardous explosions. In general, water from all gas wells often returns to the surface containing very low but measurable concentrations of radioactive elements and large salt concentration. Salts or brine can be harmful if not treated properly. Small earthquakes have been triggered in rare instances after the introduction of brine into deep wells.

Along with these regional consequences, natural gas extraction has world-wide environmental impacts, because both the methane gas that is retrieved through extraction and the carbon dioxide liberated during methane burning are greenhouse gases that add to global climate change. Recent fracking technologies foster the extraction of higher quantities of gas, which adds more to climate change than former natural gas extraction processes.

In Pennsylvania, there has been rapid development of the Marcellus Shale, a geological formation that could contain nearly 500 trillion cubic feet of gas. This amount of natural gas is considered enough to power all U.S. residences for 50 years at current rates of usage. The experience in Pennsylvania with water and soil contamination, however, is of concern. Shale gas in Pennsylvania is accessed at depths of thousands of feet, while water for drinking is removed from depths of only hundreds of feet. Nowhere in the state have fracking chemicals injected at depth been shown to contaminate drinking water. In a research study of 200 private drinking water wells in Pennsylvania fracking regions, water quality was the same before and shortly after drilling in all wells except one. Unfortunately, however, trucking and storage accidents have spilled fracking chemicals and brines, leading to contamination of water and soils that required decontamination. Also, many gas companies do not consistently reveal the composition of all fracking and drilling compounds, which makes it challenging to check for injected chemicals in surface and groundwater.

Instances of methane leaking into aquifers in regions where shale-gas drilling is ongoing have also occurred in Pennsylvania. A portion of this gas is "drift gas" that forms naturally in deposits left behind by the most recent glaciers. But occasionally methane seeps out of gas wells because linings are not structurally sound, which occurs in about 1–2 percent of the wells. The linings can be repaired to address these slight leaks, and the risk of such methane leaks could further decrease if linings were designed specifically for each geological area.

The disposal of shale gas salt/brine was originally addressed in Pennsylvania by permitting the gas industry to use municipal water treatment plants that were not equipped to manage the toxic substances. In 2011 new regulations were enacted and Pennsylvania energy companies now recycle 90 percent of the salty water by using it to frack more shale.

Overall, the experience of fracking in Pennsylvania has led to industry changes that alleviate the impact of drilling and fracking on the local environment. Though the natural gas produced by fracking does increase greenhouse gases in the atmosphere through leakage during gas extraction and carbon dioxide emitted during burning, it does hold an important environmental benefit over coal mining. Gases released from shale contain 50 percent of the carbon dioxide per unit of energy as does coal, and coal burning also releases metals such as mercury into the atmosphere that ultimately settle back into water and soil.

In Europe, there is currently an increase in reliance on coal while discouraging or restricting fracking. If Americans are going to get our energy needs mostly from fossil fuels, banning fracking while mining and burning coal appears to be a negative environmental trade-off. The question is: Should Europe and the United States support fracking or prohibit it? Many regional effects of fracking and drilling have received a lot of press but actually generated a small amount of problems, while others are more serious. Economic interests in the short term favor fracking. The Pennsylvania experience caused natural gas prices to fall and jobs were created both directly in the gas industry and indirectly as local and national economies benefit from reduced energy costs. If, however, fracked gas shifts efforts to develop cleaner energy sources without decreasing reliance on coal, the consequences of accelerated global climate change will occur.

Overall, there are both advantages and disadvantages to hydraulic fracturing. The environmental impact could be lessened as well as the risk to human health via water contamination and the increase in greenhouse gases by utilizing lessons learned from Pennsylvania. In the YES and NO selections, John Rumpler argues that we are making a mistake in thinking that fracking is worth the damage to the environment. Bruce McKenzie Everett disagrees and claims that fracking offers substantial economic benefits and its problems are relatively minor compared to the advantages.

YES ↵

John Rumpler

Fracking: Pro and Con

For some Americans, it is our energy dreams come true. To others, it is an environmental nightmare. Ever since a new drilling technology, called hydraulic fracturing or fracking, made it possible to extract natural gas from shale deposits about a mile underground, a new gold rush has been under way.

While fracking has created jobs and contributed to record-low natural gas prices, it comes with another kind of potential cost: risks to our environment and health that some say are far too high.

The fracking process begins with a bore hole drilled some 6,000 feet below ground, cutting through many geological layers and aquifers, which tend to be no more than a few hundred feet below the surface. The shaft is then lined with steel and cement casing. Monitors above ground signal when drilling should shift horizontally, boring sideways to pierce long running sections of shale bedrock.

Millions of gallons of water mixed with sand and chemicals are then blasted into the bedrock, the pressure creating cracks that release trapped natural gas from the shale. The gas and water mixture then flows back up to the surface, where the gas is separated from the water. While most of the water stays in the well bore, up to 20 percent is either reused for more fracking or injected into disposal wells thousands of feet underground.

The wellpad and related infrastructure take up to eight to nine acres of land, according to the Nature Conservancy. Fracking is currently occurring in Texas and Pennsylvania, the two largest gas-producing states, as well as in North Dakota, Arkansas, California, Colorado and New Mexico. And the oil and gas industry is eager to expand its fracking operations into New York, North Carolina, Maryland and Illinois. . . .

John Rumpler . . . argues that we are making a mistake in thinking that fracking is worth the damage to the environment. He is a senior attorney at Environment America, which is leading a national effort to restrict, regulate and ultimately end the practice of fracking. He has fought for clean air in Ohio and advocated to protect the Great Lakes and the Chesapeake Bay. This fall he is teaching the Experimental College course Fracked Out: Understanding the New Gas Rush.

Tufts Now: Is Fracking Safe?

. . .

John Rumpler: Fracking presents a staggering array of threats to our environment and our health. These range from contaminating drinking water and making families living near well sites sick to turning pristine landscapes into industrial wastelands. There are air pollution problems and earthquakes from the deep-well injections of the wastewater into the gas-producing shale, as well as significant global warming emissions.

When the industry says there has not been a single case of groundwater contamination, they mean there is not a verified instance of the fracking fluid traveling up through a mile of bedrock into the water table. What they cannot dispute is that fluid and chemicals have leached into groundwater at 421 fracking waste pits in New Mexico. What they cannot dispute is that a peer-reviewed study by Duke University linked methane in people's drinking water wells to gas-drilling operations in surrounding areas. What they cannot dispute is a University of Colorado study published earlier this year documenting that people living within a half mile of fracking and other gas-drilling operations have an increased risk of health problems, including cancer from benzene emissions.

Are There Sufficient Regulations Now in Place to Ensure Safety?

Rumpler: Is it conceivable to imagine regulatory fixes for all the various problems caused by fracking? Theoretically, perhaps. But imagine trying to implement the hundreds of different rules and regulations at thousands of oil- and gas-drilling sites across the country, and you realize there is no practical likelihood that fracking will ever be made safe.

And there are consequences that we don't even know how to regulate yet. Geologists are just beginning to think about the long-term implications of drilling down a mile and then drilling horizontally through shale rock for another mile. We don't know what happens to the structural integrity of that bedrock once you withdraw all of the gas and liquid from it. No one has the definitive answer. There's been some recent modeling that indicates a loss of stability that goes all the way up to the water table. The U.S. Geological Survey took a look at some earthquakes that occurred in the vicinity of Youngstown, Ohio, in proximity to deep-well fracking. They found that the seismic activity was most certainly manmade—and there was no manmade activity in the area except fracking.

So when you look at the whole picture—from contaminated wells to health problems to earthquakes—[you quickly come] to see that the best defense against fracking is no fracking at all.

As for the current state of regulations, it is worth noting that fracking is exempt from key provisions of our nation's environmental laws, including the Safe Drinking Water Act, the Clean Air Act, the Clean Water Act, and the Resource Conservation Recovery Act. The reason we have national environmental laws is to prevent states from "racing to the bottom of the barrel" to appease powerful industries. . . .

What Are the Economic Benefits of Fracking?

. . .

Rumpler: First of all, any discussion of economics needs to deal with costs as well as benefits. This fall, our *Costs of Fracking* report detailed the dollars drained by dirty drilling—from property damage to health-care costs to roads ruined by heavy machinery. In Pennsylvania's last extractive boom, the state was stuck with a $5 billion bill to clean up pollution from abandoned mines. What happens when the fracking boom is long gone and communities are stuck with the bill?

In contrast, energy efficiency, wind and solar all provide great economic benefits with no hidden costs. But the oversupply of cheap gas is driving wind and solar out of the market. It's long been fashionable to say that natural gas can be a bridge to clean energy, but in fact it's become a wall to clean energy, because investors don't want to put money into wind and solar when gas is so cheap.

What Danger to the Environment or the Economy Is Caused by the Billions of Gallons of Fresh Water Each Year That Are "Consumed" by Fracking Operations? How Might This Affect the Economic Benefits or Environmental Concerns?

. . .

Rumpler: Each fracking well uses millions of gallons of water. And that water mostly winds up either staying down in the well or being injected deep into the earth as wastewater. So unlike other sectors that use much more water by volume, including agriculture and residential,

the water used for fracking is mostly consumed, gone to us for ever.

Does the Current Low Price of Natural Gas Affect Fracking or Conventional Gas Production?

Rumpler: Take a look at Chesapeake Energy, which is one of the biggest fracking operators out there. By the accounts of some analysts, they are massively overextended, with too much land and too many drilling leases. With the price at $2 per million BTU, there was some risk that Chesapeake could at some point lose enough money to risk bankruptcy—and then what would happen to these communities where fracking has taken place? If not Chesapeake, it will be another driller—probably one of the smaller ones—that goes under, and the communities will be left holding the bag. And gas companies don't tell landowners leasing property that oil and gas operations are violations of most standard mortgage agreements, because that is not a risk that the lender is willing to take. Likewise, homeowners' insurance may not cover damages from fracking. Nationwide insurance announced just this summer that their standard policy does not cover damage from fracking. That tells you something. The risk analysts who did the math figured out this is not a safety winner for them. . . .

What If We Halted All Fracking Right Now?

. . .

Rumpler: There's a difference between not starting fracking in new areas and halting it everywhere immediately. If we don't open new places to fracking in New York, Pennsylvania and Texas—just stop where we are now—the impact would be minimal. As Bruce notes, there is so much gas being produced right now that some gas companies are aggressively seeking export licenses, because they want to get rid of the excess and earn a profit. We don't need it to fill energy needs.

In North Dakota they are flaring off the gas, just wasting it into the air. If we need this gas to meet our energy needs, then they should make gas flaring a federal crime and should immediately ban any and all exports of natural gas. The industry would fight tooth and nail against this.

Until we know more, the risks to our health and environment far outweigh any possible benefit to our economy or energy future.

John Rumpler is an environmentalist and attorney.

Bruce McKenzie Everett

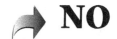

NO

Fracking: Pro and Con

For some Americans, it is our energy dreams come true. To others, it is an environmental nightmare. Ever since a new drilling technology, called hydraulic fracturing or fracking, made it possible to extract natural gas from shale deposits about a mile underground, a new gold rush has been under way. . . .

The fracking process begins with a bore hole drilled some 6,000 feet below ground, cutting through many geological layers and aquifers, which tend to be no more than a few hundred feet below the surface. The shaft is then lined with steel and cement casing. Monitors above ground signal when drilling should shift horizontally, boring sideways to pierce long running sections of shale bedrock.

Millions of gallons of water mixed with sand and chemicals are then blasted into the bedrock, the pressure creating cracks that release trapped natural gas from the shale. The gas and water mixture then flows back up to the surface, where the gas is separated from the water. While most of the water stays in the well bore, up to 20 percent is either reused for more fracking or injected into disposal wells thousands of feet underground. . . .

Bruce McKenzie Everett, F70, F72, F80, an adjunct associate professor of international business at the Fletcher School, says fracking provides substantial economic benefits and its problems are relatively small compared to those benefits. He worked at the U.S. Department of Energy from 1974 to 1980 before beginning a 20-year career with ExxonMobil, working in Hong Kong, the Middle East, Africa and Latin America. His research has included gas-to-liquid conversion technology as well as the economics of oil, gas and coal production and use. . . .

Tufts Now: Is Fracking Safe?

Bruce McKenzie Everett: Nothing in the world is entirely safe, but by the standards of industrial activity in the United States, fracking is very, very safe. Think about the airline industry. Lots of things can go wrong with airplanes, but we work very hard to make sure they don't, and as a result, flying is one of the safest activities we've got. Now, that does not mean that things can't happen. It just means that with proper attention, mistakes can be kept to an extremely low level.

The question about fracking that gets the most attention is contamination of drinking water. Aquifers, the underground rivers that provide our drinking water, are about 100 to 200 feet below the surface. The gas-producing shale rock formations tend to be 5,000 to 6,000 feet below the surface. So you need to make sure that the well you drill to pump the water and chemicals through the shale to fracture it and release the gas is sealed properly, and that's not a hard thing to do. . . .

Are There Sufficient Regulations Now in Place to Ensure Safety?

. . .

Everett: There are a lot of regulations currently in place. The question is whether they should be done at the federal or state level. For example, the state government of Pennsylvania understood that the economic activity from fracking could be very, very positive for the state. So they worked with the fracking industry and enacted numerous regulations to try to make sure that two things happened: that they eliminated the dangers to the extent that you can, but that they allowed fracking sites to go forward because the jobs and tax revenue were so positive.

In New York State, they've put a moratorium on fracking, basically saying, "I don't know what to do, so I'll study it and see what happens." I think that's unfortunate, because most of New York is quite economically depressed, and they are denying people economic opportunities.

I have taken a very strong position that it's a bad idea to federalize regulations. If you leave it at the state level, local governments will tend to strike a balance between the economic benefits and the environmental safety issues. If it is left to the federal government, you'll have the same problem you had with the Keystone oil pipeline: people who are not impacted, who will not enjoy the economic benefits, will be allowed to come in and say they don't like it.

What Are the Economic Benefits of Fracking?

Everett: It creates jobs, but that's not the most important way to measure its economic effect. The cost of everything we purchase has an energy component to it, either in its manufacture or its shipping or its packaging. So it is very important to the economy to have energy prices that are relatively low.

Natural gas has become incredibly inexpensive, way beyond what we ever thought possible. We're talking about prices going from $10 or $11 per thousand cubic feet 10 years ago down to $3.77 now, because the supply that has been released by this innovative fracking production technique is just so large. It is a simple consequence of supply and demand. These natural gas prices are the equivalent of oil prices falling to $21 per barrel from their current $86 per-barrel price. . . .

What Danger to the Environment or the Economy Is Caused by the Billions of Gallons of Fresh Water Each Year That Are "Consumed" By Fracking Operations? How Might This Affect the Economic Benefits or Environmental Concerns?

Everett: The water from fracking can be handled in one of several ways: storing, reinjecting and recycling. The real problem we have is that water is not properly priced. As a landowner, you are entitled to draw water from underground aquifers at whatever rate you wish, even if that water is only flowing through your land. We therefore tend to treat water as a free good. Putting a price on it or, alternatively, finding a way to assign property rights would probably fix this problem. As a third alternative, government could regulate it. In any case, it's a solvable problem. . . .

Does the Current Low Price of Natural Gas Affect Fracking or Conventional Gas Production?

. . .

Everett: The price of natural gas has now gotten so low that some are saying they can't produce it economically—but this is a *good* thing for all of us, because it will force them to explore new markets and uses. The United States has an open economy and is a large global trading player.

Americans pay the global price for the many things we buy and sell, and energy is one. There are several directions that natural gas production, both fracking and conventional, can take.

One is that people just stop producing it at the current rates, and the price returns to a more stable level and just stays there, likely at the $10-to-$12-dollar level of a decade ago. We could also start exporting. The world price for natural gas is $15 to $16 per thousand cubic feet. By selling it on the global market, that money would come into the U.S. economy. It would require some expensive infrastructure to support it, but the profit margin is so huge, some $12 per thousand cubic feet, that it would be well worth it and a positive impact on our economy.

We could also begin to shut down older coal-fired power plants and replace them with cleaner natural gas plants, and natural gas could find its way into the transportation sector. With engine modifications, it could be used as fuel for cars, or it could be used to produce the battery power for electric cars.

What If We Halted All Fracking Right Now?

Everett: If we stopped right now, or placed a moratorium on new fracking, the price of natural gas would go up to the previous $10 to $11, or worse case, to the global price of $15 to $16. This means electricity prices would go up, heating prices would go up, and we'd lose the economic activity the industry is generating through jobs and lower prices. Basically we would be giving up an opportunity.

Hazards can be controlled through solid regulations that include monitoring and quick responses to problems that arise. Any risks are outweighed by economic benefits. It's not even a close call. . . .

Bruce McKenzie Everett is an energy researcher and adjunct professor.

EXPLORING THE ISSUE

Will Hydraulic Fracturing (Fracking) Negatively Affect Human Health and the Environment?

Critical Thinking and Reflection

1. What are the major economic advantages to fracking?
2. What impact will fracking have on the quality of drinking water?
3. What effect will increased fracking have on the incentive to develop other cleaner energy sources including renewable?
4. Describe the health implications of fracking.

Is There Common Ground?

In the spring of 2008, filmmaker Josh Fox received an offer from a natural gas company to lease his family's land in Milanville, Pennsylvania, for $100,000 to drill for gas. Fox then set out to see how communities are being affected in the West where a natural gas drilling boom has been underway for the last 10 years. He spent time with people in their homes and on their land as they relayed their stories of natural gas drilling in Colorado, Wyoming, Utah, and Texas. Fox spoke with residents who experienced a variety of chronic health problems they claim were directly traceable to contamination of their air, of their water wells, or of surface water. In some cases, the residents report that they obtained a court injunction or settlement monies from gas companies to replace the affected water supplies with drinkable water.

The result of Fox's research was the documentary film *Gasland*. During the making of the film, Fox connected with scientists, politicians, and gas industry executives and ultimately found himself in Washington as a subcommittee was discussing the Fracturing Responsibility and Awareness of Chemicals Act, a proposed exemption for hydraulic fracturing from the Safe Drinking Water Act. While the film has both supporters and critics, it did bring publicity to the issues surrounding fracking and raised the question: Is the process safe for the environment and human health and do the economic benefits outweigh any actual or potential problems?

As the United States and Europe seek ways to reduce energy costs and reliance on imported fuels, fracking may be an opportunity to achieve these goals. It's a domestic resource that can be extracted around the country and offers jobs and cheaper energy. On the other hand, there are concerns that the fracking processes needed to extract gas may contaminate ground and surface water with toxic chemicals that could impact health and the environment.

Create Central

www.mhhe.com/createcentral

Additional Resources

Arnowitt, M. (2012). Pennsylvania's fracking land grab: Threats and opportunities. *Journal of Appalachian Studies, 18*(1/2), 44–47.

Grealy, N. (2013). Fracking is one of the best things to happen to onshore gas exploration for a century. *Engineering & Technology (17509637), 8*(1), 24.

Ratcliffe, I. (2013). Fracking is dangerous to environment and throws good energy after bad. *Engineering & Technology (17509637), 8*(1), 25.

Weinhold, B. (2012). The future of fracking. *Environmental Health Perspectives, 120*(7), A272–A279.

Wilber, T. (2012). *Under the surface: Fracking, fortunes and the fate of the Marcellus Shale*. Ithaca, NY: Cornell University Press.

Internet References . . .

Environmental Protection Agency

This site includes educational resources, information about global warming and other environmental concerns, FAQs, environmental laws, news releases, air quality by state, and links to additional resources.

www.epa.gov

Natural Gas.org

Naturalgas.org is presented as an educational website covering a variety of topics related to the natural gas industry.

www.naturalgas.org/

Hydraulic Fracturing—AmericanRivers.org

Learn how natural gas drilling is affecting your rivers and clean water and how fracking threatens clean water—FAQs on fracking.

www.americanrivers.org/fracking

Selected, Edited, and with Issue Framing Material by:
Eileen Daniel, *SUNY College at Brockport*

ISSUE

Is Breastfeeding the Best Way to Feed Babies?

YES: Jodi R. Godfrey and Ruth A. Lawrence, from "Toward Optimal Health: The Maternal Benefits of Breastfeeding," *Journal of Women's Health* (September 11, 2010)

NO: Hanna Rosin, from "The Case Against Breast-Feeding," *The Atlantic* (April 2009)

Learning Outcomes

After reading this issue, you should be able to:

- Discuss the physical benefits of breastfeeding for infants.
- Understand the maternal advantages to breastfeeding.
- Discuss why many women opt for bottle feeding.

ISSUE SUMMARY

YES: Dietitian and wellness specialist Jodi R. Godfrey and physician Ruth A. Lawrence maintain that breastfeeding is the gold standard for infant feeding and that there are significant benefits to both mother and infant.

NO: *Atlantic* magazine editor Hanna Rosin claims the data on the benefits of breastfeeding are inconclusive and suggests a more relaxed approach to the issue.

Breastfeeding is a means of providing nourishment to a baby or young child with milk directly from human breasts rather than from a bottle filled with baby formula or artificial milk. Babies have a sucking reflex that allows them to suck and swallow milk.

Most doctors, scientists, and child advocacy groups believe that human milk is the most healthful form of milk for human infants. Breastfeeding promotes health, helps to prevent disease, and reduces health care and feeding costs. In both poor and wealthy nations, bottle feeding is linked to more deaths from gastroenteritis in infants. Most doctors and scientists concur that breastfeeding is advantageous, but may disagree about the length of breastfeeding that is most valuable, and about the safety of using infant formulas.

The World Health Organization (WHO) and the American Academy of Pediatrics (AAP) suggest exclusive breastfeeding for the first 6 months of life and then breastfeeding up to 2 years or more (WHO) or at least one year of breastfeeding in total (AAP). There are many benefits to both mother and infant when the child is fed human milk. These benefits include the optimal levels of lipids, carbohydrates, water, and protein that are needed for a baby's growth and development. Breast milk also contains several anti-infective factors to help prevent disease. While there are obvious physical benefits, two initial studies also suggest some babies average seven IQ points higher if breastfed compared with babies fed cow or soy milk. Breastfeeding also appears to protect against type 1 diabetes, obesity, allergies, and celiac disease and reduced the risk of acquiring urinary tract infections in infants up to 7 months. Breastfeeding appears to decrease symptoms of upper respiratory tract infections in premature infants up to 7 months after release from the hospital. A longer period of breastfeeding is associated with a shorter duration of some middle ear infections in the first 2 years of life.

While infants appear to benefit from breastfeeding, it also positively impacts the health of nursing mothers. A recent study indicates lactation of at least 24 months is correlated with a reduced risk of heart disease, endometrial, breast, and ovarian cancer, and osteoporosis. Women who breastfeed for longer also have less chance of developing rheumatoid arthritis.

Other reasons to breastfeed include: The hormones released during breastfeeding strengthen the bond between mother and infant. Also, the fat stores which build up during pregnancy are used to produce milk, and extended breastfeeding for at least 6 months can help mothers lose weight. However, weight loss is unpredictable among nursing mothers, and diet and exercise are more dependable means of weight loss.

A lactating woman may not ovulate or have regular periods during the entire period she is nursing. The period in which ovulation is absent differs for each woman though it can be used as an imperfect form of natural contraception, with a greater than 98 percent effectiveness during the first 6 months after birth if the mother is regularly breastfeeding. It is likely, however, for some new mothers to ovulate within 2 months after birth while fully breastfeeding.

Though breastfeeding is a natural way of infant feeding, difficulties may occur. There are some situations in which breastfeeding may be harmful to the infant, including infection with the virus which causes AIDS and acute poisoning by environmental contaminants such as DDT or lead. Rarely, a mother may be unable to produce milk because of a deficiency of the hormone prolactin. In developed nations, many mothers do not breastfeed their children due to work pressures. They may need to return to work shortly after giving birth or are not able to regularly feed their babies while on the job. Other factors found to have an effect on breastfeeding are urban/nonurban residence, race, parental education, household income, neighborhood safety, familial support, maternal physical activity, and household smoking status.

While there are obvious, significant benefits to breastfeeding, many bottle-fed children grow up perfectly healthy. In the YES and NO selections, *Atlantic* editor Hanna Rosin discusses inconsistent research data on the benefits of breastfeeding. Rosin, a nursing mother, sees benefits of breastfeeding as far from conclusive, and suggests a more relaxed approach to the issue. Jodi R. Godfrey and Ruth A. Lawrence argue that there are many maternal benefits to breastfeeding and that it is the optimal way to feed babies.

YES ↙

Jodi R. Godfrey and Ruth A. Lawrence

Toward Optimal Health: The Maternal Benefits of Breastfeeding

In 2010, we can agree that breast milk is the gold standard for infant nutrition during the first 6 months of life, yet the infant formula industry has contributed to low rates of breastfeeding through a comprehensive promotional campaign that has trumped attempts to publicize the advantages of exclusive breastfeeding.[1] The result is that 71% of women in the United States initiate breastfeeding, but only 35% manage to prevail for at least 6 months.[2] In rural communities, the practice drops to 55% of women initiating breastfeeding and only 18% making it to 6 months. These data fall short of the *Healthy People 2010* goal of 50%.[3] Among urban women, breastfeeding initiation and continuation may be influenced by multiple factors, including participation in the federal Women Infants and Child (WIC) subsidy program (www.fns.usda.gov/wic/Breastfeeding/breastfeedingmainpage.HTM), support from the health system, maternal depression, and return to work or school.[4]

Women who had been working 2 months and receiving support from WIC were associated with decreased breastfeeding initiation and continuation.[4] Too few non-Caucasian women consider breastfeeding as critical or valuable, or they discontinue initial breastfeeding efforts because of discomfort, embarrassment, lack of assistance, concerns about infant weight loss or inadequate milk supply, little emotional support, and fear of concurrent breastfeeding and smoking.[4] For example, these suggest opportunities for clinicians to encourage breastfeeding more widely. There is a critical need to enhance workplace support, refocus the role of WIC, increase hospital assistance, and create a social environment in which breastfeeding is accepted as the norm.

Despite the substantial known positive outcomes of breastfeeding for both mother and child, this basic physiological opportunity continues to elude too many women. Although up to 75% of women initiate breastfeeding at childbirth, according to the Centers for Disease Control and Prevention (CDC) National Immunization Survey, the vast majority (80%) of women cease nursing before the recommended minimum of 1 year.[2,5] Furthermore, racial, ethnic, and socioeconomic disparities in breastfeeding persist at rates about 50% lower among women from ethnic groups regardless of age, income, or educational level.[4]

With the publication of the 7th edition of *Breastfeeding: A Guide for the Medical Profession*,[6] the 1st edition having been published nearly 30 years ago, the evidence basis for promoting lactation for the specific and significant long-term health benefits of the mother deserves reconsideration. Ruth A. Lawrence, M.D., focuses on the health benefits to be gained by women who commit to breastfeeding for up to 1 year, with the goal of enlisting clinicians to take a more active role in improving the rates in the coming decade.

With the publication of the 7th edition of *Breastfeeding: A Guide for the Medical Profession*, is the evidence of clinical benefits sufficient to prompt clinicians to become more actively engaged in promoting breastfeeding for almost every woman?

First, it is necessary to set the stage by acknowledging that breastfeeding is an amazingly complex and incredibly adaptive system. Breastfeeding represents an intricate process of interaction between mother and infant that is far more than nutrition. It is concerned with creating a new person, establishing an effective immune system, building brain function, developing socialization, and promoting long-term health. It is worth noting that when lactating women are exposed to a virus, the antibodies are passed to the infant through the breast milk, providing instantaneous immunity not possible with a formula.[5] Furthermore, breast milk does not reflect the mother's precise diet; rather, it is naturally reformulated to meet the growing needs of the infant, including changes in the proportion of macronutrients (e.g., proteins, carbohydrates, and fats).[4] In other words, breastfeeding is a continuously evolving system between mother and child. Another way of looking at this is that the infant develops for 9 months in the womb and then another 9–12 months out of the womb, with an intrinsic dependence on the mother for optimal sustenance. No study has identified an end point for the ideal longevity of breastfeeding, but the benefits appear to accrue for the entire duration. These findings are even more pronounced in countries and among populations with malnutrition and poor hygiene.[7,8] Although more difficult to discern in this country, the benefits remain significant for both mother and infant.[4,5,7–14]

The maternal benefits of breastfeeding are not as well studied or documented as are the advantages to the child, as long-term follow-up in numbers sufficient to quantify findings is difficult to achieve. However, the evidence is sufficient to confirm that women who breastfeed, particularly to or beyond 1 year, are known to have a reduced risk of breast cancer, type 2 diabetes, cardiovascular disease (CVD), some (reproductive) cancers, postpartum depression, and rheumatoid arthritis.[9–14] There appears to be a dose-response effect with breastfeeding and disease risk. The reduction in breast cancer risk, for which it is difficult to assess the incremental benefits of breastfeeding, has taken a long time to confirm, but the data are significant and the link is clear, which is reassuring.[9] The short lifetime duration of breastfeeding or lack thereof, typical of women in developed countries, makes a major contribution to the higher incidence of breast cancer.[9] As well, the reduction in risk of type 2 diabetes through breastfeeding is thought to be caused by the related effect of reduction in long-term obesity.[11] The data on links to other chronic diseases are described below.

Depression

Postpartum depression is among the most common antenatal complications, with devastating long-term effects. Lactation is associated with an attenuated stress response, involving cortisol and the lactogenic hormones, oxytocin and prolactin, which appear to have both antidepressant and anxiolytic effects.[12] Because reducing distress may decrease the risk of depression, parity may act as a mediator when breastfeeding is embraced in multiparous but not primiparous mothers.[12]

Coronary Heart Disease

Women who breastfed for a lifetime total of ≥2 years had a 37% lower risk of coronary heart disease (CHD).[10] With additional adjustment for early-adult adiposity, parental history, and lifestyle factors, these same women had a 23% lower risk of CHD than women who had never breastfed.[10]

Diabetes

Longer duration of breastfeeding is associated with reduced incidence of type 2 diabetes.[11] Lactation may reduce the risk of type 2 diabetes in young and middle-aged women by improving glucose homeostasis. A longer duration of breastfeeding is associated with a reduced risk of developing type 2 diabetes among parous women with no history of gestational diabetes.[13] Although lactation does not appear to offer a significant reduction in diabetes risk among women with gestational diabetes, these findings are limited to women participating in the Nurses' Health Study and are not generalizable.[11]

As for specific dosage recommendations, any breastfeeding is good, and more is better. The world consensus is that at least 6 months of exclusive breastfeeding is best for both mother and child.[7] The data follow the natural physiology of babies who are sitting at 6 months, with teeth coming in, and beginning to demand solids. The duration of breastfeeding that is best must be individualized to the family unit, however, with 1 year as a reasonable end point for the introduction of cow's milk.

Beyond the benefits of chronic disease reduction, another potential benefit of extended breastfeeding is the natural suppression of ovulation.[14,15] Prolonging postpartum anovulatory cycles is a consequence of exclusive breastfeeding, thereby serving as a natural contraceptive for up to 6 months.[14] Populations where breastfeeding is customary have been shown to have fewer births than populations in which infants are bottle fed.[4] The starting time of supplementary feeding is positively correlated with the time of the restoration of menstruation.[15]

In addition to the maternal benefits of breastfeeding, what new evidence is there about the compelling rationale for mothers to commit to breastfeeding?

Whereas the disadvantages to infants of substituting breastfeeding with bottle-fed formula are well documented, one notable risk factor recently identified is the reduced rate of sudden infant death syndrome (SIDS) in breastfed babies.[7,16] It is worth mentioning that for very low birth weight infants who are at high risk for necrotizing enterocolitis and at heightened susceptibility to a variety of infections, providing breast milk remains essential more as a medicine than as pure nourishment.[17] There are physiological and psychological maternal benefits of initiating lactation at birth, even before the infant is able to nurse, as it enables the mother's readiness to breastfeed as soon the infant is developmentally capable of nursing.[18,20]

Even among fragile premature babies, there are methods that can be effectively employed to support breastfeeding.[19,20] In contrast to a healthy term baby, the tenuous nutritional stores and immature systems of the premature newborn make it particularly vulnerable. There is a critical brief window of time in the first several days after birth when the breasts are most sensitive to frequent and effective stimulation (i.e., suckling, pumping) to ensure an adequate milk supply in the long term.[18] Providing the new mother with the support and information needed to prompt the immediate, invaluable, and demanding job of initiating milk production is essential for breastfeeding success. Breast milk remains the default choice for enteral feedings based on observational studies and meta-analyses comparing feeding with formula milk vs. donor breast milk, which support significant nonnutrient advantages of breast milk for preterm or low birth weight infants, including enhanced lifetime immunity.[17–19] Even if a third of the diet of a 2.2-pound premature baby is breast milk, the infant will leave the hospital, on average, 15 days earlier than the exclusively formula-fed baby.[18] It is worth noting that the breast milk produced after a premature delivery is different from the milk produced for a term infant. Neither formula nor even the milk from another mother can enhance the development of the brain, intestines, and immune systems as well as the infant's own mother's milk,[17] yet the number of premature infants breastfeeding successfully at discharge remains small.[3]

There are evidence-based techniques to improve the odds of premature infants breastfeeding at discharge and into the first year of life.[21,22] Among the measures available to the mother to promote the transition of the premature infant to the breast are kangaroo care, nonnutritive sucking, avoidance of bottles, and consistent and supportive staff. Similarly, guidelines for the late preterm infant, born at 34–36 weeks of gestation, are available.[21,22]

In the last decade, late preterm infants have become the fastest growing subset of preterm infants and now account for 74% of all preterm births.[21] Skin-to-skin contact, or kangaroo care, enhances the mother's capacity to synthesize specific factors that protect against the pathogenic bacteria prevalent within the hospital.[22] The intimacy of this type of care, when the mother actually wears her infant against her chest, has numerous benefits for both mother and baby, with improved milk production and infant weight gain being two overriding advantages. Beyond the quicker weight gain and decreased incidence of sepsis and necrotizing enterocolitis that account for the earlier discharge of premature infants fed breast milk, the related emotional benefits of bringing one's baby home sooner than later cannot be overestimated.[17]

Despite the available clinical evidence for chronic disease prevention in women who breastfeed, the existing information has not been acted on by the majority of practicing clinicians. What strategies might be required to prompt women's health practitioners to see breastfeeding as an appropriate clinical concern?

We are now at a point in history where the evidence about the benefits (both health and economic) of breastfeeding as a normal, natural, and optimal method of feeding is clear.[7,16,23] As clinicians, we should appreciate the physiological changes that occur in women in preparation for lactation. The endocrine system experiences a remarkable shift, with changes in pituitary production of oxytocin and pitocin, which are critical not only for the birthing process but also for initiation of breastfeeding and the shift from production of colostrum to mature milk. And that is only the beginning. Once lactation is established, it becomes a local process, an autocrine system, in which the body responds to direct demand on the breasts. If there is no demand, breast milk will cease production; conversely, nursing twins is possible because the body adjusts to meet the demand for milk. Although it may not seem relevant for clinicians to understand the minutiae of this natural process, having a better tmderstanding may inform our actions or discussions with women in practice. For example, it

may be that pacifier use may affect the infant's hormone system as well as influence the potential for breastfeeding long term.[24] Because breastfeeding is the unqualified ideal for mother (as well as baby), a heightened knowledge of all factors affecting breastfeeding may elucidate some of the common problems and strategies that better prepare clinicians to encourage women to breastfeed for a longer duration than is the current norm.

Finally, the availability of donor milk is an option primary care providers should be familiar with and prepared to recommend for circumstances in which mothers' own milk is not available, particularly for ill or at-risk newborns.[25]

For women who initially indicate a desire to breastfeed, how might clinicians approach societal barriers that occur after the baby is born to cause the dramatic dropoff in breastfeeding after a few weeks?

The debate about the relative value of breastfeeding compared with artificial means of feeding is over; the data are unequivocal in favor of breastfeeding as the ideal.[16] There is inadequate approval of breast feeding and insufficient systems to make it easier for all women to breastfeed, and the challenge must focus on establishing an appropriate environment and resources to best support women and families who are inclined to breastfeed.[23]

Despite recent progress, gaps persist between current breastfeeding practices and national breastfeeding objectives. Women experience hospital practices that are in conflict with the Baby-Friendly Hospital Initiative's guidelines for successful breastfeeding, including 74% who received free formula samples or orders, 49% whose infants were bottle fed, and 45% whose infants were given a pacifier.[26] Women who give birth in hospitals practicing 6 or 7 of the 10 recommended Baby-Friendly guidelines are more likely to achieve their goal of exclusive breastfeeding than are those whose hospitals practice no more than 1 of the steps. This suggests that hospital practices have an influence on whether women succeed at breastfeeding.[27,28] Where breastfeeding practices are suboptimal, simple one-encounter antenatal education and counseling significantly improve breastfeeding practice up to 3 months after delivery.[29] Receiving printed or audiovisual educational material is not deemed sufficient to promote breastfeeding; rather, one face-to-face encounter to discuss breastfeeding with expectant mothers before they deliver proves most efficacious long term.[29] Guidelines for hospital discharge to encourage exclusive breastfeeding, known as the Going home protocol, are available and should be introduced to pregnant women before delivery.[30]

The overwhelming medical, psychosocial, and societal benefits of breastfeeding for both mother and baby should be internalized by all clinicians and shared with every woman who indicates an intention to get pregnant, as breastfeeding education is a standard component of anticipatory guidance that addresses individual beliefs and practices in a culturally sensitive manner, resulting in a higher success rate.[27]

Even if the mother comes home intending to breast-fed, one of the greatest obstacles is creating a balance between contributing to the family economically and providing appropriate nutrition, which puts new mothers at an unfair disadvantage.[23] Given the framing of the situation as one of having to choose between work and breastfeeding suggests a larger, societal problem. Although breastfeeding is biologically possible for most women, only 11.3% of infants born in 2004 were exclusively breastfed at 6 months.[5] It is clear that maternal employment has a direct [effect] on whether and for how long women choose to breastfeed; for example, mothers working full time are less likely to be breastfeeding at 6 months than those working part-time or not at all.[24] In 2005, 49.5% of mothers with children under 1 year of age were employed, and more than two thirds were employed full-time.[31]

It is currently estimated that 1 in 3 women returning to the workforce within 3 months and 2 of 3 returning to work within 6 months continue to breastfeed.[31] These less than optimal numbers persist despite the known health benefits to both mother and baby conveyed by breastfeeding and translate into reduced costs to employers from lower healthcare costs, decreased absenteeism, heightened productivity, improved employee satisfaction, and a better corporate image.[32] Only five states in the United States provide paid pregnancy leave that can be extended for infant bonding. A maternity leave of ≤6 weeks has a 4-fold increase in failure to establish breastfeeding and increased probably of cessation after initial breastfeeding success and a 2-fold increase in cessation within 6–12 weeks after delivery relative to women who do not return to work.[24,32] Therefore, postpartum maternity leave may have a positive effect on breastfeeding among full-time workers, particularly those who hold nonmanagerial positions, lack job flexibility, or experience psychosocial distress. Clinicians should advocate in support of maternity leave and for extending paid postpartum leave and flexibility in work schedules for breastfeeding women.

A woman's health goes beyond breastfeeding her infant. Known as the ecological model of health, this approach considers the person in the context of family and how the healthcare system provides support and that the larger community is governed by policy.[33] To make a positive change in a health-promoting behavior, such as breastfeeding, requires an effort to address all these levels simultaneously. Therefore, the most challenging barriers to breastfeeding arise at the outer layers of community and policy support for women in this country.

Worksite programs, such as onsite day care, are one intervention that would permit women to continue to both breastfeed and work without unnecessary worry about the infant's well-being while remaining productive. The role of clinicians in this process is different in that efforts must shift to that of advocate. Clinicians must speak up at town hall meetings, write letters to the editor, and advocate for promoting worksite policies in favor of breastfeeding. In the doctor's office, when a woman asks for a note that prescribes appropriate lactation breaks to pump or nurse, this should be done swiftly.[30] To assist in this endeavor, there are templates (i.e., Academy of Breastfeeding Medicine) and other resources for practitioners to use to support women's willingness and desire to breastfeed.

Despite the current climate, it is feasible for women to breastfeed in many work settings.[27] Accommodating breastfeeding is not complicated, but as with other work-site issues, clarifying mutual expectations and understanding local policy will minimize misunderstandings. The key needs to foster worksite breastfeeding are basic: time (appropriate, allocated breaks); a suitable location in which to nurse, pump, or express breast milk; and employer–employee communication. When child care is on-site or nearby and schedules are supportive, breastfeeding can continue seamlessly.

Even before the workplace challenges are be considered, the birth care system as a whole continues to offer resistance to breastfeeding, and may prove more related to the pressures of clinicians. There are actions that need attention from clinicians as individuals but also as a collective profession so that when women indicate a desire to breastfeed, every possible strategy is employed to encourage success. The hospital policy on breastfeeding not only has a significant effect on whether a woman will breastfeed but also influences her initial intention.[34] The current healthcare system is quite capable of sabotaging good intentions to breastfeed. The CDC's maternal care practices survey has established concrete baseline practices at hospital and birthing centers across the country.[35] The data are shocking, given the disturbing rates at which formula feeding is imposed on women who come into the system with the intention of breastfeeding and successfully initiate nursing.[28,29,36]

Despite popular belief, there are very few contraindications to breastfeeding. Providing maternal support and structured antenatal and postpartum breastfeeding education are the most effective means of achieving breastfeeding success.[28,29] In addition, immediate skin-to-skin contact between mother and infant and early initiation of breastfeeding are shown to improve breastfeeding outcomes.[27] Once practices like this are identified and quantified, it gives us a chance to address the problems head-on and effect changes, which must gain traction from physicians as well as nurses and other allied health professionals whose function is to support women throughout the childbearing process. Just having all women's health practitioners advocating for a birthing system that is supportive of the personal choice to breastfeed can result in a favorable outcome.

Although the opportunity to effect this kind of change may not be evident in private practice, *per se*, it can be an opportunity to partner with patients and the wider community. Small, meaningful steps can be considerably effective in making a difference in maternal willingness to remain committed to breastfeeding once at home. Making sure that medical students and interns are educated about the importance of breastfeeding and having the evidence of breastfeeding benefits included in the (re)certification examination are steps in the right direction.

How do the lifestyle needs of a breastfeeding woman differ from those of a woman who is bottlefeeding, and what might the clinician do to promote proper nutrition and lifestyle management in women who are breastfeeding?

Useful resources for clinicians to share with women who are breastfeeding include MyPyramid.gov, which is a Department of Agriculture/Department of Health and Human Services program to address the specific nutritional needs of American adults. This tool can be tailored to women who are pregnant as well as those who are breastfeeding and can be accessed at: www.mypyramid.gov/mypyramidmoms. The interactive program can be used in the office setting or prescribed for home use to reinforce the healthy nutrition messages. Even better, this program can be used to customize the nutritional profile of variables common among breastfeeding women, such as accommodating for the changing age of the child along with the health status of the mother and her level of lactation (i.e., supplementation half the time vs. exclusively breastfeeding).

Another underused resource is the Academy of Breastfeeding Medicine protocols on the National Guidelines Clearinghouse website; these are evidence-based recommendations written from the clinician's perspective about what to do in specific circumstances. Of particular interest is the protocol on creating a breastfeeding-friendly office.[35] With 19 protocols, it is unlikely that every clinician can implement the full complement. The intention is to provide practice-specific suggestions that expand on the Breastfeeding-Friendly Hospital Initiative so that support and encouragement are established prenatally and can be carried on after the mother and newborn come home.

This point brings the discussion back to the concept of the ecological model.[33] Clinicians must begin to think about the importance of supporting women prenatally, during delivery, and postnatally in child care settings. Interventions may include multiple strategies, such as formal breastfeeding education for mothers and families, direct support of mothers during breastfeeding observations, and training of health professional staff about breastfeeding and techniques for breastfeeding support. Evidence suggests that interventions that include both prenatal and postnatal components may be the most effective at increasing the duration of breastfeeding duration.[27,29,30,34-36] Many successful programs include peer support, prenatal breastfeeding education, or both. The U.S. Preventive Services Task Force found that the most effective breastfeeding interventions are multifactorial, addressing different issues along the continuum.[16]

Offering support is the most important factor in assuring that women will continue to breastfeed, a concept that is worth reinforcing.[16] Beyond support, an equally important factor is watching women breastfeed and knowing the basics of latch and hold so that any problems can be identified and remedied.[27,30,34,35] As any mother who has breastfed will tell you, it does not come naturally to mother or baby.[28] It is a process that must be learned, and this process includes clinicians who should be familiar with the basics so that assistance can be given as needed.

Additional Resources

American Academy of Family Physicians. Family physicians. Supporting breastfeeding. Position paper, 2008.

World Health Organization. Infant and young child feeding: Model chapter for textbooks for medical students and allied health professionals. Geneva: WHO Press, 2009.

U.S. Department of Health and Human Services, Health Resources and Services Administration (HRSA), Maternal and Child Health Bureau. The business case for breastfeeding. Every Mother, Inc. and Rich Winter Design and Multimedia, 2008. Available at www.mchb.hrsa.gov/pregnancyandbeyondPrint

References

1. Kaplan DL, Graff KM. Breastfeeding—Reversing corporate influence on infant feeding practices. J Urban Health 2008;85:486–504.

2. Li R, Darling N, Maurice E, Barker L, Grummer-Strawn LM. Breastfeeding rates in the United States by characteristics of the child, mother, or family: The 2002 National Immunization Survey. Pediatrics 2005;115:e31–37.

3. U.S. Department of Health and Human Services. Healthy People 2010: Understanding and improving health, 2nd ed. Washington, DC: U.S. Government Printing Office, 2000.

4. Flower KB, Willoughby M, Cadigan RJ, Perrin EM, Randolph G, and The Family Life Project Investigative Team. Understanding breastfeeding initiation and continuation in rural communities: A combined qualitative/quantitative approach. Matern Child Health J 2008;12:402–414.

5. Centers for Disease Control and Prevention. Breastfeeding among U.S. children born 1999–2005, CDC National Immunization Survey, 2008.

6. Lawrence RA, Lawrence R. Breast feeding: A guide for the medical profession, 7th ed. Philadelphia: Saunders (projected publication date, August 2010).

7. WHO. Evidence on the long-term effects of breastfeeding: Systematic reviews and meta-analyses. Geneva: World Health Organization, 2007.

8. Grummer-Strawn L, Scanlon KS, Darling N, Conrey EJ. Racial and socioeconomic disparities in breastfeeding—United States, 2004. MMWR 2006;55:335–339.

9. Collaborative Group on Hormonal Factors in Breast Cancer. Breast cancer and breastfeeding: Collaborative reanalysis of individual data from 47 epidemiological studies in 30 countries, including 50,302 women with breast cancer and 96,973 women without the disease. Lancet 2002;360: 187–195.

10. Schwartz E, Ray R, Stuebe A, et al. Duration of lactation and risk factors for maternal cardiovascular disease. Obstet Gynecol 2009;113:974–982.

11. Stuebe A, Rich-Edwards J, Willett W, Manson J, Michels K. Duration of lactation and incidence of type 2 diabetes. JAMA 2005;294:2601–2610.

12. Sibolboro Mezzacappa E, Endicott J. Parity mediates the association between infant feeding method and maternal depressive symptoms in the postpartum. Arch Womens Ment Health 2007;10:259–266.

13. Bentley-Lewis R, Levkoff S, Stuebe A, Seely EW. Gestational diabetes mellitus: Postpartum opportunities for the diagnosis and prevention of type 2 diabetes mellitus. Nat Clin Pract Endocrinol Metab 2008;4:552–558.

14. Gross BA, Burger H, WHO Task Force on Methods for the Natural Regulation of Fertility. Breastfeeding patterns and return to fertility in Australian women. Aust NZ J Obstet Gynaecol 2002;42:148–154.

15. Li W, Qiu Y. Relation of supplementary feeding to resumptions of menstruation and ovulation in lactating postpartum women. Chin Med J 2007;120:868–870.

16. Chung M, Raman G. Trikalinos T, Lau J, Ip S. Interventions in primary care to promote breastfeeding: An evidence review for the U.S. Preventive Services Task Force. Ann Intern Med 2008;149:560–564.

17. Henderson G, Anthony M, McGuire W. Formula milk versus maternal breast milk for feeding preterm or low birth weight infants. Cochrane Database Syst Rev 2007;4.

18. Montgomery D, Schmutz N, Baer VL, et al. Effects of Instituting the "BEST Program" (Breast Milk Early Saves Trouble) in a Level III NICU. J Hum Lact 2008;24:248–251.

19. Nye C. Transitioning premature infants from gavage to breast. Neonatal Netw 2008;27:7–13.

20. Wall G. A premie needs his mother: First steps to breastfeeding your premature baby. Arch Pediatr Adolesc Med 2002;156:731–732.

21. Wight N. Breastfeeding the borderline (near-term) preterm infant. Pediatr Ann 2003;32:329–336.

22. Raju TNK, Higgins RD, Stark AR, Leveno KJ. Optimizing care and outcome for late preterm (near-term) infants: A summary of the workshop sponsored by the National Institute of Child Health and Human Development. Pediatrics 2006;118:1207–1214.

23. Weimer J. The economic benefits of breastfeeding: A review and analysis. In: Food and Rural Economics Division. U.S. Department of Agriculture. Food Assistance and Nutrition Research, ed. Economic Research Service, 2001;13:1–14.

24. Ryan A, Zhou W, Arensberg M. The effect of employment status on breastfeeding in the United States. Womens Health Issues 2006;16:243–251.

25. Woo K, Spatz D. Human milk donation: What do you know about it? Am J Matern Child Nurs 2007;32:150–155.

26. Philipp B, Merewood A. The Baby-Friendly way: The best breastfeeding start. Pediatr Clin North Am 2004;51:761–783.

27. Labbok M. Breastfeeding and Baby-Friendly Hospital Initiative: More important and with more evidence than ever. J Pediatr 2007;83:99–101.

28. Declercq E, Sakala C, Corry MP, Applebaum S. New mothers speak out: National survey results highlight women's postpartum experiences. New York: Childbirth Connection and Lamaze International, 2008.

29. Mattar CN, Chong Y-S, Chan Y-S, et al. Simple antenatal preparation to improve breastfeeding practice: A randomized controlled trial. Obstet Gynecol 2007;109:73–80.

30. Keister D, Roberts K, Werner S. Strategies for breastfeeding success. Am Fam Physician 2008;78:225–232.

31. U.S. Department of Labor, Bureau of Labor Statistics. Employment characteristics of families in 2006. Washington, DC: The Department of Labor, 2007: Table 6.

32. Guendelman S, Kosa JL, Pearl M, Graham S, Goodman J, Kharrazi M. Juggling work and breastfeeding: Effects of maternity leave and occupational characteristics. Pediatrics 2009;123:e38–46.

33. Tiedje L, Schiffman R, Omar M, et al. An ecological approach to breastfeeding. Am J Matern Child Nurs 2002; 27:154–161.

34. Breastfeeding-related maternity practices among hospitals and birth centers—United States, 2007. MMWR, Centers for Disease Control and Prevention, 2007.

35. Chantry CJ, Howard CR, Lawrence RA, Powers NG, Shaikh U. ABM Clinical Protocol 14: Breastfeeding-friendly physician's office, Part 1: Optimizing care for infants and children. Breastfeed Med 2006;1:115–119.

36. DiGirolamo AM, Grummer-Strawn LM, Fein SB. Effect of maternity-care practices on breastfeeding. Pediatrics 2008: 122 (Suppl):S43–S49.

JODI R. GODFREY is a health and wellness specialist in private practice and contributing editor to the *Journal of Women's Health*.

RUTH A. LAWRENCE is a physician and professor of pediatrics and obstetrics and gynecology at the University of Rochester School of Medicine in Rochester, New York. She is a founding member and past president of the Academy of Breastfeeding Medicine and is editor-in-chief of *Breastfeeding Medicine*.

Hanna Rosin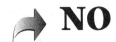

The Case Against Breast-Feeding

One afternoon at the playground last summer, shortly after the birth of my third child, I made the mistake of idly musing about breast-feeding to a group of new mothers I'd just met. This time around, I said, I was considering cutting it off after a month or so. At this remark, the air of insta-friendship we had established cooled into an icy politeness, and the mothers shortly wandered away to chase little Emma or Liam onto the slide. Just to be perverse, over the next few weeks I tried this experiment again several more times. The reaction was always the same: circles were redrawn such that I ended up in the class of mom who, in a pinch, might feed her baby mashed-up Chicken McNuggets.

In my playground set, the urban moms in their tight jeans and oversize sunglasses size each other up using a whole range of signifiers: organic content of snacks, sleekness of stroller, ratio of tasteful wooden toys to plastic. But breast-feeding is the real ticket into the club. My mother friends love to exchange stories about subversive ways they used to sneak frozen breast milk through airline security (it's now legal), or about the random brutes on the street who don't approve of breast-feeding in public. When Angelina Jolie wanted to secure her status as America's ur-mother, she posed on the cover of *W* magazine nursing one of her twins. Alt-rocker Pete Wentz recently admitted that he tasted his wife, Ashlee Simpson's, breast milk ("soury" and "weird"), after bragging that they have a lot of sex—both of which must have seemed to him markers of a cool domestic existence.

From the moment a new mother enters the obstetrician's waiting room, she is subjected to the upper-class parents' jingle: "Breast Is Best." Parenting magazines offer "23 Great Nursing Tips," warnings on "Nursing Roadblocks," and advice on how to find your local lactation consultant (note to the childless: yes, this is an actual profession, and it's thriving). Many of the stories are accompanied by suggestions from the ubiquitous parenting guru Dr. William Sears, whose Web site hosts a comprehensive list of the benefits of mother's milk. "Brighter Brains" sits at the top: "I.Q. scores averaging seven to ten points higher!" (Sears knows his audience well.) The list then moves on to the dangers averted, from infancy on up: fewer ear infections, allergies, stomach illnesses; lower rates of obesity, diabetes, heart disease. Then it adds, for good measure, stool with a "buttermilk-like odor" and "nicer skin"—benefits, in short, "more far-reaching than researchers have even dared to imagine."

In 2005, *Babytalk* magazine won a National Magazine Award for an article called "You Can Breastfeed." Given the prestige of the award, I had hoped the article might provide some respite from the relentlessly cheerful tip culture of the parenting magazines, and fill mothers in on the real problems with nursing. Indeed, the article opens with a promisingly realistic vignette, featuring a theoretical "You" cracking under the strain of having to breast-feed around the clock, suffering "crying jags" and cursing at your husband. But fear not, You. The root of the problem is not the sudden realization that your ideal of an equal marriage, with two parents happily taking turns working and raising children, now seems like a farce. It turns out to be quite simple: You just haven't quite figured out how to fit "Part A into Part B." Try the "C-hold" with your baby and some "rapid arm movement," the story suggests. Even Dr. Sears pitches in: "Think 'fish lips,'" he offers.

In the days after my first child was born, I welcomed such practical advice. I remember the midwife coming to my hospital bed and shifting my arm here, and the baby's head there, and then everything falling into place. But after three children and 28 months of breast-feeding (and counting), the insistent cheerleading has begun to grate. Buttermilk-like odor? Now Dr. Sears is selling me too hard. I may have put in fewer parenting years than he has, but I do have *some* perspective. And when I look around my daughter's second-grade class, I can't seem to pick out the unfortunate ones: "Oh, poor little Sophie, whose mother couldn't breast-feed. What dim eyes she has. What a sickly pallor. And already sprouting acne!"

I dutifully breast-fed each of my first two children for the full year that the American Academy of Pediatrics recommends. I have experienced what the *Babytalk* story calls breast-feeding-induced "maternal nirvana." This time around, *nirvana* did not describe my state of mind; I was launching a new Web site and I had two other children to care for, and a husband I would occasionally like to talk to. Being stuck at home breast-feeding as he walked out the door for work just made me unreasonably furious, at him and everyone else.

In Betty Friedan's day, feminists felt shackled to domesticity by the unreasonably high bar for housework, the endless dusting and shopping and pushing the Hoover around—a vacuum cleaner being the obligatory prop for the "happy housewife heroine," as Friedan sardonically called her. When I looked at the picture on the cover of Sears's *Breastfeeding Book*—a lady lying down, gently smiling at her baby and *still in her robe*, although the sun is well up—the scales fell from my eyes: it was not the vacuum that was keeping me and my 21st-century sisters down, but another sucking sound.

Still, despite my stint as the postpartum playground crank, I could not bring myself to stop breast-feeding—too many years of Sears's conditioning, too many playground spies. So I was left feeling trapped, like many women before me, in the middle-class mother's prison of vague discontent: surly but too privileged for pity, breast-feeding with one hand while answering the cell phone with the other, and barking at my older kids to get their own organic, 100 percent juice—the modern, multitasking mother's version of Friedan's "problem that has no name."

And in this prison I would have stayed, if not for a chance sighting. One day, while nursing my baby in my pediatrician's office, I noticed a 2001 issue of the *Journal of the American Medical Association* open to an article about breast-feeding: "Conclusions: There are inconsistent associations among breastfeeding, its duration, and the risk of being overweight in young children." Inconsistent? There I was, sitting half-naked in public for the tenth time that day, the hundredth time that month, the millionth time in my life—and the associations were *inconsistent?* The seed was planted. That night, I did what any sleep-deprived, slightly paranoid mother of a newborn would do. I called my doctor friend for her password to an online medical library, and then sat up and read dozens of studies examining breast-feeding's association with allergies, obesity, leukemia, mother-infant bonding, intelligence, and all the Dr. Sears highlights.

After a couple of hours, the basic pattern became obvious: the medical literature looks nothing like the popular literature. It shows that breast-feeding is probably, maybe, a little better; but it is far from the stampede of evidence that Sears describes. More like tiny, unsure baby steps: two forward, two back, with much meandering and bumping into walls. A couple of studies will show fewer allergies, and then the next one will turn up no difference. Same with mother-infant bonding, IQ, leukemia, cholesterol, diabetes. Even where consensus is mounting, the meta studies—reviews of existing studies—consistently complain about biases, missing evidence, and other major flaws in study design. "The studies do not demonstrate a universal phenomenon, in which one method is superior to another in all instances," concluded one of the first, and still one of the broadest, meta studies, in a 1984 issue of *Pediatrics*, "and they do not support making a mother feel that she is doing psychological harm to her child if she is unable or unwilling to breastfeed." Twenty-five years later, the picture hasn't changed all that much. So how is it that every mother I know has become a breast-feeding fascist?

Like many babies of my generation, I was never breast-fed. My parents were working-class Israelis, living in Tel Aviv in the '70s and aspiring to be modern. In the U.S., people were already souring on formula and passing out No NESTLÉ buttons, but in Israel, Nestlé formula was the latest thing. My mother had already ditched her fussy Turkish coffee for Nescafé (just mix with water), and her younger sister would soon be addicted to NesQuik. Transforming soft, sandy grains from solid to magic liquid must have seemed like the forward thing to do. Plus, my mom believed her pediatrician when he said that it was important to precisely measure a baby's food intake and stick to a schedule. (To this day she pesters me about whether I'm *sure* my breast-fed babies are getting enough to eat; the parenting magazines would classify her as "unsupportive" and warn me to stay away.) Formula grew out of a late-19th-century effort to combat atrocious rates of infant mortality by turning infant feeding into a controlled science. Pediatrics was then a newly minted profession, and for the next century, the men who dominated it would constantly try to get mothers to welcome "enlightenment from the laboratory," writes Ann Hulbert in *Raising America*. But now and again, mothers would fight back. In the U.S., the rebellion against formula began in the late '50s, when a group of moms from the Chicago suburbs got together to form a breast-feeding support group they called La Leche League. They were Catholic mothers, influenced by the Christian Family Movement, who spoke of breast-feeding as "God's plan for mothers and babies." Their role model was the biblical Eve ("Her baby came. The milk came. She nursed her baby," they wrote in their first, pamphlet edition of *The Womanly Art of Breastfeeding*, published in 1958).

They took their league's name, La Leche, from a shrine to the Madonna near Jacksonville, Florida, called Nuestra Señora de La Leche y Buen Parto, which loosely translates into "Our Lady of Happy Delivery and Plentiful Milk." A more forthright name was deemed inappropriate: "You didn't mention *breast* in print unless you were talking about Jean Harlow," said co-founder Edwina Froehlich. In their photos, the women of La Leche wear practical pumps and high-neck housewife dresses, buttoned to the top. They saw themselves as a group of women who were "kind of thinking crazy," said co-founder Mary Ann Cahill. "Everything we did was radical."

La Leche League mothers rebelled against the notion of mother as lab assistant, mixing formula for the specimen under her care. Instead, they aimed to "bring mother and baby together again." An illustration in the second edition shows a woman named Eve—looking not unlike Jean Harlow—exposed to the waist and caressing her baby, with no doctor hovering nearby. Over time the group adopted a feminist edge. A 1972 publication rallies mothers to have "confidence in themselves and their sisters rather than passively following the advice of licensed professionals." As one woman wrote in another league publication, "Yes, I want to be liberated! I want to be free! I want to be free to be a woman!"

In 1971, the Boston Women's Health Book Collective published *Our Bodies, Ourselves,* launching a branch of feminism known as the women's-health movement. The authors were more groovy types than the La Leche

League moms; they wore slouchy jeans, clogs, and ban-danas holding back waist-length hair. But the two move-ments had something in common; *Our Bodies* also grew out of "frustration and anger" with a medical establish-ment that was "condescending, paternalistic, judgmen-tal and non-informative." Teaching women about their own bodies would make them "more self-confident, more autonomous, stronger," the authors wrote. Breasts were not things for men to whistle and wink at; they were made for women to feed their babies in a way that was "sen-sual and fulfilling." The book also noted, in passing, that breast-feeding could "strengthen the infant's resistance to infection and disease"—an early hint of what would soon become the national obsession with breast milk as liquid vaccine.

Pediatricians have been scrutinizing breast milk since the late 1800s. But the public didn't pay much attention until an international scandal in the '70s over "killer baby bottles." Studies in South America and Africa showed that babies who were fed formula instead of breast milk were more likely to die. The mothers, it turned out, were using contaminated water or rationing formula because it was so expensive. Still, in the U.S., the whole episode turned breast-feeding advocates and formula makers into Crips and Bloods, and introduced the take-no-prisoners turf war between them that continues to this day.

Some of the magical thinking about breast-feeding stems from a common misconception. Even many doc-tors believe that breast milk is full of maternal antibod-ies that get absorbed into the baby's bloodstream, says Sydney Spiesel, a clinical professor of pediatrics at Yale University's School of Medicine. That is how it works for most mammals. But in humans, the process is more pedes-trian, and less powerful. A human baby is born with anti-bodies already in place, having absorbed them from the placenta. Breast milk dumps another layer of antibodies, primarily secretory IgA, directly into the baby's gastroin-testinal tract. As the baby is nursing, these extra antibodies provide some added protection against infection, but they never get into the blood.

Since the identification of sIgA, in 1961, labs have hunted for other marvels. Could the oligosaccharides in milk prevent diarrhea? Do the fatty acids boost brain development? The past few decades have turned up many promising leads, hypotheses, and theories, all sugges-tive and nifty but never confirmed in the lab. Instead, most of the claims about breast-feeding's benefits lean on research conducted outside the lab: comparing one group of infants being breast-fed against another being breast-fed less, or not at all. Thousands of such studies have been published, linking breast-feeding with healthier, happier, smarter children. But they all share one glaring flaw.

An ideal study would randomly divide a group of mothers, tell one half to breast-feed and the other not to, and then measure the outcomes. But researchers cannot ethically tell mothers what to feed their babies. Instead they have to settle for "observational" studies. These simply look for differences in two populations, one breast-fed and one not. The problem is, breast-fed infants are typically brought up in very different families from those raised on the bottle. In the U.S., breast-feeding is on the rise—69 percent of mothers initiate the practice at the hospital, and 17 percent nurse exclusively for at least six months. But the numbers are much higher among women who are white, older, and educated; a woman who attended college, for instance, is roughly twice as likely to nurse for six months. Researchers try to factor out all these "confounding variables" that might affect the babies' health and development. But they still can't know if they've missed some critical factor. "Studies about the benefits of breast-feeding are extremely difficult and com-plex because of who breast-feeds and who doesn't," says Michael Kramer, a highly respected researcher at McGill University. "There have been claims that it prevents everything—cancer, diabetes. A reasonable person would be cautious about every new amazing discovery."

The study about obesity I saw in my pediatrician's office that morning is a good example of the complexity of breast-feeding research—and of the pitfalls it contains. Some studies have found a link between nursing and slim-mer kids, but they haven't proved that one causes the other. This study surveyed 2,685 children between the ages of 3 and 5. After adjusting for race, parental education, mater-nal smoking, and other factors—all of which are thought to affect a child's risk of obesity—the study found little correlation between breast-feeding and weight. Instead, the strongest predictor of the child's weight was the moth-er's. Whether obese mothers nursed or used formula, their children were more likely to be heavy. The breast-feeding advocates' dream—that something in the milk somehow reprograms appetite—is still a long shot.

In the past decade, researchers have come up with ever more elaborate ways to tease out the truth. One 2005 paper focused on 523 sibling pairs who were fed differ-ently, and its results put a big question mark over all the previous research. The economists Eirik Evenhouse and Siobhan Reilly compared rates of diabetes, asthma, and allergies; childhood weight; various measures of mother-child bonding; and levels of intelligence. Almost all the differences turned out to be statistically insignificant. For the most part, the "long-term effects of breast feeding have been overstated," they wrote.

Nearly all the researchers I talked to pointed me to a series of studies designed by Kramer, published starting in 2001. Kramer followed 17,000 infants born in Belarus throughout their childhoods. He came up with a clever way to randomize his study, at least somewhat, without doing anything unethical. He took mothers who had already started nursing, and then subjected half of them to an intervention strongly encouraging them to nurse exclu-sively for several months. The intervention worked: many women nursed longer as a result. And extended breast-feeding did reduce the risk of a gastrointestinal infection by 40 percent. This result seems to be consistent with the protection that sIgA provides; in real life, it adds up to about four out of 100 babies having one less incident of diarrhea or vomiting. Kramer also noted some reduction in infant rashes. Otherwise, his studies found very few significant differences: none, for instance, in weight, blood pressure, ear infections, or allergies—some of the most commonly cited benefits in the breast-feeding literature.

Both the Kramer study and the sibling study did turn up one interesting finding: a bump in "cognitive ability" among breast-fed children. But intelligence is tricky to measure, because it's subjective and affected by so many factors. Other recent studies, particularly those that have factored out the mother's IQ, have found no difference at all between breast-fed and formula-fed babies. In Kramer's study, the mean scores varied widely and mysteriously from clinic to clinic. What's more, the connection he found "could be banal," he told me—simply the result of "breast-feeding mothers' interacting more with their babies, rather than of anything in the milk."

The IQ studies run into the central problem of breast-feeding research: it is impossible to separate a mother's decision to breast-feed—and everything that goes along with it—from the breast-feeding itself. Even sibling studies can't get around this problem. With her first child, for instance, a mother may be extra cautious, keeping the neighbor's germy brats away and slapping the nurse who gives out the free formula sample. By her third child, she may no longer breast-feed—giving researchers the sibling comparison that they crave—but many other things may have changed as well. Maybe she is now using day care, exposing the baby to more illnesses. Surely she is not noticing that kid No. 2 has the baby's pacifier in his mouth, or that the cat is sleeping in the crib (trust me on this one). She is also not staring lovingly into the baby's eyes all day, singing songs, reading book after infant book, because she has to make sure that the other two kids are not drowning each other in the tub. On paper, the three siblings are equivalent, but their experiences are not.

What does all the evidence add up to? We have clear indications that breast-feeding helps prevent an extra incident of gastrointestinal illness in some kids—an unpleasant few days of diarrhea or vomiting, but rarely life-threatening in developed countries. We have murky correlations with a whole bunch of long-term conditions. The evidence on IQs is intriguing but not all that compelling, and at best suggests a small advantage, perhaps five points; an individual kid's IQ score can vary that much from test to test or day to day. If a child is disadvantaged in other ways, this bump might make a difference. But for the kids in my playground set, the ones whose mothers obsess about breast-feeding, it gets lost in a wash of Baby Einstein videos, piano lessons, and the rest. And in any case, if a breast-feeding mother is miserable, or stressed out, or alienated by nursing, as many women are, if her marriage is under stress and breast-feeding is making things worse, surely that can have a greater effect on a kid's future success than a few IQ points.

So overall, yes, breast is probably best. But not so much better that formula deserves the label of "public health menace," alongside smoking. Given what we know so far, it seems reasonable to put breast-feeding's health benefits on the plus side of the ledger and other things—modesty, independence, career, sanity—on the minus side, and then tally them up and make a decision. But in this risk-averse age of parenting, that's not how it's done.

In the early '90s, a group of researchers got together to revise the American Academy of Pediatrics' policy statement on breast-feeding. They were of the generation that had fought the formula wars and had lived through the days when maternity wards automatically gave women hormone shots to stop the flow of breast milk. The academy had long encouraged mothers to make "every effort" to nurse their newborns, but the researchers felt the medical evidence justified a stronger statement. Released in 1997, the new policy recommended exclusive breast-feeding for six months, followed by six more months of partial breast-feeding, supplemented with other foods. The National Organization for Women complained that this would tax working mothers, but to no avail. "The fact that the major pediatric group in the country was taking a definitive stance made all the difference," recalls Lawrence Gartner, a pediatrician and neonatologist at the University of Chicago, and the head of the committee that made the change. "After that, every major organization turned the corner, and the popular media changed radically."

In 2004, the Department of Health and Human Services launched the National Breastfeeding Awareness Campaign. The ads came out just after my second child was born, and were so odious that they nearly caused me to wean him on the spot. One television ad shows two hugely pregnant women in a logrolling contest, with an audience egging them on. "You wouldn't take risks before your baby is born," reads the caption. "Why start after?" The screen then flashes: "Breastfeed exclusively for 6 months." A second spot shows a pregnant woman—this time African American—riding a mechanical bull in a bar while trying to hold on to her huge belly. She falls off the bull and the crowd moans.

To convey the idea that failing to breast-feed is harmful to a baby's health, the print ads show ordinary objects arranged to look like breasts: two dandelions (respiratory illness), two scoops of ice cream with cherries on top (obesity), two otoscopes (ear infections). Plans were made to do another ad showing rubber nipples on top of insulin syringes (suggesting that bottle-feeding causes diabetes), but then someone thought better of it. The whole campaign is so knowing, so dripping with sexual innuendo and condescension, that it brings to mind nothing so much as an episode of *Mad Men*, where Don Draper and the boys break out the whiskey at day's end to toast another victory over the enemy sex.

What's most amazing is how, 50 years after La Leche League's founding, "enlightenment from the laboratory"—judgmental and absolutist—has triumphed again. The seventh edition of *The Womanly Art*, published in 2004, has ballooned to more than 400 pages, and is filled with photographs in place of the original hand drawings. But what's most noticeable is the shift in attitude. Each edition of the book contains new expert testimony about breast milk as an "arsenal against illness." "The resistance to disease that human milk affords a baby cannot be duplicated in any other way," the authors scold. The experience of reading the 1958 edition is like talking with your bossy but charming neighbor, who has some motherly advice to share. Reading the latest edition is like being trapped in the office of a doctor who's haranguing you about the choices you make.

In her critique of the awareness campaign, Joan Wolf, a women's-studies professor at Texas A&M University, chalks up the overzealous ads to a new ethic of "total motherhood." Mothers these days are expected to "optimize every dimension of children's lives," she writes. Choices are often presented as the mother's selfish desires versus the baby's needs. As an example, Wolf quotes *What to Expect When You're Expecting,* from a section called the "Best-Odds Diet," which I remember quite well: "Every bite counts. You've got only nine months of meals and snacks with which to give your baby the best possible start in life. . . . Before you close your mouth on a forkful of food, consider, 'Is this the best bite I can give my baby?' If it will benefit your baby, chew away. If it'll only benefit your sweet tooth or appease your appetite put your fork down." To which any self-respecting pregnant woman should respond: "I am carrying 35 extra pounds and my ankles have swelled to the size of a life raft, and now I would like to eat some coconut-cream pie. So you know what you can do with this damned fork."

About seven years ago, I met a woman from Montreal, the sister-in-law of a friend, who was young and healthy and normal in every way, except that she refused to breast-feed her children. She wasn't working at the time. She just felt that breast-feeding would set up an unequal dynamic in her marriage—one in which the mother, who was responsible for the very sustenance of the infant, would naturally become responsible for everything else as well. At the time, I had only one young child, so I thought she was a kooky Canadian—and selfish and irresponsible. But of course now I know she was right. I recalled her with sisterly love a few months ago, at three in the morning, when I was propped up in bed for the second time that night with my new baby (note the *my*). My husband acknowledged the ripple in the nighttime peace with a grunt, and that's about it. And why should he do more? There's no use in both of us being a wreck in the morning. Nonetheless, it's hard not to seethe.

The Bitch in the House, published in 2002, reframed *The Feminine Mystique* for my generation of mothers. We were raised to expect that co-parenting was an attainable goal. But who were we kidding? Even in the best of marriages, the domestic burden shifts, in incremental, mostly unacknowledged ways, onto the woman. Breast-feeding plays a central role in the shift. In my set, no husband tells his wife that it is her womanly duty to stay home and nurse the child. Instead, both parents together weigh the evidence and then make a rational, informed decision that she should do so. Then other, logical decisions follow: she alone fed the child, so she naturally knows better how to comfort the child, so she is the better judge to pick a school for the child and the better nurse when the child is sick, and so on. Recently, my husband and I noticed that we had reached the age at which friends from high school and college now hold positions of serious power. When we went down the list, we had to work hard to find any women. Where had all our female friends strayed? Why had they disappeared during the years they'd had small children?

The debate about breast-feeding takes place without any reference to its actual context in women's lives. Breast-feeding exclusively is not like taking a prenatal vitamin. It is a serious time commitment that pretty much guarantees that you will not work in any meaningful way. Let's say a baby feeds seven times a day and then a couple more times at night. That's nine times for about a half hour each, which adds up to more than half of a working day, every day, for at least six months. This is why, when people say that breast-feeding is "free," I want to hit them with a two-by-four. It's only free if a woman's time is worth nothing.

That brings us to the subject of pumping. Explain to your employer that while you're away from your baby, "you will need to take breaks throughout the day to pump your milk," suggest the materials from the awareness campaign. Demand a "clean, quiet place" to pump, and a place to store the milk. A clean, quiet place. So peaceful, so spa-like. Leave aside the preposterousness of this advice if you are, say, a waitress or a bus driver. Say you are a newspaper reporter, like I used to be, and deadline is approaching. Your choices are (a) leave your story to go down to the dingy nurse's office and relieve yourself; or (b) grow increasingly panicked and sweaty as your body continues on its merry, milk-factory way, even though the plant shouldn't be operating today and the pump is about to explode. And then one day, the inevitable will happen. You will be talking to a male colleague and saying to yourself, "Don't think of the baby. Please don't think of the baby." And then the pump *will* explode, and the stigmata will spread down your shirt as you rush into the ladies' room.

This year alone I had two friends whose babies could not breast-feed for one reason or another, so they mostly had to pump. They were both first-time mothers who had written themselves dreamy birth plans involving hot baths followed by hours of intimate nursing. When that didn't work out, they panicked about their babies' missing out on the milky elixir. One of them sat on my couch the other day hooked up to tubes and suctions and a giant deconstructed bra, looking like some fetish ad, or a footnote from the Josef Mengele years. Looking as far as humanly possible from Eve in her natural, feminine state.

In his study on breast-feeding and cognitive development, Michael Kramer mentions research on the long-term effects of mother rats' licking and grooming their pups. Maybe, he writes, it's "the physical and/or emotional act of breastfeeding" that might lead to benefits. This is the theory he prefers, he told me, because "it would suggest something the formula companies can't reproduce." No offense to Kramer, who seems like a great guy, but this gets under my skin. If the researchers just want us to lick and groom our pups, why don't they say so? We can find our own way to do that. In fact, by insisting that milk is some kind of vaccine, they make it less likely that we'll experience nursing primarily as a loving maternal act—"pleasant and relaxing," in the words of *Our Bodies, Ourselves* and more likely that we'll view it as, well, dispensing medicine.

I continue to breast-feed my new son some of the time—but I don't do it slavishly. When I am out for the day working, or out with friends at night, he can have all the formula he wants, and I won't give it a second thought. I'm not really sure why I don't stop entirely. I know it has nothing to do with the science; I have no grandiose illusions that I'm making him lean and healthy and smart with my milk. Nursing is certainly not pure pleasure, either; often I'm tapping my foot impatiently, waiting for him to finish. I do it partly because I can get away with breast-feeding part-time. I work at home and don't punch a clock, which is not the situation of most women. Had I been more closely tied to a workplace, I would have breast-fed during my maternity leave and then given him formula exclusively, with no guilt.

My best guess is something I can't quite articulate. Breast-feeding does not belong in the realm of facts and hard numbers; it is much too intimate and elemental. It contains all of my awe about motherhood, and also my ambivalence. Right now, even part-time, it's a strain. But I also know that this is probably my last chance to feel warm baby skin up against mine, and one day I will miss it.

HANNA ROSIN is a senior editor of *The Atlantic* magazine.

EXPLORING THE ISSUE

Is Breastfeeding the Best Way to Feed Babies?

Critical Thinking and Reflection

1. What are the physical advantages for breastfeeding mothers?
2. Why is breast milk better for babies?
3. Describe some of the reasons why breastfeeding does not work for all women.

Is There Common Ground?

Most authorities believe that breastfeeding provides optimal nutrition for infants and is associated with a decreased risk for infant mortality. Breastfed babies may have fewer allergies, fewer ear infections, and higher IQs. Nursing mothers are more likely to lose weight gained during pregnancy and may have a reduced risk of breast and other cancers. Breast milk is also less costly than formula. There are, however, woman who should not breastfeed. For instance, women who use and/or abuse alcohol, nicotine, and other drugs should choose formula feeding. Alcohol enters breast milk and can affect its production, volume, and composition plus overwhelm a baby's ability to break down the alcohol. Drug abusers can take in such high doses that their babies can become addicted via breast milk. Smoking mothers produce less milk and milk with abnormal fat levels. As a result, their infants gain weight more slowly than infants of nonsmoking mothers. Nursing mothers who smoke also transfer nicotine and other harmful substances in their milk as well as expose their babies to secondhand smoke.

Other contraindications to breastfeeding include environmental contaminants. A woman may hesitate to nurse because of warnings about contaminants in water, freshwater fish, or other foods may enter her milk and have a negative effect on her child. Although some contaminants enter breast milk, others may be filtered out. Formula-fed infants may also be exposed to contaminants in the water used to dilute the formula.

If a woman has a minor illness such as a head cold, she can continue nursing without worry. If she has certain other illnesses, breastfeeding is contraindicated. Active, untreated tuberculosis is an example along with HIV/AIDS. The virus responsible for causing AIDS can be transmitted from an infected mother to her infant during pregnancy, at the time of birth, or via breast feeding, particularly during the early months of life. Overall, women who have tested positive for HIV should not breastfeed their babies.

While there are contraindications to breastfeeding, experts generally agree that there are significant benefits, especially in infancy. The long-term benefits are less clear. In "Breast Is Best: The Evidence (*Early Human Development*,

November 2010), the author discusses the benefits of breastfeeding in reducing illness and death from gastrointestinal and respiratory infections and sudden infant death syndrome. While these benefits are well established, long-term health effects are less clear. The evidence is controversial concerning the effect of breastfeeding in protecting against child obesity, elevated cholesterol, hypertension, and type 2 diabetes. Cognitive development has been associated with breastfeeding in many studies, although doubts remain about the results due to cognitive and behavioral differences between mothers who breastfeed (or those who breastfeed for a longer duration or more exclusively) and those who do not. In "What Research Does and Doesn't Say about Breastfeeding: A Critical Review" (*Early Child Development & Care*, July 2010), the authors review the research literature on breastfeeding benefits. It appears that while nursing offers many advantages to infants and mothers, the authors deduce that breastfeeding promotion initiatives sometimes exaggerate or misrepresent what the research actually supports. Psychological or cognitive benefits, particularly for full-term healthy infants, may be overemphasized. In some studies, variables such as income, education, and mother's IQ are not adequately taken into account. Studies that do address these variables often find little or no relationship between breastfeeding and cognitive outcomes except in the case of premature or low-birth weight infants. That view is not completely shared by the authors of "The Risks and Benefits of Infant Feeding Practices for Women and Their Children" (*Journal of Perinatology*, March 2010). They have determined that infant feeding decisions impact both mother and child health outcomes. The decision to bottle feed can harm maternal health by increasing the risk of pre-menopausal breast cancer, ovarian cancer, type 2 diabetes, hypertension, elevated cholesterol, and cardiovascular disease. Practitioners who advise pregnant women about the health impact of infant feeding and provide evidence-based care to enhance successful breast-feeding can maximize both the short- and long-term health of both mothers and babies.

Create Central

www.mhhe.com/createcentral

Additional Resources

Chadha, A. (2011). Encouraging breastfeeding on the national agenda. *Nation's Health, 41*(2), 7.

Saunders, J. B. (2011). Got milk? *State Legislatures, 37*(9), 25–28.

Savage, L. H. (2011). On breastfeeding, shame, and whether we've come to expect too much from mothers. *Maclean's, 124*(1), 16–19.

Wolf, J. B. (2011). *Is breast best? Taking on the breastfeeding experts and the new high stakes of motherhood.* New York, NY: New York University Press.

Internet References . . .

La Leche League International

Their mission is to help mothers worldwide to breastfeed through mother-to-mother support, encouragement, information, and education, and to promote a better understanding of breastfeeding as an important element in the healthy development of the baby and mother.

www.llli.org/

HealthyChildren.org—Breastfeeding

Information on infant feeding and nutrition.

www.healthychildren.org

Centers for Disease Control and Prevention: Breastfeeding

Information about the benefits of breastfeeding with numerous links.

www.cdc.gov/breastfeeding/

Selected, Edited, and with Issue Framing Material by:
Eileen Daniel, *SUNY College at Brockport*

ISSUE

Are Restrictions on Sugar and Sugary Beverages Justified?

YES: Gary Taubes and Cristin Kearns Couzens, from "Sweet Little Lies," *Mother Jones* (November/December 2012)

NO: Kenneth W. Krause, from "Saving Us from Sweets: This Is Science and Government on Sugar," *Skeptical Inquirer* (September/October 2012)

Learning Outcomes
After reading this issue, you should be able to: • Discuss the nutritional risk factors associated with the consumption of sugar and sugary beverages.   • Understand the role sugar and sugary beverages may play in the current obesity epidemic.   • Assess the need for government restrictions on the sale of sugar and sugar beverages.

ISSUE SUMMARY

YES: Writers Gary Taubes and Cristin Kearns Couzens maintain that added sugars and sweeteners pose dangers to health and that the sugar industry continually campaigns to enhance its image.

NO: Journalist Kenneth W. Krause argues that individuals have the ability to make decisions about sugar consumption themselves and that government should not restrict our access to sugar and sugar-containing food products.

The per capita consumption of refined sugar in the United States has varied between 60 and 100 pounds in the last 40 years. In 2008, American per capita total consumption of sugar and sweeteners, exclusive of artificial sweeteners, equaled 136 pounds per year. This consisted of 65.4 pounds of refined sugar and 68.3 pounds of corn-derived sweeteners per person. Granulated sugars are used at the table to sprinkle on foods and to sweeten hot drinks and in home baking to add sweetness and texture to cooked products. From a dietary perspective, the top five contributors to added sugars in our food supply are sugar-sweetened sodas, grain-based desserts and snacks such as cakes and cookies, fruit drinks, dairy-based desserts including ice cream, and puddings and candy.

There are numerous studies linking sugar to a variety of health concerns including diabetes and obesity. Studies on the relationship between sugars and diabetes are inconsistent since some propose that consuming large quantities of sugar does not directly increase the risk of diabetes. The extra calories, however, from eating excessive amounts of sugar can lead to obesity, which may itself increase the risk of developing this diabetes. Other studies show a relationship between refined sugar consumption and the onset

of diabetes. These included a 2010 analysis of 11 studies involving over 300,000 participants. Researchers found that sugar-sweetened beverages may increase the risk of developing type 2 diabetes through obesity and other metabolic abnormalities linked to sugar consumption.

To address the increasing rates of obesity and its link to diabetes and other diseases, the New York City Board of Health approved a ban on the sale of large sodas and other sugary drinks at restaurants, street carts, and movie theaters, the first restriction of its kind in the country, in the fall of 2012. The measure, promoted by Mayor Michael R. Bloomberg, is likely to strengthen a growing national debate about soft drinks and obesity, and it could prompt other cities to follow suit, despite the fact that many New Yorkers appear uncomfortable with the ban. The measure, which bars the sale of many sweetened drinks in containers larger than 16 ounces, was to take effect in March 2013. The vote by the Board of Health was the only regulatory approval needed to make the ban binding in the city, but the American soft drink industry has campaigned strongly against the measure and promised to fight it through other means, possibly in the courts. The soft drink industry argued that to single out one food item and claim it is the cause of obesity is inappropriate. While a state judge blocked the law in March 2013, the mayor vowed to continue his fight against mounting obesity by encouraging a ban on super large sized soft drinks.

Soft drink and other food manufacturers, like all companies, advertise and promote their products in order to maximize sales. Many non-nutritious foods are presented to the public in a misleading way for that purpose. For instance, low fiber, high sugar breakfast cereals may be sprinkled with vitamins and marketed as a low fat, nutritious breakfast. Some school districts, working with food manufacturers and producers, sell fast food items in school cafeterias. Soft drink companies have provided monies and other support to schools who promote their products. Non-nutritious foods including sugary breakfast cereals, fast food, and candy are heavily advertised on television shows catering to children.

Ethical and legal standards for the food industry, mandated by the government, could address some of these concerns. For instance, clearer food labels, which allow consumers to better understand what they're eating, might help reduce excessive consumption of calories, fat, and sugar. Many non-nutritious food labels seem to have incredibly small or unrealistic serving sizes. A more accurate serving size might be beneficial to consumers. A ban on the advertising of junk foods in public schools, specifically soft drinks, candy, and other items with high sugar content, could also be enacted as well as increased taxes on these foods. Alcohol and tobacco advertisements are not allowed on children's television, so it would seem reasonable to ban the promotion of foods that encourage overeating and obesity. In addition, non-nutritious foods could have health warnings similar to the warnings on cigarette packs or bottles of alcoholic beverages.

On the other hand, the proposed ban on the sale of large containers of soft drinks, while well intentioned, is controversial as some consumers wonder just how far the government should go to protect us from ourselves. To promote public health, New York City currently restricts smoking in public parks and bans trans fats from food served in restaurants. But Mayor Bloomberg's proposal raises questions about government's role in shaping and restricting individual choices. If government officials can limit the size of sodas, next it could decide to restrict portion sizes of restaurant food or the size of pre-made meals sold at supermarkets. If government is within its rights to restrict behavior to protect health, many other limits could be imposed in the name of health promotion. As many ponder the role of government in restricting the individual freedom to eat what one wants in whatever quantity, the rate of obesity in this country remains a serious health issue.

In addressing the question of whether or not restrictions on sugar and sugary beverages are justified, Gary Taubes and Cristin Kearns Couzens believe that added sugars and sweeteners pose a threat to health by increasing the risk for diabetes and heart disease. In countering with a NO answer, Kenneth W. Krause argues that individuals have the ability to make decisions about sugar consumption themselves and that government should not restrict our access to sugar or sugar-containing foods.

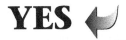

Taubes and Couzens

Sweet Little Lies

Inside an industry's campaign to frost its image, hold regulators at bay, and keep scientists from asking: **Does sugar kill?**

On a brisk spring Tuesday in 1976, a pair of executives from the Sugar Association stepped up to the podium of a Chicago ballroom to accept the Oscar of the public relations world, the Silver Anvil award for excellence in "the forging of public opinion." The trade group had recently pulled off one of the greatest turnarounds in PR history. For nearly a decade, the sugar industry had been buffeted by crisis after crisis as the media and the public soured on sugar and scientists began to view it as a likely cause of obesity, diabetes, and heart disease. Industry ads claiming that eating sugar helped you lose weight had been called out by the Federal Trade Commission, and the Food and Drug Administration had launched a review of whether sugar was even safe to eat. Consumption had declined 12 percent in just two years, and producers could see where that trend might lead. As John "JW" Tatem Jr. and Jack O'Connell Jr., the Sugar Association's president and director of public relations, posed that day with their trophies, their smiles only hinted at the coup they'd just pulled off.

Their winning campaign, crafted with the help of the prestigious public relations firm Carl Byoir & Associates, had been prompted by a poll showing that consumers had come to see sugar as fattening, and that most doctors suspected it might exacerbate, if not cause, heart disease and diabetes. With an initial annual budget of nearly $800,000 ($3.4 million today) collected from the makers of Dixie Crystals, Domino, C&H, Great Western, and other sugar brands, the association recruited a stable of medical and nutritional professionals to allay the public's fears, brought snack and beverage companies into the fold, and bankrolled scientific papers that contributed to a "highly supportive" FDA ruling, which, the Silver Anvil application boasted, made it "unlikely that sugar will be subject to legislative restriction in coming years."

The story of sugar, as Tatem told it, was one of a harmless product under attack by "opportunists dedicated to exploiting the consuming public." Over the subsequent decades, it would be transformed from what the *New York Times* in 1977 had deemed "a villain in disguise" into a nutrient so seemingly innocuous that even the American Heart Association and the American Diabetes Association approved it as part of a healthy diet. Research on the suspected links between sugar and chronic disease largely ground to a halt by the late 1980s, and scientists came to view such pursuits as a career dead end. So effective were the Sugar Association's efforts that, to this day, no consensus exists about sugar's potential dangers. The industry's PR campaign corresponded roughly with a significant rise in Americans' consumption of "caloric sweeteners," including table sugar (sucrose) and high-fructose corn syrup (HFCS). This increase was accompanied, in turn, by a surge in the chronic diseases increasingly linked to sugar. (See chart below.) Since 1970, obesity rates in the United States have more than doubled, while the incidence of diabetes has more than tripled.

Precisely how did the sugar industry engineer its turnaround? The answer is found in more than 1,500 pages of internal memos, letters, and company board reports we discovered buried in the archives of now-defunct sugar companies as well as in the recently released papers of deceased researchers and consultants who played key roles in the industry's strategy. They show how Big Sugar used Big Tobacco-style tactics to ensure that government agencies would dismiss troubling health claims against their products. Compared to the tobacco companies, which knew for a fact that their wares were deadly and spent billions of dollars trying to cover up that reality, the sugar industry had a relatively easy task. With the jury still out on sugar's health effects, producers simply needed to make sure that the uncertainty lingered. But the goal was the same: to safeguard sales by creating a body of evidence companies could deploy to counter any unfavorable research.

This decades-long effort to stack the scientific deck is why, today, the USDA's dietary guidelines only speak of sugar in vague generalities. ("Reduce the intake of calories from solid fats and added sugars.") It's why the FDA insists that sugar is "generally recognized as safe" despite considerable evidence suggesting otherwise. It's why some scientists' urgent calls for regulation of sugary products have been dead on arrival, and it's why—absent any federal leadership—New York City Mayor Michael Bloomberg felt compelled to propose a ban on oversized sugary drinks that passed in September.

In fact, a growing body of research suggests that sugar and its nearly chemically identical cousin, HFCS, may very well cause diseases that kill hundreds of thousands of Americans every year, and that these chronic conditions would be far less prevalent if we significantly dialed

Taubes, Gary and Couzens, Cristin Kearns. From *Mother Jones*, November/December 2012, pp. 35–40, 68–69. Copyright © 2012 by Mother Jones. Reprinted by permission of the Foundation for National Progress.

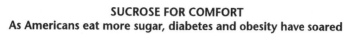

SUCROSE FOR COMFORT
As Americans eat more sugar, diabetes and obesity have soared

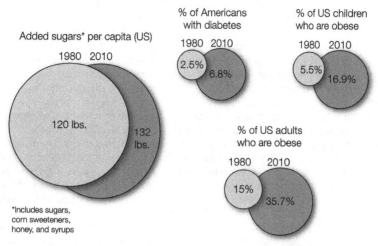

Added sugars* per capita (US)

1980   2010

120 lbs.

132 lbs.

*Includes sugars, corn sweeteners, honey, and syrups

% of Americans with diabetes

1980   2010

2.5%   6.8%

% of US children who are obese

1980   2010

5.5%   16.9%

% of US adults who are obese

1980   2010

15%   35.7%

Sources: USDA, CDC, US Census Bureau

back our consumption of added sugars. Robert Lustig, a leading authority on pediatric obesity at the University of California-San Francisco (whose arguments Gary explored in a 2011 *New York Times Magazine* cover story), made this case last February in the prestigious journal *Nature*. In an article titled "The Toxic Truth About Sugar," Lustig and two colleagues observed that sucrose and HFCS are addictive in much the same way as cigarettes and alcohol, and that overconsumption of them is driving worldwide epidemics of obesity and type 2 diabetes (the type associated with obesity). Sugar-related diseases are costing America around $150 billion a year, the authors estimated, so federal health officials need to step up and consider regulating the stuff.

The Sugar Association dusted off what has become its stock response: The Lustig paper, it said, "lacks the scientific evidence or consensus" to support its claims, and its authors were irresponsible not to point out that the full body of science "is inconclusive at best." This inconclusiveness, of course, is precisely what the Sugar Association has worked so assiduously to maintain. "In confronting our critics," Tatem explained to his board of directors back in 1976, "we try never to lose sight of the fact that no confirmed scientific evidence links sugar to the death-dealing diseases. This crucial point is the lifeblood of the association."

The Sugar Association's earliest incarnation dates back to 1943, when growers and refiners created the Sugar Research Foundation to counter World War II sugar-rationing propaganda—"How Much Sugar Do You Need? None!" declared one government pamphlet. In 1947, producers rechristened their group the Sugar Association and launched a new PR division, Sugar Information Inc., which

before long was touting sugar as a "sensible new approach to weight control." In 1968, in the hope of enlisting foreign sugar companies to help defray costs, the Sugar Association spun off its research division as the International Sugar Research Foundation. "Misconceptions concerning the causes of tooth decay, diabetes, and heart problems exist on a worldwide basis," explained a 1969 ISRF recruiting brochure.

As early as 1962, internal Sugar Association memos had acknowledged the potential links between sugar and chronic diseases, but at the time sugar executives had a more pressing problem: Weight-conscious Americans were switching in droves to diet sodas—particularly Diet Rite and Tab—sweetened with cyclamate and saccharin. From 1963 through 1968, diet soda's share of the soft-drink market shot from 4 percent to 15 percent. "A dollar's worth of sugar," ISRF vice president and research director John Hickson warned in an internal review, "could be replaced with a dime's worth" of sugar alternatives. "If anyone can undersell you nine cents out of 10," Hickson told the *New York Times* in 1969, "you'd better find some brickbat you can throw at him."

By then, the sugar industry had doled out more than $600,000 (about $4 million today) to study every conceivable harmful effect of cyclamate sweeteners, which are still sold around the world under names like Sugar Twin and Sucaryl. In 1969, the FDA banned cyclamates in the United States based on a study suggesting they could cause bladder cancer in rats. Not long after, Hickson left the ISRF to work for the Cigar Research Council. He was described in a confidential tobacco industry memo as a "supreme scientific politician who had been successful in condemning cyclamates, on behalf of the [sugar industry], on somewhat shaky evidence." It later emerged that the evidence suggesting that cyclamates caused cancer in rodents was not relevant to humans, but by then the case was officially closed. In 1977, saccharin, too, was nearly banned on the basis of animal results that would turn out to be meaningless in people.

Meanwhile, researchers had been reporting that blood lipids—cholesterol and triglycerides in particular—were a risk factor in heart disease. Some people had high cholesterol but normal triglycerides, prompting health experts to recommend that they avoid animal fats. Other people were deemed "carbohydrate sensitive," with normal cholesterol but markedly increased triglyceride levels. In these individuals, even moderate sugar consumption could cause a spike in triglycerides. John Yudkin, the United Kingdom's leading nutritionist, was making headlines with claims that sugar, not fat, was the primary cause of heart disease.

In 1967, the Sugar Association's research division began considering "the rising tide of implications of sucrose in atherosclerosis." Before long, according to a confidential 1970 review of industry-funded studies, the newly formed ISRF was spending 10 percent of its research budget on the link between diet and heart disease. Hickson, the ISRF's vice president, urged his member corporations to keep the results of the review under wraps. Of particular concern was the work of a University of Pennsylvania researcher on "sucrose sensitivity," which sugar executives feared was "likely to reveal evidence of harmful effects." One ISRF consultant recommended that sugar companies get to the truth of the matter by sponsoring a full-on study. In what would become a pattern, the ISRF opted not to follow his advice. Another ISRF-sponsored study, by biochemist Walter Pover of the University of Birmingham, in England, had uncovered a possible mechanism to explain how sugar raises triglyceride levels. Pover believed he was on the verge of demonstrating this mechanism "conclusively" and that 18 more weeks of work would nail it down. But instead of providing the funds, the ISRF nixed the project, assessing its value as "nil."

The industry followed a similar strategy when it came to diabetes. By 1973, links between sugar, diabetes, and heart disease were sufficiently troubling that Sen. George McGovern of South Dakota convened a hearing of his Select Committee on Nutrition and Human Needs to address the issue. An international panel of experts—including Yudkin and Walter Mertz, head of the Human Nutrition Institute at the Department of Agriculture—testified that variations in sugar consumption were the best explanation for the differences in diabetes rates between populations, and that research by the USDA and others supported the notion that eating too much sugar promotes dramatic population-wide increases in the disease. One panelist, South African diabetes specialist George Campbell, suggested that anything more than 70 pounds per person per year—about half of what is sold in America today—would spark epidemics.

In the face of such hostile news from independent scientists, the ISRF hosted its own conference the following March, focusing exclusively on the work of researchers who were skeptical of a sugar/diabetes connection. "All those present agreed that a large amount of research is still necessary before a firm conclusion can be arrived at," according to a conference review published in a prominent diabetes journal. In 1975, the foundation reconvened in Montreal to discuss research priorities with its consulting scientists. Sales were sinking, Tatem reminded the gathered sugar execs, and a major factor was "the impact of consumer advocates who link sugar consumption with certain diseases."

Following the Montreal conference, the ISRF disseminated a memo quoting Errol Marliss, a University of Toronto diabetes specialist, recommending that the industry pursue "well-designed research programs" to establish sugar's role in the course of diabetes and other diseases. "Such research programs *might* produce an answer that sucrose is bad in certain individuals," he warned. But the studies "should be undertaken in a sufficiently comprehensive way as to produce results. A gesture rather than full support is unlikely to produce the sought-after answers."

A gesture, however, is what the industry would offer. Rather than approve a serious investigation of the purported links between sucrose and disease, American sugar companies quit supporting the ISRF's research projects. Instead, via the Sugar Association proper, they would spend roughly $655,000 between 1975 and 1980 on 17 studies designed, as internal documents put it, "to maintain research as a main prop of the industry's defense." Each proposal was vetted by a panel of industry-friendly scientists and a second committee staffed by representatives from sugar companies and "contributing research members" such as Coca-Cola, Hershey's, General Mills, and Nabisco. Most of the cash was awarded to researchers whose studies seemed explicitly designed to exonerate sugar. One even proposed to explore whether sugar could be shown to boost serotonin levels in rats' brains, and thus "prove of therapeutic value, as in the relief of depression," an internal document noted.

At best, the studies seemed a token effort. Harvard Medical School professor Ron Arky, for example, received money from the Sugar Association to determine whether sucrose has a different effect on blood sugar and other diabetes indicators if eaten alongside complex carbohydrates like pectin and psyllium. The project went nowhere, Arky told us recently. But the Sugar Association "didn't care."

In short, rather than do definitive research to learn the truth about its product, good or bad, the association stuck to a PR scheme designed to "establish with the broadest possible audience—virtually everyone is a consumer—the safety of sugar as a food." One of its first acts was to establish a Food & Nutrition Advisory Council consisting of a half-dozen physicians and two dentists willing to defend sugar's place in a healthy diet, and set aside roughly $60,000 per year (more than $220,000 today) to cover its cost.

Working to the industry's recruiting advantage was the rising notion that cholesterol and dietary fat—especially saturated fat—were the likely causes of heart disease. (Tatem even suggested, in a letter to the *Times Magazine*, that some "sugar critics" were motivated merely by wanting "to keep the heat off saturated fats.") This was the brainchild of nutritionist Ancel Keys, whose University of Minnesota laboratory had received financial support from the sugar industry as early as 1944. From the 1950s through the 1980s, Keys remained the most outspoken proponent of the fat hypothesis, often clashing publicly with Yudkin, the most vocal supporter of the sugar hypothesis—the two men "shared a good deal of loathing," recalled one of Yudkin's colleagues.

So when the Sugar Association needed a heart disease expert for its Food & Nutrition Advisory Council, it approached Francisco Grande, one of Keys' closest colleagues. Another panelist was University of Oregon nutritionist William Connor, the leading purveyor of the notion that it is dietary cholesterol that causes heart disease. As its top diabetes expert, the industry recruited Edwin Bierman of the University of Washington, who believed that diabetics need not pay strict attention to their sugar intake so long as they maintained a healthy weight by burning off the calories they consumed. Bierman also professed an apparently unconditional faith that it was dietary fat (and *being* fat) that caused heart disease, with sugar having no meaningful effect.

It is hard to overestimate Bierman's role in shifting the diabetes conversation away from sugar. It was primarily Bierman who convinced the American Diabetes Association to liberalize the amount of carbohydrates (including sugar) it recommended in the diets of diabetics, and focus more on urging diabetics to lower their fat intake, since diabetics are particularly likely to die from heart disease. Bierman also presented industry-funded studies when he coauthored a section on potential causes for a National Commission on Diabetes report in 1976; the document influences the federal diabetes research agenda to this day. Some researchers, he acknowledged, had "argued eloquently" that consumption of refined carbohydrates (such as sugar) is a precipitating factor in diabetes. But then Bierman cited five studies—two of them bankrolled by the ISRF—that were "inconsistent" with that hypothesis. "A review of all available laboratory and epidemiologic evidence," he concluded, "suggests that the most important dietary factor in increasing the risk of diabetes is total calorie intake, irrespective of source."

The point man on the industry's food and nutrition panel was Frederick Stare, founder and chairman of the department of nutrition at the Harvard School of Public Health. Stare and his department had a long history of ties to Big Sugar. An ISRF internal research review credited the sugar industry with funding some 30 papers in his department from 1952 through 1956 alone. In 1960, the department broke ground on a new $5 million building funded largely by private donations, including a $1 million gift from General Foods, the maker of Kool-Aid and Tang.

By the early 1970s, Stare ranked among the industry's most reliable advocates, testifying in Congress about the wholesomeness of sugar even as his department kept raking in funding from sugar producers and food and beverage giants such as Carnation, Coca-Cola, Gerber, Kellogg, and Oscar Mayer. His name also appears in tobacco documents, which show that he procured industry funding for a study aimed at exonerating cigarettes as a cause of heart disease.

The first act of the Food & Nutrition Advisory Council was to compile "Sugar in the Diet of Man," an 88-page white paper edited by Stare and published in 1975 to "organize existing scientific facts concerning sugar." It was a compilation of historical evidence and arguments that sugar companies could use to counter the claims of Yudkin, Stare's Harvard colleague Jean Mayer, and other researchers whom Tatem called "enemies of sugar." The document was sent to reporters—the Sugar Association circulated 25,000 copies—along with a press release headlined "Scientists dispel sugar fears." The report neglected to mention that it was funded by the sugar industry, but internal documents confirm that it was.

The Sugar Association also relied on Stare to take its message to the people: "Place Dr. Stare on the AM America Show" and "Do a 3½ minute interview with Dr. Stare for 200 radio stations," note the association's meeting minutes. Using Stare as a proxy, internal documents explained, would help the association "make friends with the networks" and "keep the sugar industry in the background." By the time Stare's copious conflicts of interest were finally revealed—in "Professors on the Take," a 1976 exposé by the Center for Science in the Public Interest—Big Sugar no longer needed his assistance. The industry could turn to an FDA document to continue where he'd left off.

While Stare and his colleagues had been drafting "Sugar in the Diet of Man," the FDA was launching its first review of whether sugar was, in the official jargon, generally recognized as safe (GRAS), part of a series of food-additive reviews the Nixon administration had requested of the agency. The FDA subcontracted the task to the Federation of American Societies of Experimental Biology, which created an 11-member committee to vet hundreds of food additives from acacia to zinc sulfate. While the mission of the GRAS committee was to conduct unbiased reviews of the existing science for each additive, it was led by biochemist George W. Irving Jr., who had previously served two years as chairman of the scientific advisory board of the International Sugar Research Foundation. Industry documents show that another committee member, Samuel Fomon, had received sugar-industry funding for three of the five years prior to the sugar review.

The FDA's instructions were clear: To label a substance as a potential health hazard, there had to be "credible evidence of, or reasonable grounds to suspect, adverse biological effects"—which certainly existed for sugar at the time. But the GRAS committee's review would depend heavily on "Sugar in the Diet of Man" and other work by its authors. In the section on heart disease, committee members cited 14 studies whose results were "conflicting," but 6 of those bore industry fingerprints, including Francisco Grande's chapter from "Sugar in the Diet of Man" and 5 others that came from Grande's lab or were otherwise funded by the sugar industry.

The diabetes chapter of the review acknowledged studies suggesting that "long term consumption of sucrose can result in a functional change in the capacity to metabolize carbohydrates and thus lead to diabetes mellitus," but it went on to cite five reports contradicting that notion. All had industry ties, and three were authored by Ed Bierman, including his chapter in "Sugar in the Diet of Man."

In January 1976, the GRAS committee published its preliminary conclusions, noting that while sugar probably contributed to tooth decay, it was not a "hazard to the public." The draft review dismissed the diabetes link as "circumstantial" and called the connection to cardiovascular disease "less than clear," with fat playing a greater role. The only cautionary note, besides cavities, was that all bets were off if sugar consumption were to increase significantly. The committee then thanked the Sugar Association for contributing "information and data." (Tatem would later remark that while he was "proud of the credit line . . . we would probably be better off without it.")

The committee's perspective was shared by many researchers, but certainly not all. For a public hearing on the draft review, scientists from the USDA's Carbohydrate Nutrition Laboratory submitted what they considered "abundant evidence that sucrose is one of the dietary factors responsible for obesity, diabetes, and heart disease." As they later explained in the *American Journal of Clinical Nutrition,* some portion of the public—perhaps 15 million Americans at that time—clearly could not tolerate a diet rich in sugar and other carbohydrates. Sugar consumption, they said, should come down by "a minimum of 60 percent," and the government should launch a national campaign "to inform the populace of the hazards of excessive sugar consumption." But the committee stood by its conclusions in the final version of its report presented to the FDA in October 1976.

For the sugar industry, the report was gospel. The findings "should be memorized" by the staff of every company associated with the sugar industry, Tatem told his membership. "In the long run," he said, the document "cannot be sidetracked, and you may be sure we will push its exposure to all comers of the country."

The association promptly produced an ad for newspapers and magazines exclaiming "Sugar is Safe!" It "does not cause death-dealing diseases," the ad declared, and "there is no substantiated scientific evidence indicating that sugar causes diabetes, heart disease or any other malady. . . . The next time you hear a promoter attacking sugar, beware the ripoff. Remember he can't substantiate his charges. Ask yourself what he's promoting or what he is seeking to cover up. If you get a chance, ask him about the GRAS Review Report. Odds are you won't get an answer. Nothing stings a nutritional liar like scientific facts."

The Sugar Association would soon get its chance to put the committee's sugar review to the test. In 1977, McGovern's select committee—the one that had held the 1973 hearings on sugar and diabetes—blindsided the industry with a report titled "Dietary Goals for the United States," recommending that Americans lower their sugar intake by 40 percent. The association "hammered away" at the McGovern report using the GRAS review "as our scientific Bible," Tatem told sugar executives.

McGovern held fast, but Big Sugar would prevail in the end. In 1980, when the USDA first published its own set of dietary guidelines, it relied heavily on a review written for the American Society of Clinical Nutrition by none other than Bierman, who used the GRAS committee's findings to bolster his own. "Contrary to widespread opinion, too much sugar does not seem to cause diabetes," the USDA guidelines concluded. They went on to counsel that people should "avoid too much sugar," without bothering to explain what that meant.

In 1982, the FDA once again took up the GRAS committee's conclusion that sugar was safe, proposing to make it official. The announcement resulted in a swarm of public criticism, prompting the agency to reopen its case. Four years later, an agency task force concluded, again leaning on industry-sponsored studies, that "there is no conclusive evidence . . . that demonstrates a hazard to the general public when sugars are consumed at the levels that are now current." (Walter Glinsmann, the task force's lead administrator, would later become a consultant to the Corn Refiners Association, which represents producers of high-fructose corn syrup.)

The USDA, meanwhile, had updated its own dietary guidelines. With Fred Stare now on the advisory committee, the 1985 guidelines retained the previous edition's vague recommendation to "avoid too much" sugar but stated unambiguously that "too much sugar in your diet does not cause diabetes." At the time, the USDA's own Carbohydrate Nutrition Laboratory was still generating evidence to the contrary and supporting the notion that "even low sucrose intake" might be contributing to heart disease in 10 percent of Americans.

By the early 1990s, the USDA's research into sugar's health effects had ceased, and the FDA's take on sugar had become conventional wisdom, influencing a generation's worth of key publications on diet and health. Reports from the surgeon general and the National Academy of Sciences repeated the mantra that the evidence linking sugar to chronic disease was inconclusive, and then went on to equate "inconclusive" with "nonexistent." They also ignored a crucial caveat: The FDA reviewers had deemed added sugars—those in excess of what occurs naturally in our diets—safe at "current" 1986 consumption levels.

But the FDA's consumption estimate was 43 percent lower than that of its sister agency, the USDA. By 1999, the average American would be eating more than double the amount the FDA had deemed safe—although we have cut back by 13 percent since then.

Asked to comment on some of the documents described in this article, a Sugar Association spokeswoman responded that they are "at this point historical in nature and do not necessarily reflect the current mission or function" of the association. But it is clear enough that the industry still operates behind the scenes to make sure regulators never officially set a limit on the amount of sugar Americans can safely consume. The authors of the 2010 USDA dietary guidelines, for instance, cited two scientific reviews as evidence that sugary drinks don't make adults fat. The first was written by Sigrid Gibson, a nutrition consultant whose clients included the Sugar Bureau (England's version of the Sugar Association) and the World Sugar Research Organization (formerly the ISRF). The second review was authored by Carrie Ruxton, who served as research manager of the Sugar Bureau from 1995 to 2000.

The Sugar Association has also worked its connections to assure that the government panels making dietary recommendations—the USDA's Dietary Guidelines Advisory Committee, for instance—include researchers sympathetic to its position. One internal newsletter boasted in 2003 that for the USDA panel, the association had "worked diligently to achieve the nomination of another expert wholly through third-party endorsements."

In the few instances when governmental authorities have sought to reduce people's sugar consumption, the industry has attacked openly. In 2003, after an expert panel convened by the World Health Organization recommended that no more than 10 percent of all calories in people's diets should come from added sugars—nearly 40 percent less than the USDA's estimate for the average American—current Sugar Association president Andrew Briscoe wrote the WHO'S director general warning that the association would "exercise every avenue available to expose the dubious nature" of the report and urge "congressional appropriators to challenge future funding" for the WHO. Larry Craig (R-Idaho, sugar beets) and John Breaux (D-La., sugarcane), then co-chairs of the Senate Sweetener Caucus, wrote a letter to Secretary of Health and Human Services Tommy Thompson, urging his "prompt and favorable attention" to prevent the report from becoming official WHO policy. (Craig had received more than $36,000 in sugar industry contributions in the previous election cycle.) Thompson's people responded with a 28-page letter detailing "where the US Government's policy recommendations and interpretation of the sci-

ence differ" with the WHO report. Not surprisingly, the organization left its experts' recommendation on sugar intake out of its official dietary strategy.

In recent years, the scientific tide has begun to turn against sugar. Despite the industry's best efforts, researchers and public health authorities have come to accept that the primary risk factor for both heart disease and type 2 diabetes is a condition called metabolic syndrome, which now affects more than 75 million Americans, according to the Centers for Disease Control and Prevention. Metabolic syndrome is characterized by a cluster of abnormalities—some of which Yudkin and others associated with sugar almost 50 years ago—including weight gain, increased insulin levels, and elevated triglycerides. It also has been linked to cancer and Alzheimer's disease. "Scientists have now established causation," Lustig said recently. "Sugar causes metabolic syndrome."

Newer studies from the University of California-Davis have even reported that LDL cholesterol, the classic risk factor for heart disease, can be raised significantly in just *two weeks* by drinking sugary beverages at a rate well within the upper range of what Americans consume—four 12-ounce glasses a day of beverages like soda, Snapple, or Red Bull. The result is a new wave of researchers coming out publicly against Big Sugar.

During the battle over the 2005 USDA guidelines, an internal Sugar Association newsletter described its strategy toward anyone who had the temerity to link sugar consumption with chronic disease and premature death: "Any disparagement of sugar," it read, "will be met with forceful, strategic public comments and the supporting science." But since the latest science is anything but supportive of the industry, what happens next?

"At present," Lustig ventures, "they have absolutely no reason to alter any of their practices. The science is in—the medical and economic problems with excessive sugar consumption are clear. But the industry is going to fight tooth and nail to prevent that science from translating into public policy."

Like the tobacco industry before it, the sugar industry may be facing the inexorable exposure of its product as a killer—science will ultimately settle the matter one way or the other—but as Big Tobacco learned a long time ago, even the inexorable can be held up for a very long time.

Gary Taubes is a science writer and journalist.

Cristin Kearns Couzens is a senior consultant at the University of Colorado Center for Health Administration and an acting instructor at the University of Washington School of Dentistry.

Kenneth W. Krause

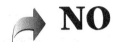

Saving Us from Sweets: This Is Science and Government on Sugar

I've carried an intense personal grudge against "sugar" for decades. No, not the mostly benign, unrefined types packed into blueberries, green beans, and pumpernickels, for example. And no, not *only* the sickly sweet stuff shamelessly dumped into sodas, pastries, and swirling coffee froths either. I truly despise every pale-ish, pure and innocent looking slice of bread, wedge of potato, and grain of rice, and, I promise you, no pasta noodle, cracker, or corn flake will ever again bamboozle its way into my ever-shriveling food pantry.

At emotionally critical moments, my well-intentioned mother told me I was "husky" or "big-boned," which, by the way, is never true if it needs to be said. I was just plain F-A-T—obese, actually, just like more than a third of Americans today—until my junior year of high school. At that fateful point, I got fed up and decided to take matters into my own ignorant yet determined hands. Thanks to vigorous exercise and a dramatically reformed diet, I dropped seventy pounds in about three months. From then on, my world just got bigger and brighter.

Even now, at age forty-seven, I can relish every exhilaration my aging body will tolerate. In fact, I've recently given up weight lifting and jogging for power lifting, plyometrics, and high-intensity intervals. Last month, I look up mountain biking (the initial wounds should heal well before publication) because road cycling just wasn't exciting enough anymore.

I'm not bragging. Truth he told, I'm not particularly good at any of it. The point, rather, is that I love it all, and that I should have enjoyed an even richer physical life as a kid. In some tragic measure, I squandered the most dynamic years of my life guzzling and gobbling the same general strain of refuse that farmers use every day to fatten their cattle for slaughter. Yes, I'm a little bitter about sugar.

And I'm clearly not alone. "Clean-eating" advocates now dominate the nutrition world, and most of us agree generally with food guru Michael Pollan that we should eat less and that our diets should consist of mostly plants. Nevertheless, others in our ranks have lately embraced a more militant and less scientifically defensible approach to the problem.

Take, for example, Robert Lustig, Laura Schmidt, and Claire Brindis, three public health experts from the University or California, San Francisco. In a recent issue of *Nature*, they compared the "deadly effect" of added sugars (high-fructose corn syrup and sucrose) to that of alcohol. When consumed to excess, they observe, both substances cause a host of dreadful maladies, including hypertension, myocardial infarction, dyslipidemia, pancreatitis, obesity, malnutrition, hepatic dysfunction, and habituation (if not addiction).[1]

Far from mere "empty calories," they add, sugar is potentially "toxic." It alters metabolism, raises blood pressure, causes hormonal chaos, and damages our livers. Like both tobacco and alcohol (a distillation of sugar), it affects our brains, encouraging us to increase consumption. Indeed, they say, worldwide sugar consumption has tripled in the last fifty years.

Thus, Lustig et al. infer that sugar is at least partly responsible tor thirty-five million deaths every year from chronic, non-communicable diseases, which according to the United Nations now pose a greater health risk worldwide than their infectious counterparts. The authors also point out that Americans waste $65 billion in lost productivity and $150 billion on health-care related resources annually vis-à-vis illnesses linked to sugar-induced metabolic syndrome.

At the risk of piling on, I should emphasise that 17 percent of U.S. children are now obese too, and that the average American consumes more than forty pounds of high-fructose corn syrup per year. Recent investigations suggest that sugar might also impair our cognition. For example, in a new study from the University of California, Los Angeles, physiologist Fernando Gomez-Pinilla concludes that dicts consistently high in fructose can slow brain functions and weaken memory and learning in rats.

All of this reinforces my already firm personal resolve. But apparently many accomplished scientists lack not only confidence in our abilities as individuals to educate or control ourselves, but also respect for our rights to disagree or to make informed but less than perfectly rational decisions regarding our private consumption habits. As such, Lustig et al. urge Americans especially to support restrictions on their own liberty in the form of government-imposed regulation of sugar.

To support their cause, Lustig et al. rely on four criteria, "now largely accepted by the public health community,"

Krause, Kenneth W. From *Skeptical Inquirer*, September/October 2012, pp. 24–25, 59. Copyright © 2012 by Skeptical Inquirer. Reprinted by permission. www.csicop.org

originally offered by social psychologist Thomas Babor in 2003 to justify the regulation of alcohol. The target substance must be toxic and unavoidable (or pervasive), and it must have a negative impact on society and a potential for abuse. Sugar satisfies each requirement, they contend, and is thus analogous to alcohol in terms of demanding bureaucratic imposition.

In a letter to me, Gomez-Pinilla echoed their concerns. Diabetes and obesity, he specified, come with greatly increased risks of several neurological and psychiatric disorders. In light of both the human and economic costs, he opined broadly, "it is in the general public concern to regulate high-sugar products as well as other unhealthy aspects of diet and lifestyle."

Unsurprisingly, the *Nature* paper inspired a flurry of defiant correspondences. Observers close to the sugar industry quickly took issue with both the researchers' facts and their logic. Richard Cottrell from the World Sugar Research Organisation in London first disputed the San Franciscans' calculation of worldwide sugar consumption. Because global population has more than doubled since 1960, he corrected, intake has increased only by 60 percent, not 300 percent. Moreover, he added, consumption in the United States, the United Kingdom, and Canada has risen only marginally as a proportion of total food-energy intake.

Judging metabolic syndrome a "controversial concept" in itself, Cottrell then cited analyses from the United Nations, the United States, and Europe that found no evidence of typical sugar consumption's contribution to any non-dental disease. On the other hand, he chided, "Overconsumption of anything is harmful, including water and air."

Ron Boswell, a senator from Queensland, Australia, noted that while the overweight population in his country has doubled and the incidence of diabetes has tripled since 1980, sugar consumption has actually dropped 23 percent during the same period. To describe sugar as "toxic," he continued, "is extreme, as is its ludicrous comparison with alcohol." The senator then scolded Lustig et al. for risking "damage to the livelihoods of thousands of people working in the sugar industry worldwide."

Other writers were no less reproachful. Christiani Jeyakumar Henry, a nutrition researcher in Singapore, criticized the *Nature* piece for its exclusive emphasis on sugar. Several foods with high glycemic indices, he noted, including wheat, rice, and potatoes, also contribute to both obesity and diabetes. Finally, writing from the University of Vermont, Burlington, Saleem Ali criticized the San Franciscans' "misleading" comparison of sugar to alcohol and tobacco, the former of which causes neither behavioral intoxication nor second-hand contamination.

But David Katz, MD, renowned nutritionist and founding director of the Yale University Prevention Research Center, has long contested Lustig's claims. Last spring, for example, Katz characterized the researcher's dualistic, good vs. evil attacks on sugar as fanatical "humbug." "It is

the overall quality and quantity of our diet that matters," be reasoned, "not just one villainous or virtuous nutrient du jour."

Refreshingly, Katz reassessed the subject from a broader, more reliable perspective based on evolutionary science. "We like sweet," he appreciated, "because mammals who like sweet are more apt to survive than mammals who don't. Period." Why should it shock and abhor so many of us that sugar is addictive? The real surprise, Katz answered, is not that high-energy food is habit-forming, "but rather that anything else is."

Katz's subsequent response to the *Nature* article, however, sends a frustratingly abstruse and well-mixed message. On the one hand, he recognizes that "Regulating nutrients, *per se*, is a slippery slope." Good intentions, he wisely if somewhat vaguely counsels, "could bog us down in conflict that forestalls all progress, distort the relative importance of just one nutrient relative to overall nutrition," and lead us to "unintended consequences."

On the other hand, Katz expressly defends some of Lustig et al.'s proposed governmental intrusions, Most reasonably, he favors restrictions on the sale of sugary products to kids where their attendance is officially compelled. "There is no reason," he argues, "why schools should be propagating the consumption of solid or liquid candy by students." Many locales have already seen fit to install such policies.

Far less noble, however, is the good doctor's support for punitive taxes on sugary drinks. "There is no inalienable right to afford soda in the Constitution," he observes. Those of lesser means, Katz resolves, "should perhaps consider that they can't afford to squander such limited funds on the empty calories of soda." Indeed they should, but Katz never explains how people can make decisions already made on their behalf.

But—in the name of science, most regrettably— Lustig et al. advocate considerably more intrusive schemes decorously styled "gentle, supply-side" controls. Unsatisfied with a soda tax, they favor a similar penalty on "processed foods that contain any form of added sugars." That means ketchup, salsa, jam, deli meat, frozen fruit, many breads, and chocolate milk (now highly rated as a recovery drink following intense exercise). Ideally, the trio adds, such tariffs would be accompanied by an outright "ban" on television advertisements.

The San Franciscans would like to "limit availability" as well, by "reducing the hours that retailers are open, controlling the location and density of retail markets and limiting who can legally purchase the products." Alluding to a cadre of parents in South Philadelphia who recently blocked children from entering nearby convenience stores for snacks, Lustig et al. inquired, "Why couldn't a public health directive do the same?"

In late May of this year, New York City Mayor Michael Bloomberg announced the first plan in U.S. history to outlaw the sale of large sugary drinks—anything over sixteen fluid ounces—in all restaurants, movie theaters, sports arenas, and even from street carts. If approved by the Bloomberg-appointed Board of Health, the ban could take effect next March.

Sugar can be bad; most of us get that. But even the most impassioned personal grudge against potentially harmful food is just that—personal. Science, like government, is valued beyond calculation insofar as it expands personal choice. But the appropriate boundaries of science are almost always exceeded when it attempts to join with government to first judge the masses incompetent and then restrict their personal choices.

I grow particularly nervous when even the most distinguished researchers transcend their callings to campaign for product taxes and bans or, most egregiously, to vaguely advocate for the regulation of "unhealthy aspects of diet and lifestyle." Science's time-tested authority springs vibrantly from its practitioners' exacting and impartial roles as explorers, skeptics, and even teachers. But never has it spawned from the deluded cravings of some to act as our parents or priests.

Notes

1. The authors dispute the common assertion that these diseases are caused by obesity. Rather, they argue, obesity is merely "a marker for metabolic dysfunction, which is even more prevalent." In support, they cite statistics showing that 20 percent of obese people have normal metabolism and that 40 percent of normal-weight people develop metabolic syndrome.
2. Neither "inalienable" nor "unalienable" rights are listed in the Constitution, of course. But three of the latter—life, liberty, and the pursuit of happiness—are enshrined in the Declaration of Independence. Katz and others might wish to reexamine their historical and philosophical significance.

KENNETH W. KRAUSE is a contributing editor, book editor, and "The Good Book" columnist for *The Humanist* and a contributing editor and columnist for *Skeptical Inquirer*.

EXPLORING THE ISSUE

Are Restrictions on Sugar and Sugary Beverages Justified?

Critical Thinking and Reflection

1. What impact would restriction of sugar and sugary beverages have on our right to make individual choices?
2. Do the health risks of sugar warrant bans on the sale of large sized sugary beverages?
3. Describe the role government should play in regards to prevention of obesity.

Is There Common Ground?

Jacob Sullum, in "The War on Fat: Is the Size of Your Butt the Government's Business?" (*Reason*, August/September 2004), grants that while obesity is a health problem, it should not be a government issue. Despite Sullum's views, Americans have been steadily gaining weight over the past 30 years. Children, in particular, have grown heavier for a variety of reasons including less physical activity, more eating away from home, and increased portion sizes. Food manufacturers advertise an increasing array of non-nutritious foods to children while schools offer these foods in the cafeteria. With the success of the antismoking forces, some nutritionists see the government as the answer to the obesity problem. Increased taxes on junk food, warning labels on non-nutritious food packages, and restrictions on advertising have all been discussed as a means of improving the nation's nutritional status. In "The Perils of Ignoring History: Big Tobacco Played Dirty and Millions Died. How Similar Is Big Food?" (*Milbank Quarterly*, March 2009), the authors discussed how in 1954 the tobacco industry paid to publish the "Frank Statement to Cigarette Smokers" in hundreds of U.S. newspapers. It stated that the public's health was the industry's concern above all others and promised a variety of good-faith changes. What followed were years of lies and actions that cost countless lives. The tobacco industry had a script that focused on personal responsibility, paying scientists who delivered research that instilled doubt, criticizing the "junk" science that found risks associated with smoking, making self-regulatory pledges, lobbying with massive resources to stifle government action, introducing "safer" products, and simultaneously manipulating and denying both the addictive nature of their products and their marketing to children. The script of the food industry is both similar to and different from the tobacco industry script. Food is quite different from tobacco, and the food industry differs from tobacco companies in other ways, but there are also major similarities in the actions that these two industries have taken in response to concern that their products cause disease. Because obesity is now a major global problem, the world cannot afford a repeat of the tobacco history. If sugary food advertisements were banned from children's television, less might be consumed.

Other proposals to improve Americans' diets include levying a tax on sugary foods such as soft drinks, candy, and sugared cereals and the ban on trans fats in New York City. While many states already tax these items if purchased in a restaurant or grocery store, proponents argue that these foods should be taxed regardless of where purchased. While this may seem to be a reasonable approach to address the problem, it is not approved by all. The food industry, understandably, is not in favor of any of these measures.

Create Central

www.mhhe.com/createcentral

Additional Resources

Is a Ban on Large Sodas the Answer to Obesity? (2012, June 18). *New York Times*, p. 22.

Grynbaum, M. M. (2012, July 24). Fighting ban on big sodas with appeals to patriotism. *New York Times*, p. 18.

Lustig, R. H., Schmidt, L. A., & Brindis, C. D. (2012). The toxic truth about sugar. *Nature, 482,* 27–29.

Sullum, J. (2012). Bloomberg's big beverage ban. *Reason, 44*(5), 8.

Zmuda, N. & Morrison, M. (2012). Sugary-drink ban would trim bottom lines. *Advertising Age, 83*(23), 2–19.

Internet References . . .

The American Dietetic Association

www.eatright.org

Center for Science in the Public Interest (CSPI)

www.cspinet.org

Food and Nutrition Information Center

www.nalusda.gov/fnic/index.html

The Sugar Association, Inc.

www.sugar.org

Unit 6

Consumer Health

A shift is occurring in medical care toward informed self-care. People are starting to reclaim their autonomy, and the relationship between doctor and patient is changing. Many patients are asking more questions of their physicians, considering a wider range of medical options, accessing medical information online, focusing on prevention, and in general, becoming more educated about what determines their health. They are also concerned about the quality of numerous consumer health products, drugs, and services available to them. This unit addresses consumer issues and initiatives that empower consumers to make decisions and take actions that improve personal, family, and community health.

Selected, Edited, and with Issue Framing Material by:
Eileen Daniel, *SUNY College at Brockport*

ISSUE

Is Weight-Loss Maintenance Possible?

YES: **Barbara Berkeley,** from "The Fat Trap: My Response" (December 29, 2011) www.refusetoregain.com/2011/12/the-fat-trap-my-response.html

NO: **Tara Parker-Pope,** from "The Fat Trap," *The New York Times Magazine* (January 1, 2012)

Learning Outcomes
After reading this issue, you should be able to: • Discuss why it is so difficult for many people to maintain weight loss.   • Discuss the argument that weight-loss maintenance is not possible for most people.   • Discuss the risk factors associated with obesity and overweight.

ISSUE SUMMARY

YES: Physician Barbara Berkeley believes that weight maintenance is not easy but possible as long as people separate themselves from the world of typical American eating. She also claims that some individuals are heavy because they are susceptible to the modern diet or because they use food for comfort.

NO: Journalist Tara Parker-Pope disagrees and maintains that there are biological imperatives that cause people to regain all the weight they lose and for those genetically inclined to obesity, it's almost impossible to maintain weight loss.

While the number of Americans who diet varies, depending on the source, the Boston Medical Center indicates that approximately 45 million Americans diet each year and spend $33 billion on weight-loss products in their pursuit of a trimmer, fitter body. Currently, about two-thirds of American adults are overweight including more than one-third who are classified as obese. This is almost 20 percent more than 20 years ago. Obesity can double mortality and can reduce life expectancy by 10–20 years. If current trends continue, the average American's life expectancy will actually begin to decline by 5 years. Obesity is linked to unhealthy blood fat levels including cholesterol and heart disease. Other health risks associated with obesity include high blood pressure, some cancers, diabetes, gallbladder and kidney disease, sleep disorders, arthritis, and other bone and joint disorders. Obesity is also linked to complications of pregnancy, stress incontinence, and elevated surgical risk. The risks from obesity rise with its severity, and they are much more likely to occur among people more than double their recommended body weight. Obesity can impact psychological as well as physical well-being. Being obese can contribute to psychological problems including depression, anxiety, and low self-esteem.

Since 1990, the prevalence of overweight and obesity has been rising in the United States. Despite public health campaigns, the trend shows little sign of changing. A 2006 campaign conducted by Ogden et al. ("Prevalence of Overweight and Obesity in the US 1999–2004," *JAMA*, vol. 295, 2006) reported that during the 6-year period from 1999 to 2004, the prevalence of overweight in children and adolescents increased significantly, as did the prevalence of obesity in men. Along with these rising rates of obesity come increased rates of obesity-related health issues. There has been a 60 percent rise in type 2 diabetes since 1990. Inactivity and overweight may be responsible for as many as 112,000 premature deaths each year in the United States, second only to smoking-related deaths.

According to the U.S. Department of Agriculture (USDA), the average American has increased his/her caloric intake by more than 500 calories per day while levels of physical activity have decreased. This is related to more meals eaten away from the home, which typically are higher in calories, fat, sugar, and salt. Restaurants also tend to serve larger portions than home-cooked meals. Many Americans are also sleep deprived. Lack of sleep appears to trigger weight gain. Finally, Americans are more engaged in sedentary activities and less likely to engage in physical activity on a regular basis. Whatever the cause of obesity, its incidence and prevalence appear to be rising and it is linked to multiple health concerns.

Because of health and appearance concerns, many Americans attempt to lose weight by dieting and/or exercise. Types of weight-loss diets typically include reduced calories or a reduction of a major nutrient such as fat or carbohydrates. Interestingly, most studies find no difference between the main diet types and subsequent weight loss. However, long-term studies of dieting indicate that the majority of individuals who lose weight regain virtually all of the weight that was lost after dieting, regardless of whether they maintain their diet or exercise program.

The YES and NO selections address whether it is possible to diet, lose weight, and actually maintain that weight loss. Barbara Berkeley maintains that while it's not easy to maintain lost pounds, it is certainly possible. Tara Parker-Pope disagrees and believes that our biological make-up causes us to regain weight and for most people, it's almost impossible to maintain a weight loss.

YES ↵

Barbara Berkeley

The Fat Trap: My Response

Once a month, in a small room off the lobby of Lake West Hospital in Willoughby, Ohio, a special group convenes. For someone observing the group and unaware of its purpose, it might appear to be a simple mix of everyday people . . . young, old, racially diverse. The members would seem to be old friends but with a particular seriousness of purpose, perhaps a community group attending a lecture or learning some new skill together. What a casual observer would not guess is that each of these people was once obese, some having weighed over 100 pounds more than they do today.

Our Refuse to Regain group is an experiment, a safe haven for maintainers who have lost weight in many different ways and now face the reality of reconstructing their lives. We've had people from Weight Watchers, people who've undergone bariatric surgery, people I've treated in my practice and others who simply did it on their own. A weight loss diet is no different than emptying the trash. It doesn't matter which technique you use to toss out the garbage. But learning how to avoid the reaccumulation of unwanted junk is a completely different skill. There are many basics in this process that will be the same for everyone. There are also many specifics that will vary from person to person and which must be individually discovered. Here's some of what we've learned so far:

1. Weight maintenance is possible. There is nothing in our group experience (or in my personal clinical experience) to suggest that the body "forces" one to regain.
2. Weight maintenance requires a separation from the world of "normal" American eating . . . which is not normal at all.
3. Some people are heavy simply because they are susceptible to the modern diet, no more no less. Others are heavy because they use food for soothing or sedation. Most people are a mix of both. If psychological issues are a *major* part of weight gain—significantly beyond the common enjoyment of food for pleasure, they need to be addressed during the maintenance phase.
4. Weight maintainers are special people who live on a kind of food island. It's really nice to know that the island is inhabited, often with fascinating, determined people just like you. Rarely do maintainers get to meet and talk with one another.

This week, I gave my group a reading assignment. That was a first. I asked everyone to read Tara Parker Pope's article on weight maintenance called *The Fat Trap*. This article is currently online and will appear in Sunday's *New York Times Magazine*. Our group will be discussing it at our January meeting, but I'll give you a preview of my reaction here. Many of you may be reading our blog because you read The Fat Trap and discovered Lynn Haraldson, my blogging partner on this site. The fact that you got here likely means that you are interested in knowing whether we are bound to regain the weight we lose, so please, read on . . . leave comments and join the discussion.

For those of you who are new to this blog, you should know that I am a physician who has specialized in weight management since the late 1980s. This is the only thing I do and that's unusual. Why? Because most doctors are not particularly interested in obesity, and certainly weren't back in the 80s. Over the past twenty years, a continuing source of frustration for me has been the willingness of doctors and the general public to accept "truths" about weight loss that are the beliefs of everyone *except* those who actually work with overweight people.

Scientific research needs to square with what we see in clinical practice. If it doesn't, we should question its validity. "The Fat Trap" is an article that starts with a single, small research study and builds around it. Its point? That there are inevitable biological imperatives that cause people to regain all the weight they lose.

I don't buy it.

Here is the opening paragraph of Ms. Parker Pope's article:

> For 15 years, Joseph Proietto has been helping people lose weight. When these obese patients arrive at his weight-loss clinic in Australia, they are determined to slim down. And most of the time, he says, they do just that, sticking to the clinic's program and dropping excess pounds. But then, almost without exception, the weight begins to creep back. In a matter of months or years, the entire effort has come undone, and the patient is fat again.

At one time, this was my experience too. But things have changed. After years of focusing my practice much more on weight maintenance, writing a book about it, and trying to figure out how to teach and encourage it, I no longer see patients with an "entire effort come undone." Instead, I see more and more people learning how to become successfully anchored at their new weight. And these POWs (previous overweight people) are not from my practice alone. They are people like Lynn Haraldson and her friends "The Maintaining Divas." They are the long term POWs who write to me via this blog, on Facebook and on Twitter. They are the people I hear about with increasing frequency every day.

I admire Ms. Parker Pope for acknowledging her own struggles with weight, but as someone who has not yet solved the maintenance problem I would submit that she is not the best person to rationally evaluate evidence that says that regain is inevitable. After talking to a number of scientists who believe that the body fights weight loss, her concluding paragraph says:

> For me, understanding the science of weight loss has helped make sense of my own struggles to lose weight, as well as my mother's endless cycle of dieting, weight gain and despair. I wish she were still here so I could persuade her to finally forgive herself for her dieting failures. While I do, ultimately, blame myself for allowing my weight to get out of control, it has been somewhat liberating to learn that there are factors other than my character at work when it comes to gaining and losing weight.

Those of us who come from families which struggle with obesity can believe one of two things. We can believe that biological and metabolic factors doom us to fatness or we can believe that we come from families who are very sensitive to the current food environment and perhaps need to live in a new and more creative way. It has been my experience that all successful maintainers have learned how to live a life that exists outside the current food norms. For some, this is a daily and difficult challenge and for others it becomes a simple and treasured way of life, but either way, it is not about some inevitable biological destiny. Rather, these maintainers have come to terms with the fact that they are ancient bodies and souls living in a modern environment and that our food culture is capable of killing them. Controlling that environment is their choice and their challenge.

Where I do agree with "The Fat Trap" is in its assertion that obesity is much more difficult to deal with once it is established. We would do well to focus intense and constant attention on healthful nutrition during pregnancy and in childhood. I believe that we can do this much more easily than we believe, if we would only adopt the idea that we should eat more like we did originally as hunter-gatherers. It has been my clinical experience that elimination (or major curtailment) of starches and sugars (including whole grains and the things that come from them, by the way) simply works. And this clinical observation makes sense, since the ancestors whose genes we carry were not exposed to the large amounts of starch and sugar we now eat. Along with consumption of real food . . . not things in boxes, cans, or packages . . . this easy concept can change lives. We could make things so much easier by teaching this lesson to kids rather than endlessly focusing them on per cents of fat, protein and carbs and on counting calories.

But such approaches to weight maintenance are not easily sold. It's far simpler to believe that weight must be regained. I'm fond of using this example for patients: If you were to tell your friends that you are becoming vegetarian and that you will no longer touch a drop of red meat, fish, or poultry, no one would blink an eye. You'd probably be encouraged and congratulated. If, on the other hand, you announced that you were giving up sugar and grain, the same friends would be horrified. "You mean you're never going to have another piece of bread???"

I believe that the resistance to finding the maintenance solution comes from the addictive nature of starch and sugar foods. I also believe that most of America and other SAD (standard American diet) countries are operating "under the influence" of addictive carbs. Life without them, or even with LESS of them, is too awful to contemplate.

But I digress. To return to my original point, I want to forcefully say that we must stop finding reasons we can't maintain and start getting much, much better at teaching people how to do it. Support networks, communication between maintainers, and many more books, advocates, and techniques that focus on maintenance are key.

I believe I may scream if I see yet another book with a catchy title that touts yet another weight loss approach without ever talking about what happens in the after-diet world. January is the month for those glossy little productions.

Time to get serious. Maintenance can be done, and if you want to meet the people who are doing it, hang around this blog.

BARBARA BERKELEY is a physician and diplomate of the American Board of Internal Medicine and the American Board of Obesity Medicine. She has specialized in the care of overweight and obese patients since 1988.

Tara Parker-Pope

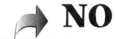 **NO**

The Fat Trap

For 15 years, Joseph Proietto has been helping people lose weight. When these obese patients arrive at his weight-loss clinic in Australia, they are determined to slim down. And most of the time, he says, they do just that, sticking to the clinic's program and dropping excess pounds. But then, almost without exception, the weight begins to creep back. In a matter of months or years, the entire effort has come undone, and the patient is fat again. "It has always seemed strange to me," says Proietto, who is a physician at the University of Melbourne. "These are people who are very motivated to lose weight, who achieve weight loss most of the time without too much trouble and yet, inevitably, gradually, they regain the weight."

Anyone who has ever dieted knows that lost pounds often return, and most of us assume the reason is a lack of discipline or a failure of willpower. But Proietto suspected that there was more to it, and he decided to take a closer look at the biological state of the body after weight loss.

Beginning in 2009, he and his team recruited 50 obese men and women. The men weighed an average of 233 pounds; the women weighed about 200 pounds. Although some people dropped out of the study, most of the patients stuck with the extreme low-calorie diet, which consisted of special shakes called Optifast and two cups of low-starch vegetables, totaling just 500 to 550 calories a day for eight weeks. Ten weeks in, the dieters lost an average of 30 pounds.

At that point, the 34 patients who remained stopped dieting and began working to maintain the new lower weight. Nutritionists counseled them in person and by phone, promoting regular exercise and urging them to eat more vegetables and less fat. But despite the effort, they slowly began to put on weight. After a year, the patients already had regained an average of 11 of the pounds they struggled so hard to lose. They also reported feeling far more hungry and preoccupied with food than before they lost the weight.

While researchers have known for decades that the body undergoes various metabolic and hormonal changes while it's losing weight, the Australian team detected something new. A full year after significant weight loss, these men and women remained in what could be described as a biologically altered state. Their still-plump bodies were acting as if they were starving and were working overtime to regain the pounds they lost. For instance, a gastric hormone called ghrelin, often dubbed the

"hunger hormone," was about 20 percent higher than at the start of the study. Another hormone associated with suppressing hunger, peptide YY, was also abnormally low. Levels of leptin, a hormone that suppresses hunger and increases metabolism, also remained lower than expected. A cocktail of other hormones associated with hunger and metabolism all remained significantly changed compared to pre-dieting levels. It was almost as if weight loss had put their bodies into a unique metabolic state, a sort of post-dieting syndrome that set them apart from people who hadn't tried to lose weight in the first place. "What we see here is a coordinated defense mechanism with multiple components all directed toward making us put on weight," Proietto says. "This, I think, explains the high failure rate in obesity treatment."

While the findings from Proietto and colleagues, published this fall in *The New England Journal of Medicine,* are not conclusive—the study was small and the findings need to be replicated—the research has nonetheless caused a stir in the weight-loss community, adding to a growing body of evidence that challenges conventional thinking about obesity, weight loss and willpower. For years, the advice to the overweight and obese has been that we simply need to eat less and exercise more. While there is truth to this guidance, it fails to take into account that the human body continues to fight against weight loss long after dieting has stopped. This translates into a sobering reality: once we become fat, most of us, despite our best efforts, will probably stay fat.

I have always felt perplexed about my inability to keep weight off. I know the medical benefits of weight loss, and I don't drink sugary sodas or eat fast food. I exercise regularly—a few years ago, I even completed a marathon. Yet during the 23 years since graduating from college, I've lost 10 or 20 pounds at a time, maintained it for a little while and then gained it all back and more, to the point where I am now easily 60 pounds overweight.

I wasn't overweight as a child, but I can't remember a time when my mother, whose weight probably fluctuated between 150 and 250 pounds, wasn't either on a diet or, in her words, cheating on her diet. Sometimes we ate healthful, balanced meals; on other days dinner consisted of a bucket of Kentucky Fried Chicken. As a high-school cross-country runner, I never worried about weight, but in college, when my regular training runs were squeezed out by studying and socializing, the numbers on the scale slowly began to move up. As adults, my three sisters and

I all struggle with weight, as do many members of my extended family. My mother died of esophageal cancer six years ago. It was her great regret that in the days before she died, the closest medical school turned down her offer to donate her body because she was obese.

It's possible that the biological cards were stacked against me from the start. Researchers know that obesity tends to run in families, and recent science suggests that even the desire to eat higher-calorie foods may be influenced by heredity. But untangling how much is genetic and how much is learned through family eating habits is difficult. What is clear is that some people appear to be prone to accumulating extra fat while others seem to be protected against it.

In a seminal series of experiments published in the 1990s, the Canadian researchers Claude Bouchard and Angelo Tremblay studied 31 pairs of male twins ranging in age from 17 to 29, who were sometimes overfed and sometimes put on diets. (None of the twin pairs were at risk for obesity based on their body mass or their family history.) In one study, 12 sets of the twins were put under 24-hour supervision in a college dormitory. Six days a week they ate 1,000 extra calories a day, and one day they were allowed to eat normally. They could read, play video games, play cards and watch television, but exercise was limited to one 30-minute daily walk. Over the course of the 120-day study, the twins consumed 84,000 extra calories beyond their basic needs.

That experimental binge should have translated into a weight gain of roughly 24 pounds (based on 3,500 calories to a pound). But some gained less than 10 pounds, while others gained as much as 29 pounds. The amount of weight gained and how the fat was distributed around the body closely matched among brothers, but varied considerably among the different sets of twins. Some brothers gained three times as much fat around their abdomens as others, for instance. When the researchers conducted similar exercise studies with the twins, they saw the patterns in reverse, with some twin sets losing more pounds than others on the same exercise regimen. The findings, the researchers wrote, suggest a form of "biological determinism" that can make a person susceptible to weight gain or loss.

But while there is widespread agreement that at least some risk for obesity is inherited, identifying a specific genetic cause has been a challenge. In October 2010, the journal *Nature Genetics* reported that researchers have so far confirmed 32 distinct genetic variations associated with obesity or body-mass index. One of the most common of these variations was identified in April 2007 by a British team studying the genetics of Type 2 diabetes. According to Timothy Frayling at the Institute of Biomedical and Clinical Science at the University of Exeter, people who carried a variant known as FTO faced a much higher risk of obesity—30 percent higher if they had one copy of the variant; 60 percent if they had two.

This FTO variant is surprisingly common; about 65 percent of people of European or African descent and an estimated 27 to 44 percent of Asians are believed to carry at least one copy of it. Scientists don't understand how the FTO variation influences weight gain, but studies in children suggest the trait plays a role in eating habits. In one 2008 study led by Colin Palmer of the University of Dundee in Scotland, Scottish schoolchildren were given snacks of orange drinks and muffins and then allowed to graze on a buffet of grapes, celery, potato chips and chocolate buttons. All the food was carefully monitored so the researchers knew exactly what was consumed. Although all the children ate about the same amount of food, as weighed in grams, children with the FTO variant were more likely to eat foods with higher fat and calorie content. They weren't gorging themselves, but they consumed, on average, about 100 calories more than children who didn't carry the gene. Those who had the gene variant had about four pounds more body fat than noncarriers.

I have been tempted to send in my own saliva sample for a DNA test to find out if my family carries a genetic predisposition for obesity. But even if the test came back negative, it would only mean that my family doesn't carry a known, testable genetic risk for obesity. Recently the British television show "Embarrassing Fat Bodies" asked Frayling's lab to test for fat-promoting genes, and the results showed one very overweight family had a lower-than-average risk for obesity.

A positive result, telling people they are genetically inclined to stay fat, might be self-fulfilling. In February, *The New England Journal of Medicine* published a report on how genetic testing for a variety of diseases affected a person's mood and health habits. Over all, the researchers found no effect from disease-risk testing, but there was a suggestion, though it didn't reach statistical significance, that after testing positive for fat-promoting genes, some people were more likely to eat fatty foods, presumably because they thought being fat was their genetic destiny and saw no sense in fighting it.

While knowing my genetic risk might satisfy my curiosity, I also know that heredity, at best, would explain only part of why I became overweight. I'm much more interested in figuring out what I can do about it now.

The National Weight Control Registry tracks 10,000 people who have lost weight and have kept it off. "We set it up in response to comments that nobody ever succeeds at weight loss," says Rena Wing, a professor of psychiatry and human behavior at Brown University's Alpert Medical School, who helped create the registry with James O. Hill, director of the Center for Human Nutrition at the University of Colorado at Denver. "We had two goals: to prove there were people who did, and to try to learn from them about what they do to achieve this long-term weight loss." Anyone who has lost 30 pounds and kept it off for at least a year is eligible to join the study, though the average member has lost 70 pounds and remained at that weight for six years.

Wing says that she agrees that physiological changes probably do occur that make permanent weight loss difficult, but she says the larger problem is environmental, and that people struggle to keep weight off because they are surrounded by food, inundated with food messages and constantly presented with opportunities to eat. "We live in an environment with food cues all the time," Wing says. "We've taught ourselves over the years that one of the ways to reward yourself is with food. It's hard to change the environment and the behavior."

There is no consistent pattern to how people in the registry lost weight—some did it on Weight Watchers, others with Jenny Craig, some by cutting carbs on the Atkins diet and a very small number lost weight through surgery. But their eating and exercise habits appear to reflect what researchers find in the lab: to lose weight and keep it off, a person must eat fewer calories and exercise far more than a person who maintains the same weight naturally. Registry members exercise about an hour or more each day—the average weight-loser puts in the equivalent of a four-mile daily walk, seven days a week. They get on a scale every day in order to keep their weight within a narrow range. They eat breakfast regularly. Most watch less than half as much television as the overall population. They eat the same foods and in the same patterns consistently each day and don't "cheat" on weekends or holidays. They also appear to eat less than most people, with estimates ranging from 50 to 300 fewer daily calories.

Kelly Brownell, director of the Rudd Center for Food Policy and Obesity at Yale University, says that while the 10,000 people tracked in the registry are a useful resource, they also represent a tiny percentage of the tens of millions of people who have tried unsuccessfully to lose weight. "All it means is that there are rare individuals who do manage to keep it off," Brownell says. "You find these people are incredibly vigilant about maintaining their weight. Years later they are paying attention to every calorie, spending an hour a day on exercise. They never don't think about their weight."

Janice Bridge, a registry member who has successfully maintained a 135-pound weight loss for about five years, is a perfect example. "It's one of the hardest things there is," she says. "It's something that has to be focused on every minute. I'm not always thinking about food, but I am always aware of food." Bridge, who is 66 and lives in Davis, Calif., was overweight as a child and remembers going on her first diet of 1,400 calories a day at 14. At the time, her slow pace of weight loss prompted her doctor to accuse her of cheating. Friends told her she must not be paying attention to what she was eating. "No one would believe me that I was doing everything I was told," she says. "You can imagine how tremendously depressing it was and what a feeling of rebellion and anger was building up."

After peaking at 330 pounds in 2004, she tried again to lose weight. She managed to drop 30 pounds, but then her weight loss stalled. In 2006, at age 60, she joined a medically supervised weight-loss program with her husband, Adam, who weighed 310 pounds. After nine months on an 800-calorie diet, she slimmed down to 165 pounds. Adam lost about 110 pounds and now weighs about 200.

During the first years after her weight loss, Bridge tried to test the limits of how much she could eat. She used exercise to justify eating more. The death of her mother in 2009 consumed her attention; she lost focus and slowly regained 30 pounds. She has decided to try to maintain this higher weight of 195, which is still 135 pounds [less] than her heaviest weight.

"It doesn't take a lot of variance from my current maintenance for me to pop on another two or three pounds," she says. "It's been a real struggle to stay at this weight, but it's worth it, it's good for me, it makes me feel better. But my body would put on weight almost instantaneously if I ever let up."

So she never lets up. Since October 2006 she has weighed herself every morning and recorded the result in a weight diary. She even carries a scale with her when she travels. In the past six years, she made only one exception to this routine: a two-week, no-weigh vacation in Hawaii.

She also weighs everything in the kitchen. She knows that lettuce is about 5 calories a cup, while flour is about 400. If she goes out to dinner, she conducts a Web search first to look at the menu and calculate calories to help her decide what to order. She avoids anything with sugar or white flour, which she calls her "gateway drugs" for cravings and overeating. She has also found that drinking copious amounts of water seems to help; she carries a 20-ounce water bottle and fills it five times a day. She writes down everything she eats. At night, she transfers all the information to an electronic record. Adam also keeps track but prefers to keep his record with pencil and paper.

"That transfer process is really important; it's my accountability," she says. "It comes up with the total number of calories I've eaten today and the amount of protein. I do a little bit of self-analysis every night."

Bridge and her husband each sought the help of therapists, and in her sessions, Janice learned that she had a tendency to eat when she was bored or stressed. "We are very much aware of how our culture taught us to use food for all kinds of reasons that aren't related to its nutritive value," Bridge says. Bridge supports her careful diet with an equally rigorous regimen of physical activity. She exercises from 100 to 120 minutes a day, six or seven days a week, often by riding her bicycle to the gym, where she takes a water-aerobics class. She also works out on an elliptical trainer at home and uses a recumbent bike to "walk" the dog, who loves to run alongside the low, three-wheeled machine. She enjoys gardening as a hobby but allows herself to count it as exercise on only those occasions when she needs to "garden vigorously." Adam is also a committed exerciser, riding his bike at least two hours a day, five days a week.

Janice Bridge has used years of her exercise and diet data to calculate her own personal fuel efficiency. She knows that her body burns about three calories a minute during gardening, about four calories a minute on the recumbent bike and during water aerobics and about five a minute when she zips around town on her regular bike.

"Practically anyone will tell you someone biking is going to burn 11 calories a minute," she says. "That's not my body. I know it because of the statistics I've kept."

Based on metabolism data she collected from the weight-loss clinic and her own calculations, she has discovered that to keep her current weight of 195 pounds, she can eat 2,000 calories a day as long as she burns 500 calories in exercise. She avoids junk food, bread and pasta and many dairy products and tries to make sure nearly a third of her calories come from protein. The Bridges will occasionally share a dessert, or eat an individual portion of Ben and Jerry's ice cream, so they know exactly how many calories they are ingesting. Because she knows errors can creep in, either because a rainy day cuts exercise short or a mismeasured snack portion adds hidden calories, she allows herself only 1,800 daily calories of food. (The average estimate for a similarly active woman of her age and size is about 2,300 calories.)

Just talking to Bridge about the effort required to maintain her weight is exhausting. I find her story inspiring, but it also makes me wonder whether I have what it takes to be thin. I have tried on several occasions (and as recently as a couple weeks ago) to keep a daily diary of my eating and exercise habits, but it's easy to let it slide. I can't quite imagine how I would ever make time to weigh and measure food when some days it's all I can do to get dinner on the table between finishing my work and carting my daughter to dance class or volleyball practice. And while I enjoy exercising for 30- or 40-minute stretches, I also learned from six months of marathon training that devoting one to two hours a day to exercise takes an impossible toll on my family life.

Bridge concedes that having grown children and being retired make it easier to focus on her weight. "I don't know if I could have done this when I had three kids living at home," she says. "We know how unusual we are. It's pretty easy to get angry with the amount of work and dedication it takes to keep this weight off. But the alternative is to not keep the weight off. "

"I think many people who are anxious to lose weight don't fully understand what the consequences are going to be, nor does the medical community fully explain this to people," Rudolph Leibel, an obesity researcher at Columbia University in New York, says. "We don't want to make them feel hopeless, but we do want to make them understand that they are trying to buck a biological system that is going to try to make it hard for them."

Leibel and his colleague Michael Rosenbaum have pioneered much of what we know about the body's response to weight loss. For 25 years, they have meticulously tracked about 130 individuals for six months or longer at a stretch. The subjects reside at their research clinic where every aspect of their bodies is measured. Body fat is determined by bone-scan machines. A special hood monitors oxygen consumption and carbon-dioxide output to precisely measure metabolism. Calories burned during digestion are tracked. Exercise tests measure maximum heart rate, while blood tests measure hormones and brain chemicals. Muscle biopsies are taken to analyze their metabolic efficiency. (Early in the research, even stool samples were collected and tested to make sure no calories went unaccounted for.) For their trouble, participants are paid $5,000 to $8,000.

Eventually, the Columbia subjects are placed on liquid diets of 800 calories a day until they lose 10 percent of their body weight. Once they reach the goal, they are subjected to another round of intensive testing as they try to maintain the new weight. The data generated by these experiments suggest that once a person loses about 10 percent of body weight, he or she is metabolically different than a similar-size person who is naturally the same weight.

The research shows that the changes that occur after weight loss translate to a huge caloric disadvantage of about 250 to 400 calories. For instance, one woman who entered the Columbia studies at 230 pounds was eating about 3,000 calories to maintain that weight. Once she dropped to 190 pounds, losing 17 percent of her body weight, metabolic studies determined that she needed about 2,300 daily calories to maintain the new lower weight. That may sound like plenty, but the typical 30-year-old 190-pound woman can consume about 2,600 calories to maintain her weight—300 more calories than the woman who dieted to get there.

Scientists are still learning why a weight-reduced body behaves so differently from a similar-size body that has not dieted. Muscle biopsies taken before, during and after weight loss show that once a person drops weight, their muscle fibers undergo a transformation, making them more like highly efficient "slow twitch" muscle fibers. A result is that after losing weight, your muscles burn 20 to 25 percent fewer calories during everyday activity and moderate aerobic exercise than those of a person who is naturally at the same weight. That means a dieter who thinks she is burning 200 calories during a brisk half-hour walk is probably using closer to 150 to 160 calories.

Another way that the body seems to fight weight loss is by altering the way the brain responds to food. Rosenbaum and his colleague Joy Hirsch, a neuroscientist also at Columbia, used functional magnetic resonance imaging to track the brain patterns of people before and after weight loss while they looked at objects like grapes, Gummi Bears, chocolate, broccoli, cellphones and yo-yos. After weight loss, when the dieter looked at food, the scans showed a bigger response in the parts of the brain associated with reward and a lower response in the areas associated with control. This suggests that the body, in order to get back to its pre-diet weight, induces cravings by making the person feel more excited about food and giving him or her less willpower to resist a high-calorie treat.

"After you've lost weight, your brain has a greater emotional response to food," Rosenbaum says. "You want it more, but the areas of the brain involved in restraint are less active." Combine that with a body that is now burning fewer calories than expected, he says, "and you've created the perfect storm for weight regain." How long this state lasts isn't known, but preliminary research at Columbia suggests that for as many as six years after weight loss, the body continues to defend the old, higher weight by burning off far fewer calories than would be expected. The problem could persist indefinitely. (The same phenomenon occurs when a thin person tries to drop about 10 percent of his or her body weight—the body defends the higher weight.) This doesn't mean it's impossible to lose weight and keep it off; it just means it's really, really difficult.

Lynn Haraldson, a 48-year-old woman who lives in Pittsburgh, reached 300 pounds in 2000. She joined Weight Watchers and managed to take her 5-foot-5 body down to 125 pounds for a brief time. Today, she's a member of the National Weight Control Registry and maintains about 140 pounds by devoting her life to weight maintenance. She became a vegetarian, writes down what she eats every day, exercises at least five days a week and blogs about the challenges of weight maintenance. A former journalist and antiques dealer, she returned to school for a two-year program on nutrition and health; she plans to become a dietary counselor. She has also come to accept that she can never stop being "hypervigilant" about what she eats. "Everything has to change," she says. "I've been up and down the scale so many times, always thinking I can go back to 'normal,' but I had to establish a new normal. People don't like hearing that it's not easy."

What's not clear from the research is whether there is a window during which we can gain weight and then lose it without creating biological backlash. Many people experience transient weight gain, putting on a few extra pounds during the holidays or gaining 10 or 20 pounds during the first years of college that they lose again. The actor Robert De Niro lost weight after bulking up for his performance in "Raging Bull." The filmmaker Morgan Spurlock also lost the weight he gained during the making of "Super Size Me." Leibel says that whether these temporary pounds became permanent probably depends on a person's genetic risk for obesity and, perhaps, the length of time a person carried the extra weight before trying to lose it. But researchers don't know how long it takes for the body to reset itself permanently to a higher weight. The good news is that it doesn't seem to happen overnight.

"For a mouse, I know the time period is somewhere around eight months," Leibel says. "Before that time, a fat mouse can come back to being a skinny mouse again without too much adjustment. For a human we don't know, but I'm pretty sure it's not measured in months, but in years."

Nobody wants to be fat. In most modern cultures, even if you are healthy—in my case, my cholesterol and blood pressure are low and I have an extraordinarily healthy heart—to be fat is to be perceived as weak-willed and lazy. It's also just embarrassing. Once, at a party, I met a well-respected writer who knew my work as a health writer.

"You're not at all what I expected," she said, eyes widening. The man I was dating, perhaps trying to help, finished the thought. "You thought she'd be thinner, right?" he said. I wanted to disappear, but the woman was gracious. "No," she said, casting a glare at the man and reaching to warmly shake my hand. "I thought you'd be older."

If anything, the emerging science of weight loss teaches us that perhaps we should rethink our biases about people who are overweight. It is true that people who are overweight, including myself, get that way because they eat too many calories relative to what their bodies need. But a number of biological and genetic factors can play a role in determining exactly how much food is too much for any given individual. Clearly, weight loss is an intense struggle, one in which we are not fighting simply hunger or cravings for sweets, but our own bodies.

While the public discussion about weight loss tends to come down to which diet works best (Atkins? Jenny Craig? Plant-based? Mediterranean?), those who have tried and failed at all of these diets know there is no simple answer. Fat, sugar and carbohydrates in processed foods may very well be culprits in the nation's obesity problem. But there is tremendous variation in an individual's response.

The view of obesity as primarily a biological, rather than psychological, disease could also lead to changes in the way we approach its treatment. Scientists at Columbia have conducted several small studies looking at whether injecting people with leptin, the hormone made by body fat, can override the body's resistance to weight loss and help maintain a lower weight. In a few small studies, leptin injections appear to trick the body into thinking it's still fat. After leptin replacement, study subjects burned more calories during activity. And in brain-scan studies, leptin injections appeared to change how the brain responded to food, making it seem less enticing. But such treatments are still years away from commercial development. For now, those of us who want to lose weight and keep it off are on our own.

One question many researchers think about is whether losing weight more slowly would make it more sustainable than the fast weight loss often used in scientific studies. Leibel says the pace of weight loss is unlikely to make a difference, because the body's warning system is based solely on how much fat a person loses, not how quickly he or she loses it. Even so, Proietto is now conducting a study using a slower weight-loss method and following dieters for three years instead of one.

Given how hard it is to lose weight, it's clear, from a public-health standpoint, that resources would best be focused on preventing weight gain. The research underscores the urgency of national efforts to get children to exercise and eat healthful foods.

But with a third of the U.S. adult population classified as obese, nobody is saying people who already are very overweight should give up on weight loss. Instead, the solution may be to preach a more realistic goal. Studies suggest that even a 5 percent weight loss can lower a person's risk for diabetes, heart disease and other health problems associated with obesity. There is also speculation that the body is more willing to accept small amounts of weight loss.

But an obese person who loses just 5 percent of her body weight will still very likely be obese. For a 250-pound woman, a 5 percent weight loss of about 12 pounds probably won't even change her clothing size. Losing a few pounds may be good for the body, but it does very little for the spirit and is unlikely to change how fat people feel about themselves or how others perceive them.

So where does that leave a person who wants to lose a sizable amount of weight? Weight-loss scientists say they believe that once more people understand the genetic and biological challenges of keeping weight off, doctors and patients will approach weight loss more realistically and more compassionately. At the very least, the science may compel people who are already overweight to work harder to make sure they don't put on additional pounds. Some people, upon learning how hard permanent weight loss can be, may give up entirely and return to overeating. Others may decide to accept themselves at their current weight and try to boost their fitness and overall health rather than changing the number on the scale.

For me, understanding the science of weight loss has helped make sense of my own struggles to lose weight, as well as my mother's endless cycle of dieting, weight gain and despair. I wish she were still here so I could persuade her to finally forgive herself for her dieting failures. While I do, ultimately, blame myself for allowing my weight to get out of control, it has been somewhat liberating to learn that there are factors other than my character at work when it comes to gaining and losing weight. And even though all the evidence suggests that it's going to be very, very difficult for me to reduce my weight permanently, I'm surprisingly optimistic. I may not be ready to fight this battle this month or even this year. But at least I know what I'm up against.

TARA PARKER-POPE is an author of books on health topics and a columnist for *The New York Times,* where she edits the Well blog.

EXPLORING THE ISSUE

Is Weight-Loss Maintenance Possible?

Critical Thinking and Reflection

1. Why is it so difficult for most people to maintain their weight loss?
2. What role does the typical American diet play in overweight and obesity?
3. Describe the biological mechanisms that make weight-loss maintenance so challenging.
4. What role does genetics play in the onset of obesity?

Is There Common Ground?

Although genetics and metabolism may elevate the risk for overweight and obesity, they don't explain the rising rate of obesity seen in the United States. Our genetic background has not changed significantly in the past 40 years, during which time the rate of obesity among Americans has more than doubled. The causes can be linked to changing eating habits and a decline in physical activity.

While dieting is a common means of losing weight, there is an overall belief that even if one loses weight, virtually no one succeeds in long-term maintenance of weight loss. However, research has shown that approximately 20 percent of overweight people are successful at long-term weight loss (defined as losing at least 10 percent of initial body weight and maintaining the loss for at least 1 year). The National Weight Control Registry provides information about the approaches used by successful weight-loss maintainers to attain and sustain long-term weight loss. To maintain their weight loss, the successful report high levels of physical activity, eating a low-calorie, low-fat diet, eating breakfast regularly, self-monitoring weight, and maintaining a consistent eating pattern across weekdays and weekends. In addition, weight-loss maintenance may get less challenging over time. After individuals have successfully maintained their weight loss for over 2 years, the chance of longer-term success greatly increases. Continuing to diet and exercise is also associated with long-term success. National Weight Control Registry members provide evidence that long-term weight-loss maintenance is possible and helps identify the specific approaches associated with long-term success (Wing and Phelan, 2005).

The same tactics that help people lose weight don't necessarily help them keep it off. A recent study, which appears in the August 2011 issue of the *American Journal of Preventive Medicine*, suggests that successful losers need to rethink their eating and exercise practices to maintain their weight loss. Researchers interviewed nearly 1,200 adults about 36 specific behaviors to find out which of these practices were associated with weight loss and more important, weight-loss maintenance.

From the study results, it appears that different skill sets and behaviors are involved with weight loss and weight maintenance. Participating in a weight-loss program, restricting sugar, eating healthy snacks, and not skipping meals may help people initially lose weight, but these practices don't appear to be effective in maintaining the loss.

Eating low-fat sources of protein, following a consistent exercise routine, and using rewards for maintaining these behaviors were linked to maintaining weight loss.

Create Central

www.mhhe.com/createcentral

Reference

Wing, R. R. & Phelan, S. (2005). Long term weight loss maintenance. *American Journal of Clinical Nutrition, 82*, 2225–2255.

Additional Resources

Schusdziarra, V., Hausmann, M., Wiedemann, C., Hess, J., Barth, C., Wagenpfeil, S., & Erdmann, J. (2011). Successful weight loss and maintenance in everyday clinical practice with an individually tailored change of eating habits on the basis of food energy density. *European Journal of Nutrition, 50*(5), 351–361.

Sciamanna, C. N., Kiernan, M., & Rolls, B. J., et al. (2011). Practices associated with weight loss versus weight-loss maintenance: Results of a national survey. *American Journal of Preventive Medicine, 41*(2), 159–166.

Sherwood, N. E., Crain, A., Martinson, B. C., Anderson, C. P., Hayes, M. G., Anderson, J. D., & Jeffery, R. W. (2013). Enhancing long-term weight loss maintenance: 2-Year results from the Keep It Off randomized controlled trial. *Preventive Medicine, 56*(3/4), 171–177.

Stubbs, R. J. & Lavin, J. H. (2013). The challenges of implementing behavior changes that lead to sustained weight management. *Nutrition Bulletin, 38*(1), 5–22.

Internet References . . .

The American Dietetic Association

www.eatright.org

National Weight Control Registry

www.nwcr.ws/

Center for Science in the Public Interest (CSPI)

www.cspinet.org

Food and Nutrition Information Center

www.nalusda.gov/fnic/index.html

Shape Up America!

www.shapeup.org

Selected, Edited, and with Issue Framing Material by:
Eileen Daniel, *SUNY College at Brockport*

ISSUE

Are Energy Drinks with Alcohol Dangerous Enough to Ban?

YES: Don Troop, from "Four Loko Does Its Job with Efficiency and Economy, Students Say," *The Chronicle of Higher Education* (November 1, 2010)

NO: Jacob Sullum, from "Loco Over Four Loko," *Reason Magazine* (March 2011)

Learning Outcomes

After reading this issue, you should be able to:

- Discuss the health implications of energy drinks.
- Discuss the argument that energy drinks should be banned from sale and distribution.
- Assess the reason for the drink's popularity among college students.

ISSUE SUMMARY

YES: *The Chronicle of Higher Education* journalist Don Troop argues that the combination of caffeine and alcohol is extremely dangerous and should not be sold or marketed to college students and young people.

NO: Journalist and editor of *Reason Magazine* Jacob Sullum disagrees and claims that alcoholic energy drinks should not have been targeted and banned since many other products are far more dangerous.

Energy drinks such as Four Loko are alcoholic beverages that originally also contained caffeine and other stimulants. These products have been the object of legal, ethical, and health concerns related to companies supposedly marketing them to underaged consumers and the alleged danger of combining alcohol and caffeine. After the beverage was banned in several states, a product reintroduction in December 2010 removed caffeine and the malt beverage is no longer marketed as an energy drink.

In 2009, companies that produced and sold caffeinated alcohol beverages were investigated, on the grounds that their products were being inappropriately advertised to an underage audience and that the drinks had possible health risks by masking feelings of intoxication due to the caffeine content. Energy drinks came under major fire in 2010, as colleges and universities across the United States began to see injuries and blackouts related to the drink's consumption. Colleges such as the University of Rhode Island banned this product from their campus that year. The state of Washington banned Four Loko after nine university students, all under 20, from Central Washington University became ill after consuming the beverage at a nearby house party. The Central Washington

college students were hospitalized and one student, with extremely high blood alcohol content, nearly died.

Following the hospitalization of 17 students and 6 visitors in 2010, Ramapo College of New Jersey banned the possession and consumption of Four Loko on its campus. Several other colleges also prohibited the sale of the beverages. Many colleges and universities sent out notices informing their students to avoid the drinks because of the risk associated with their consumption.

Other efforts to control the use of energy drinks have been under way. The Pennsylvania Liquor Control Board sent letters to all liquor stores urging distributors to discontinue the sale of the drink. The PLCB also sent letters to all colleges and universities warning them of the dangers of the product. While the board has stopped short of a ban, it has asked retailers to stop selling the drink until U.S. Food and Drug Administration (FDA) findings prove the products are safe. Several grocery chains have voluntarily removed energy beverages from their stores. In Oregon, the sale of the restricted products carried a penalty of 30-day suspension of liquor license.

The U.S. FDA issued a warning letter in 2010 to four manufacturers of caffeinated alcohol beverages stating that the caffeine added to their malt alcoholic beverages is an "unsafe food additive" and said that further action, including seizure of their products, may occur under federal law. The FDA determined that beverages that combine caffeine with alcohol, such as Four Loco energy drinks, are a "public health concern" and couldn't stay on the market in their current form. The FDA also stated that concerns have been raised that caffeine can mask some of the sensory cues individuals might normally rely on to determine their level of intoxication. Warning letters were issued to each of the four companies requiring them to provide to the FDA in writing within 15 days of the specific steps the firms will be taking. Prior to the FDA ruling, many consumers bought and hoarded large quantities of the beverage. This buying frenzy created a black market for energy drinks, with some sellers charging inflated prices. A reformulated version of the drink was put on shelves in late 2010. The new product had exactly the same design as the original, but the caffeine had been removed.

Effective February 2013, cans of Four Loko carry an "Alcohol Facts" label. The label change is part of a final settlement between the Federal Trade Commission and Phusion Projects, the manufacturer of Four Loko. The company still disagrees with the commission's allegations, but said in a statement that the agreement provides a practical way for the company to move ahead. The FTC claimed that ads for Four Loko inaccurately claimed that a 23.5-ounce can contain the alcohol equivalent of one to two cans of beer. In fact, the FTC says, it's more like four to five beers. In the YES and NO selections, Don Troop argues that the combination of caffeine and alcohol is extremely dangerous and should not be sold or marketed to college students and young people. Journalist and editor of *Reason Magazine* Jacob Sullum disagrees and claims that alcoholic energy drinks should not have been targeted and banned since many other products are far more dangerous.

YES ↵

Don Troop

Four Loko Does Its Job with Efficiency and Economy, Students Say

It's Friday night in this steep-hilled college town, and if anyone needs an excuse to party, here are two: In 30 minutes the Mountaineers football team will kick off against the UConn Huskies in East Hartford, Conn., and tonight begins the three-day Halloween weekend.

A few blocks from the West Virginia University campus, young people crowd the aisles of Ashebrooke Liquor Outlet, an airy shop that is popular among students. One rack in the chilled-beverage cooler is nearly empty, the one that is usually filled with 23.5-ounce cans of Four Loko, a fruity malt beverage that combines the caffeine of two cups of coffee with the buzz factor of four to six beers.

"That's what everyone's buying these days," says a liquor store employee, "Loko and Burnett's vodka," a line of distilled spirits that are commonly mixed with nonalcoholic energy drinks like Red Bull and Monster to create fruity cocktails with a stimulating kick.

Four Loko's name comes from its four primary ingredients—alcohol (12 percent by volume), caffeine, taurine, and guarana. Although it is among dozens of caffeinated alcoholic drinks on the market, Four Loko has come to symbolize the dangers of such beverages because of its role in binge-drinking incidents this fall involving students at New Jersey's Ramapo College and at Central Washington University. Ramapo and Central Washington have banned Four Loko from their campuses, and several other colleges have sent urgent e-mail messages advising students not to drink it. But whether Four Loko is really "blackout in a can" or just the highest-profile social lubricant of the moment is unclear.

Just uphill from Ashebrooke Liquor Outlet, four young men stand on a porch sipping cans of Four Loko—fruit punch and cranberry-lemonade. All are upperclassmen except for one, Philip Donnachie, who graduated in May. He says most Four Loko drinkers he knows like to guzzle a can of it at home before meeting up with friends, a custom that researchers in the field call "predrinking."

"Everyone that's going to go out for the night, they're going to start with a Four Loko first," Mr. Donnachie says, adding that he generally switches to beer.

A student named Tony says he paid $5.28 at Ashebrooke for two Lokos—a bargain whether the goal is to get tipsy or flat-out drunk. Before the drink became infamous, he says, he would see students bring cans of it into classrooms. "The teachers didn't know what it was," Tony says, and if they asked, the student would casually reply, "It's an energy drink."

Farther uphill, on the sidewalk along Grant Avenue, the Tin Man from *The Wizard of Oz* carries a Loko—watermelon flavor, judging by its color. Down the block a keg party spills out onto the front porch, where guests sprawl on a sofa and flick cigarette ashes over the railing. No one here is drinking Four Loko, but most are eager to talk about the product because they've heard that it could be banned by the federal government as a result of the student illnesses.

Research Gap

That's not likely to happen anytime soon, according to the Food and Drug Administration.

"The FDA's decision regarding the regulatory status of caffeine added to various alcoholic beverages will be a high priority for the agency," Michael L. Herndon, an FDA spokesman, wrote in an e-mail message. "However, a decision regarding the use of caffeine in alcoholic beverages could take some time." The FDA does not consider such drinks to be "generally recognized as safe." A year ago the agency gave 27 manufacturers 30 days to provide evidence to the contrary, if it existed. Only 19 of the companies have responded.

Dennis L. Thombs is chairman of the Department of Social and Behavioral Sciences at the University of North Texas Health Science Center, in Fort Worth. He knows a great deal about the drinking habits of young people.

Last year he was the lead author on a paper submitted to the journal *Addictive Behaviors* that described his team's study of bar patrons' consumption of energy drinks and alcohol in the college town of Gainesville, Fla. After interviewing 802 patrons and testing their blood-alcohol content, Mr. Thombs and his fellow researchers concluded that energy drinks' labels should clearly describe the ingredients, their amounts, and the potential risks involved in using the products.

But Mr. Thombs says the government should have more data before it decides what to do about alcoholic energy drinks.

"There's still a big gap in this research," he says. "We need to get better pharmacological measures in natural drinking environments" like bars.

He says he has submitted a grant application to the National Institutes of Health in hopes of doing just that.

"Liquid Crack"

Back at the keg party in Morgantown, a student wearing Freddy Krueger's brown fedora and razor-blade glove calls Four Loko "liquid crack" and says he prefers not to buy it for his underage friends. "I'll buy them something else," he says, "but not Four Loko."

Dipsy from the *Teletubbies* says the people abusing Four Loko are younger students, mostly 17- and 18-year-olds. He calls the students who became ill at Ramapo and Central Washington "a bunch of kids that don't know how to drink."

Two freshmen at the party, Gabrielle and Meredith, appear to confirm that assertion.

"I like Four Loko because it's cheap and it gets me drunk," says Gabrielle, 19, who seems well on her way to getting drunk tonight, Four Loko or not. "Especially for concerts. I drink two Four Lokos before going, and then I don't have to spend $14 on a couple drinks at the stadium."

Meredith, 18 and equally intoxicated, says that although she drinks Four Loko, she favors a ban. "They're 600 calories, and they're gross."

An interview with Alex, a 19-year-old student at a religiously affiliated college in the Pacific Northwest, suggests one reason that the drink might be popular among a younger crowd. In his state and many others, the laws that govern the sale of Four Loko and beer are less stringent than those for hard liquor.

That eases the hassle for older friends who buy for Alex. These days that's not a concern, though. He stopped drinking Four Loko because of how it made him feel the next day.

"Every time I drank it I got, like, a blackout," says Alex. "Now I usually just drink beer."

DON TROOP is a senior editor of the *Chronicles of Higher Education*, which covers state policy, as well as economic development, town-and-gown relations, fund raising and endowments, and other financial issues at the campus level.

Jacob Sullum

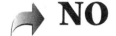 **NO**

Loco Over Four Loko: How a Fruity, Brightly Colored Malt Beverage Drove Politicians to Madness in Two Short Years

In a column at the end of October, *The New York Times* restaurant critic Frank Bruni looked down his nose at Four Loko, a fruity, bubbly, brightly colored malt beverage with a lower alcohol content than Chardonnay and less caffeine per ounce than Red Bull. "It's a malt liquor in confectionery drag," Bruni wrote, "not only raising questions about the marketing strategy behind it but also serving as the clearest possible reminder that many drinkers aren't seeking any particular culinary or aesthetic enjoyment. They're taking a drug. The more festively it's dressed and the more vacuously it goes down, the better."

Less than two weeks after Bruni panned Four Loko and its déclassé drinkers, he wrote admiringly of the "ambition and thought" reflected in hoity-toity coffee cocktails offered by the Randolph at Broome, a boutique bar in downtown Manhattan. He conceded that "there is a long if not entirely glorious history of caffeine and alcohol joining forces, of whiskey or liqueurs poured into after-dinner coffee by adults looking for the same sort of effect that Four Loko fans seek: an extension of the night without a surrender of the buzz."

Like Bruni's distaste for Four Loko, the moral panic that led the Food and Drug Administration (FDA) to ban the beverage and others like it in November, just two years after it was introduced, cannot be explained in pharmacological terms. As Brum admitted and as the drink's Chicago-based manufacturer, Phusion Projects, kept pointing out to no avail, there is nothing new about mixing alcohol with caffeine. What made this particular formulation intolerable—indeed "adulterated," according to the FDA—was not its chemical composition but its class connotations: the wild and crazy name, the garish packaging, the low cost, the eight color-coded flavors, and the drink's popularity among young partiers who see "blackout in a can" as a recommendation. Those attributes made Four Loko offensive to the guardians of public health and morals in a way that Irish coffee, rum and cola, and even Red Bull and vodka never were.

The FDA itself conceded that the combination of alcohol and caffeine, a feature of many drinks, that remain legal, was not the real issue. Rather, the agency complained that "the marketing of the caffeinated versions of this class of alcoholic beverage appears to be specifically

directed to young adults," who are "especially vulnerable" to "combined ingestion of caffeine and alcohol."

Because Four Loko was presumed to be unacceptably hazardous, the FDA did not feel a need to present much in the way of scientific evidence. A grand total of two studies have found that college-students who drink alcoholic beverages containing caffeine (typically bar- or home-mixed cocktails unaffected by the FDA's ban) tend to drink more and are more prone to risky behavior than college students who drink alcohol by itself. Neither study clarified whether the differences were due to the psychoactive effects of caffeine or to the predispositions of hearty partiers attracted to drinks they believe will help keep them going all night. But that distinction did not matter to panic-promoting politicians and their publicists in the press, who breathlessly advertised Four Loko while marveling at its rising popularity.

This dual function of publicity about an officially condemned intoxicant is familiar to anyone who has witnessed or read about previous scare campaigns against stigmatized substances, ranging from absinthe to *Salvia divinorum*. So is the evidentiary standard employed by Four Loko alarmists: If something bad happens and Four Loko is anywhere in the vicinity, blame Four Loko.

The National Highway Traffic Safety Administration counted 13,800 alcohol-related fatalities in 2008. It did not place crashes involving Four Loko drinkers in a special category. But news organizations around the country, primed to perceive the drink as unusually dangerous, routinely did. Three days before the FDA declared Four Loko illegal, a 14-year-old stole his parents' SUV and crashed it into a guardrail on Interstate 35 in Denton, Texas. His girlfriend, who was not wearing a seat belt, was ejected from the car and killed. Police, who said they found a 12-pack of beer and five cans of Four Loko in the SUV, charged the boy with intoxication manslaughter. Here is how the local Fox station headlined its story: "'Four Loko' Found in Deadly Teen Crash."

Likewise, college students were getting sick after drinking too much long before Four Loko was introduced in August 2008. According to the federal government's Drug Abuse Warning Network, more than 100,000 18-to-20-year-olds make alcohol-related visits to American emergency rooms every year. Yet 15 students at two colleges who were treated for alcohol poisoning after consuming excessive amounts of Four Loko were repeatedly held up as examples of the drink's unique dangers.

If all alcoholic beverages had to satisfy the reckless college student test, all of them would be banned. In a sense, then, we should be grateful for the government's inconsistency. With Four Loko, as with other taboo tipples and illegal drugs, there is little logic to the process by which the scapegoat is selected, but there are noticeable patterns. Once an intoxicant has been identified with a disfavored group—in this case, heedless, hedonistic "young adults"—everything about it is viewed in that light. Soon the wildest charges seem plausible: Four Loko is "a recipe for disaster," "a death wish disguised as an energy drink," a "witch's brew" that drives you mad, makes you shoot yourself in the head, and compels you to steal vehicles and crash them into things.

The timeline that follows shows how quickly a legal product can be transformed into contraband once it becomes the target of such over-the-top opprobrium. Although it's too late for Four Loko, lessons gleaned from the story of its demise could help prevent the next panicky prohibition by scaremongers who criminalize first and ask questions later.

June 2008: Anheuser-Busch, under pressure from 11 attorneys general who are investigating the brewing giant for selling the caffeinated malt beverages Tilt and Bud Extra, agrees to decaffeinate the drinks. "Drinking is not a sport, a race, or an endurance test," says New York Attorney General Andrew Cuomo, who will later be elected governor. "Adding alcohol to energy drinks sends exactly the wrong message about responsible drinking, most especially to young people."

August 2008: Phusion Projects, a Chicago company founded in 2005 by three recent graduates of Ohio State University, introduces Four Loko, which has an alcohol content of up to 12 percent (depending on state regulations); comes in brightly colored, 23.5-ounce cans; contains the familiar energy-drink ingredients caffeine, guarana, and taurine; and is eventually available in eight fruity, neon-hued varieties.

September 2008: The Center for Science in the Public Interest (CSPI), a pro-regulation group that is proud of being known as "the food police," sues MillerCoors Brewing Company over its malt beverage Sparks, arguing that the caffeine and guarana in the drink are additives that have not been approved by the FDA. "Mix alcohol and stimulants with a young person's sense of invincibility," says CSPI's George Hacker, "and you have a recipe for disaster. Sparks is a drink designed to mask feelings of drunkenness and to encourage people to keep drinking past the point at which they otherwise would have stopped. The end result is more drunk driving, more injuries, and more sexual assaults."

December 2008: In a deal with 13 attorneys general and the city of San Francisco, MillerCoors agrees to reformulate Sparks, removing the caffeine, guarana, taurine, and ginseng. Cuomo says caffeinated alcoholic beverages are "fundamentally dangerous and put drinkers of all ages at risk."

July 2009: *The Wall Street Journal* reports that Cuomo, Connecticut Attorney General Richard Blumenthal (now a U.S. senator), California Attorney General Jerry Brown (now governor), and their counterparts in several other states are investigating Four Loko and Joose, a close competitor. The National Association of Convenience Stores says the two brands are growing fast now that Tilt and Sparks have left the caffeinated malt beverage market.

August 2009: To demonstrate the threat that Four Loko poses to the youth of America, Blumenthal cites an online testimonial from a fan of the drink: "You just gotta drink it and drink it and drink it and drink it and not even worry about it because it's awesome and you're just partying and having fun and getting wild and drinking it." *The Chicago Tribune* cannot locate that particular comment on Phusion Projects' website, but it does find this: "I'm having a weird reaction to Four that makes me want to dance in my bra and panties. Please advise."

September 2009: Eighteen attorneys general ask the FDA to investigate the safety of alcoholic beverages containing caffeine.

November 2009: The FDA sends letters to 27 companies known to sell caffeinated alcoholic beverages, warning them that the combination has never been officially approved and asking them to submit evidence that it is "generally recognized as safe," as required by the Food, Drug, and Cosmetic Act. In addition to Phusion Projects, the recipients include Joose's manufacturer, United Brands; Charge Beverages, which sells similar products; the PINK Spirits Company, which makes caffeinated vodka, rum, gin, whiskey, and sake; and even the Ithaca Beer Company, which at one point made a special-edition stout brewed with coffee. "I continue to be very concerned that these drinks are extremely dangerous," says Illinois Attorney General Lisa Madigan, "especially in the hands of young people."

February 2010: In a feature story carried by several newspapers under headlines such as "Alcopops Only Look Innocent and Can Hook Kids," Kim Hone-McMahan of the *Akron Beacon Journal* outlines one scenario in which these extremely dangerous drinks might end up in tiny hands: "Intentionally or by accident, a child could grab an alcoholic beverage that looks like an energy drink, and hand it to Mom to pay for at the register. Without taking a closer look at the label, Mom may think it's just another brand of nonalcoholic energy beverage." It does seem like the sort of mistake that Hone-McMahan, who confuses fermented malt beverages with distilled spirits and warns parents about an alcoholic energy drink that was never actually introduced, might make. She explains that the combination of alcohol and caffeine "can confuse the nervous system," producing "wired, wide-awake drunks."

July 12, 2010: Sen. Charles Schumer (D-N.Y.) urges the Federal Trade Commission to investigate Four Loko and products like it. "It is my understanding that caffeine-infused, flavored malt beverages are becoming increasingly popular among teenagers," he writes. "The style and promotion of these products is extremely troubling." Schumer complains that the packaging of Joose and Four Loko is "designed to appear hip with flashy colors and funky designs that could appeal to younger consumers."

July 29, 2010: Schumer, joined by Sens. Dianne Feinstein (D-Calif.), Amy Klobuchar (D-Minn.), and Jeff Merkley (D-Ore.), urges the FDA to complete its investigation. "The FDA needs to determine once and for all if these drinks are safe, and if they're not, they ought to be banned," says Schumer, right before telling the FDA the conclusion it should reach: "Caffeine and alcohol are a dangerous mix, especially for young people."

August 1, 2010: After a crash in St. Petersburg, Florida, that kills four visitors from Orlando, police arrest 20-year-old Demetrius Jordan and charge him with drunk driving and manslaughter. The *St. Petersburg Times* reports that Jordan, who "had been drinking liquor and a caffeinated alcoholic beverage and smoking marijuana prior to the crash," "may have been going in excess of 80 mph when he crashed into the other vehicle." It notes that a "can of Four Loko was found on the floor of the back seat."

August 5, 2010: In a follow-up story, the *St. Petersburg Times* reports that "Four Loko, the caffeine-fueled malt liquor that police say Demetrius Jordan downed before he was accused of driving drunk and killing four people, is part of a new breed of beverages stirring controversy across the country." It quotes Bruce Goldberger, a toxicologist at the University of Florida, who declares, "I don't think there's a place for these beverages in the marketplace." The headline: "Alcohol, Caffeine: A Deadly Combo?"

August 12, 2010: The *Orlando Sentinel*, catching up with the *St. Petersburg Times*, shows it can quote Goldberger too. "It's a very bad combination having alcohol, plus caffeine, plus the brain of a young person," he says. "It's like a perfect storm." The headline: "Did High-Octane Drink Fuel Deadly Crash?"

September 2010: Peter Mercer, president of Ramapo College in Mahwah, New Jersey, bans Four Loko and other caffeinated malt beverages from campus after several incidents in which a total of 23 students were hospitalized for alcohol poisoning. Just six of the students were drinking Four Loko. Mercer later tells the Associated Press, "There's no redeeming social purpose to be served by having the beverage."

October 9, 2010: In a story about nine gang members who tied up and tortured a gay man after luring him to an abandoned building in the Bronx by telling him they were having a party, the *New York Daily News* plays up the detail that they "forced him to guzzle four cans" of the Four Loko he had brought with him. "The sodomized man couldn't give police a clear account of what he'd gone through," the paper reports, "possibly because of the Four Loko he was forced to drink."

October 10, 2010: In a follow-up story, the *Daily News* reports that Four Loko, a "wild drink full of caffeine and booze," "is causing controversy from coast to coast," citing the deadly crash in St. Petersburg.

October 13, 2010: Police in New Port Richey, Florida, arrest Justin Barker, 21, after he breaks into an old woman's home, trashes the place, strips naked, defecates on the floor, and then breaks into another house, where he falls asleep on the couch. Barker says Four Loko made him do it.

October 15, 2010: Calling Four Loko "a quick and intense high that has been dubbed 'blackout in a can,'" the Passaic County, New Jersey, *Herald News* notes the Ramapo College ban and quotes Mahwah Police Chief James Batelli. "The bottom line on the product is it gets you very drunk, very quick," he says. "To me, Four Loko is just a dangerous substance." The "blackout in a can" sobriquet, obviously hyperbolic when applied to a beverage that contains less alcohol per container than a bottle of wine, originated with Four Loko fans who considered it high praise; one of their Facebook pages is titled "four lokos are blackouts in a can and the end of my morals."

October 19, 2010: Bruce Goldberger, who co-authored one of the two studies linking caffeinated alcohol to risky behavior, tells the *Pittsburgh Post-Gazette* "the science is clear that consumption of alcohol with caffeine leads to risky behaviors." Mary Claire O'Brien, the Wake Forest University researcher who co-authored the other study, expresses her anger at the FDA. "I'm mad as a hornet that they didn't do something in the first place," she says, "and I'm mad as a hornet that they haven't done anything yet."

October 20, 2010: Based on a single case of a 19-year-old who came to Temple University Hospital in Philadelphia with chest pains after drinking Four Loko, ABC News warns that the stuff, which contains about one-third as much caffeine per ounce as coffee, can cause fatal heart attacks in perfectly healthy people. "That was the only explanation we had," says the doctor who treated the 19-year-old, before extrapolating further from his sample of one: "This is a dangerous product from what we've seen. It doesn't have to be chronic use. I think it could happen to somebody on a first-time use."

October 25, 2010: Citing the hospitalization of nine Central Washington University students for alcohol poisoning following an October 8 party in Roslyn where they drank Four Loko along with beer, rum, and vodka, Washington Attorney General Rob McKenna calls for a ban on caffeinated malt liquor. "The wide availability of the alcoholic energy drinks means that a single mistake can be deadly," he says. "They're marketed to kids by using fruit flavors that mask the taste of alcohol, and they have such high levels of stimulants that people have no idea how inebriated they really are." McKenna's office cites Ken Briggs, chairman of the university's physical education department, who says Four Loko is known as "liquid cocaine" as well as "blackout in a can," and with good reason, since it is "a binge drinker's dream."

October 26, 2010: McKenna's reaction to college students who drank too much Four Loko, like Peter Mercer's at Ramapo, attracts national attention. A Pennsylvania E.R. doctor quoted by *The New York Times* calls Four Loko "a recipe for disaster" and "one of the most dangerous new alcohol concoctions I have ever seen."

November 1, 2010: The Pennsylvania Liquor Control Board asks retailers to stop selling Four Loko, which is produced at the former Rolling Rock brewery in Latrobe, because it may "pose a significant threat to the health of all Pennsylvanians." State Rep. Robert Donatucci (D-Philadelphia) says "there is overriding circumstantial evidence that this combination may be very dangerous," and "until we can determine its effect on people and what kind of danger it may present, it should be yanked from the shelves."

November 3, 2010: Two Chicago aldermen propose an ordinance that would ban Four Loko from the city where its manufacturer is based. "I think it is completely irresponsible," says one, "to manufacture and market a product that can make young people so intoxicated so fast."

November 4, 2010: The Michigan Liquor Control Commission bans 55 "alcohol energy drinks," including Four Loko, Joose, a "hard" iced tea that no longer exists, a cola-flavored variety of Jack Daniel's Country Cocktails, and an India pale ale brewed with yerba mate. "With all the things that are happening, it's very alarming," explains commission chairwoman Nida Samona. "It's more serious than any of us ever imagined."

November 8, 2010: Oklahoma's Alcoholic Beverage Laws Enforcement Commission bans Four Loko from the state "in light of the growing scientific evidence against alcohol energy drinks, and the October 8th incident involving Four Loko in Roslyn, Washington."

November 9, 2010: NPR quotes Washington State University student Jarod Franklin as an authority on Four Loko's effects. "We would start to lose those inhibitions," he says, "and then [it would be like], 'How did you get a broken knuckle?' 'Oh, I punched through a three-inch layer of ice [because] you bet me I couldn't.'"

November 10, 2010: The Washington State Liquor Control Board bans beverages that "combine beer, strong beer, or malt liquor with caffeine, guarana, taurine, or other similar substances." Gov. Christine Gregoire, who recommended the ban, explains her reasoning: "I was particularly concerned that these drinks tend to target young people. Reports of inexperienced or underage drinkers consuming them in reckless amounts have given us cause for concern. . . . By taking these drinks off the shelves we are saying 'no' to irresponsible drinking and taking steps to prevent incidents like the one that made these college students so ill."

Sen. Schumer urges the New York State Liquor Authority to "immediately ban caffeinated alcoholic beverages." He says drinks like Four Loko "are a toxic, dangerous mix of caffeine and alcohol, and they are spreading like a plague across the country." Schumer claims "studies have shown that caffeinated alcoholic beverages raise unique and disturbing safety concerns, especially for younger drinkers." While they "can be extremely hazardous for teens and adults alike," he says, they "pose a unique danger because they target young people" with their "vibrantly colored aluminum can colors and funky designs."

November 12, 2010: A CBS station in Baltimore reports that two cans of Four Loko caused a 21-year-old Maryland woman to "lose her mind," steal a friend's pickup truck, and crash it into a telephone pole, killing herself.

A CBS station in Philadelphia reports that a middle-aged suburban dad "spiraled into a hallucinogenic frenzy" featuring "nightmarish delusions" after drinking a can and a half of Four Loko. "It was like he was stuck inside a horror movie and he couldn't get out and I couldn't get him out," the man's wife says. "In his mind, he had harmed all of our kids and he had to kill me and kill himself so that we could go to heaven to take care of them. Next thing I know, he was having convulsions [and] making gurgling sounds as if someone were choking him, and then he stopped breathing."

Connecticut Attorney General Blumenthal urges the FDA to "impose a nationwide ban on these dangerous and potentially deadly drinks."

November 14, 2010: Under pressure from Gov. David Paterson and the state liquor authority, Phusion Projects agrees to stop shipping Four Loko to New York. "We have an obligation to keep products that are potentially hazardous off the shelves," says the liquor authority's chairman.

Bruce Goldberger tells the *New Haven Register* Four Loko is "a very significant problem" for the "instant gratification generation." The kids today, he says, "text, they have iPhones, and they can access the Internet any minute of their life. And now, they can get drunk for literally less than $5, and they can get drunk very rapidly."

November 15, 2010: WBZ, the CBS affiliate in Boston, reports that the Massachusetts Alcoholic Beverages Control Commission plans to ban Four Loko. According to WBZ, commission officials say the drink—a fermented malt beverage with an alcohol content of 12 percent, compared to 40 percent or more for distilled spirits—"is really not a malt liquor, but a much more potent form of hard liquor, like vodka." The commission's chairman explains that the ban is aimed at protecting consumers who cannot read: "We are concerned that people who are drinking these alcoholic beverages are not aware of the ingredients which are contained in them."

The New York Times reports that Four Loko "has been blamed for several deaths over the last several months," including that of a 20-year-old sophomore at Florida State University in Tallahassee who "started playing with a gun and fatally shot himself after drinking several cans of Four Loko over a number of hours." Richard Blumenthal tells the *Times* "there's just no excuse for the delay in applying standards that clearly should bar this kind of witch's brew." Mary Claire O'Brien argues that Four Loko is guilty until proven innocent: "The addition of the caffeine impairs the ability of the drinker to tell when they're drunk. What is the level at which it becomes dangerous? We don't know that, and until we can figure it out, the answer is that no level is safe."

November 16, 2010: Phusion Projects says it will reformulate Four Loko, removing the caffeine, guarana, and taurine. "We have repeatedly contended—and still believe, as do many people throughout the country—that the combination of alcohol and caffeine is safe," the company's founders say. "We are taking this step after trying—unsuccessfully—to navigate a difficult and politically charged regulatory environment at both the state and federal levels."

The Arizona Republic reports that an "extremely intoxicated" 18-year-old from Mesa crashed her SUV into a tree after "playing 'beer pong' with the controversial caffeinated alcoholic beverage Four Loko." The headline: "Caffeine, Alcohol Drink Tied to Crash."

Reporting on a lawsuit against Phusion Projects by the parents of the FSU student who shot himself after drinking Four Loko, ABC News quotes Schumer, who avers, "It's almost a death wish disguised as an energy drink."

November 17, 2010: The FDA and the Federal Trade Commission send warning letters to Phusion Projects, United Brands, Charge Beverages, and New Century Brewing Company, which makes a caffeinated lager called Moonshot. The agency says their products are "adulterated," and therefore illegal under the Food, Drug, and Cosmetic Act, because they contain an additive, caffeine, that is not generally recognized as safe in this context. But the FDA does not conclude that all beverages combining alcohol and caffeine are inherently unsafe. It focuses on these particular companies because they "seemingly target the young adult user." Federal drug czar Gil Kerlikowske approves the FDA's marketing-based definition of adulteration, saying "these products are designed, branded, and promoted to encourage binge drinking."

NPR correspondent Tovia Smith reports that "many college students say they agree with the FDA that alcoholic energy drinks do result in more risky behavior, like drunk driving or sexual assaults." Smith presents one such student, Ali Burak of Boston College, who says "it seems like every time someone wakes up in the morning and regrets the night before it's usually because they had Four Loko."

November 20, 2010: In a *Huffington Post* essay, David Katz, director of Yale University's Prevention Research Center, explains why "anyone who is for sanity and safety in marketing" should welcome the FDA's ban. "Combining alcohol and caffeine is—in one word—crazy," he writes. "Don't do it! It has an excellent chance of hurting you, and a fairly good chance of killing you." His evidence: the Maryland car crash in which a woman who had been drinking Four Loko died after colliding with a telephone pole. "It's hard to imagine any argument for such products," Katz concludes. "It's also hard to imagine anyone objecting to a ban of such products."

JACOB SULLUM is a journalist and editor of *Reason Magazine*.

EXPLORING THE ISSUE

Are Energy Drinks with Alcohol Dangerous Enough to Ban?

Critical Thinking and Reflection

1. Why were energy drinks with caffeine banned?
2. Why are caffeinated energy drinks so popular among college students?
3. Describe why the drinks are dangerous and how they contributed to deaths among some college students.

Is There Common Ground?

Four Loco and other energy drinks provide the effects of caffeine and sugar, but there is little or no evidence that a wide variety of other ingredients have any impact on the body. A variety of physiological and psychological effects, however, have been blamed on energy drinks and their components. Excess use of energy drinks may produce mild-to-moderate euphoria primarily due to the stimulant properties of caffeine. The drinks may also cause agitation, anxiety, irritability, and sleeplessness.

Ingestion of a single energy drink will not lead to excessive caffeine intake, but consumption of two or more drinks over the course of a day can. Ginseng, guarana, and other stimulants are often added to energy drinks and may bolster the effects of caffeine. Negative effects associated with caffeine consumption in amounts greater than 400 mg include nervousness, irritability, sleeplessness, increased urination, abnormal heart rhythms, and upset stomach. By comparison, a cup of drip coffee contains about 150 mg of caffeine. Caffeine in energy drinks can cause the excretion of water from the body to dilute high concentrations of sugar entering the blood stream, leading to dehydration.

In the United States, energy drinks have been linked with reports of emergency room visits due to heart palpitations and anxiety. The beverages have been associated with seizures due to the crash following the high energy that occurs after ingestion. In the United States, caffeine dosage is not required to be on the product label for food, unlike drugs, but some advocates are urging the FDA to change this practice.

Drinking one 24-ounce can of Four Loko provides the alcoholic kick of four beers and the caffeine buzz of a strong cup of coffee. Drinking one quickly makes someone pretty drunk and reasonably awake, and able to drink more. As a result, college students seem particularly drawn to it, which has landed some in hospitals. But should Four Loko be banned state-by-state as a result? Banning Four Loko might prevent some people, especially some college students, from hurting themselves or others. But does it improve people's judgment or otherwise empower them to protect themselves?

Create Central

www.mhhe.com/createcentral

Additional Resources

The party's over. (2010, November 25). *Nature, 475.*

Siegel, S. (2011). The Four-Loko effect. *Perspectives on Psychological Science, 6*(4), 357–362.

Wood, D. B. (2010, November 19). Four Loko: Does FDA's caffeinated alcoholic beverage ban go too far? *Christian Science Monitor,* p. N.PAG.

Internet References . . .

Energy Drinks—American Association of Poison Control Centers

www.aapcc.org/alerts/energy-drinks

Food and Drug Administration

www.fda.gov

National Institute on Drug Abuse (NIDA)

www.nida.nih.gov